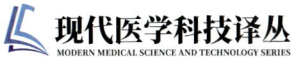

现代医学科技译丛

阿尔茨海默病
生物标志物、大数据及治疗学解析

Alzheimer's Disease
Understanding Biomarkers, Big Data, and Therapy

主编

[澳] 艾哈迈德·A. 穆斯塔法（Ahmed A. Moustafa）

主审

陈晓春　罗跃嘉

主译

陈仰昆

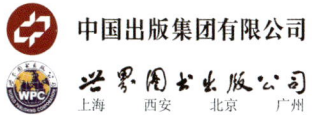

图书在版编目(CIP)数据

阿尔茨海默病:生物标志物、大数据及治疗学解析/(澳)艾哈迈德·A.穆斯塔法主编;陈仰昆译. --上海:上海世界图书出版公司, 2025.4.--ISBN 978-7-5232-1812-9

Ⅰ. R749.1

中国国家版本馆CIP数据核字第20242RE352号

书　　名	阿尔茨海默病：生物标志物、大数据及治疗学解析 Aercihaimo Bing Shengwu Biaozhiwu Dashuju ji Zhiliaoxue Jiexi
主　　编	[澳] 艾哈迈德·A. 穆斯塔法
主　　译	陈仰昆
策　　划	曹高腾
责任编辑	芮晴舟
出 版 人	唐丽芳
出版发行	上海世界图书出版公司
地　　址	上海市广中路88号 9-10楼
邮　　编	200083
网　　址	http://www.wpcsh.com
经　　销	新华书店
印　　刷	运河（唐山）印务有限公司
开　　本	787 mm × 1092 mm　1/16
印　　张	15
字　　数	220千字
版　　次	2025年4月第1版　2025年4月第1次印刷
版权登记	图字 09-2024-0272 号
书　　号	ISBN 978-7-5232-1812-9 / R·757
定　　价	130.00元

版权所有　翻印必究
如发现印装质量问题，请与印刷厂联系
（质检科电话：022-59658568）

Alzheimer's Disease : Understanding Biomarkers, Big Data, and Therapy

Ahmed A. Moustafa

ISBN: 9780128213346

Copyright © 2022 Elsevier Inc. All rights reserved.

Authorized Chinese translation published by World Publishing Shanghai Corporation Limited.

阿尔茨海默病：生物标志物、大数据及治疗学解析（陈仰昆 主译）

ISBN: 9787523218129

Copyright © Elsevier Inc. and World Publishing Shanghai Corporation Limited. All rights reserved.

No part of this publication may be reproduced or transmitted in any form or by any means, electronic or mechanical, including photocopying, recording, or any information storage and retrieval system, without permission in writing from Elsevier Inc. Details on how to seek permission, further information about the Elsevier's permissions policies and arrangements with organizations such as the Copyright Clearance Center and the Copyright Licensing Agency, can be found at our website: www.elsevier.com/permissions. This book and the individual contributions contained in it are protected under copyright by Elsevier Inc. and World Publishing Shanghai Corporation Limited. (other than as may be noted herein).

This edition of Alzheimer's Disease : Understanding Biomarkers, Big Data, and Therapy is published by World Publishing Shanghai Corporation Limited. under arrangement with ELSEVIER INC.

This edition is authorized for sale in China only, excluding Hong Kong, Macau and Taiwan. Unauthorized export of this edition is a violation of the Copyright Act. Violation of this Law is subject to Civil and Criminal Penalties.

本版由ELSEVIER INC. 授权世界图书出版上海有限公司在中国大陆地区（不包括香港、澳门以及台湾地区）出版发行。

本版仅限在中国大陆地区（不包括香港、澳门以及台湾地区）出版及标价销售。未经许可之出口，视为违反著作权法，将受民事及刑事法律之制裁。

本书封底贴有Elsevier防伪标签，无标签者不得销售。

> **注意**
>
> 本书涉及领域的知识和实践标准在不断变化。新的研究和经验拓展我们的理解，因此须对研究方法、专业实践或医疗方法作出调整。从业者和研究人员必须始终依靠自身经验和知识来评估和使用本书中提到的所有信息、方法、化合物或本书中描述的实验。在使用这些信息或方法时，他们应注意自身和他人的安全，包括注意他们负有专业责任的当事人的安全。在法律允许的最大范围内，爱思唯尔、译文的原文作者、原文编辑及原文内容提供者均不对因产品责任、疏忽或其他人身或财产伤害及/或损失承担责任，亦不对由于使用或操作文中提到的方法、产品、说明或思想而导致的人身或财产伤害及/或损失承担责任。

审译者名单

主　审　陈晓春　福建医科大学附属协和医院
　　　　　罗跃嘉　北京师范大学

主　译　陈仰昆　南方医科大学第十附属医院（东莞市人民医院）

副主译　刘勇林　南方医科大学第十附属医院（东莞市人民医院）
　　　　　翁汉育　南方医科大学第十附属医院（东莞市人民医院）
　　　　　赵江浩　南方医科大学第十附属医院（东莞市人民医院）
　　　　　屈剑锋　南方医科大学第十附属医院（东莞市人民医院）

译　者（按姓氏笔画排序）
　　　　　王　凤　南方医科大学第十附属医院（东莞市人民医院）
　　　　　王铭子　南方医科大学第一临床医学院
　　　　　卢志豪　南方医科大学第十附属医院（东莞市人民医院）
　　　　　丘东海　南方医科大学第十附属医院（东莞市人民医院）
　　　　　成蔚阳　南方医科大学第十附属医院（东莞市人民医院）
　　　　　向智滔　广东医科大学
　　　　　刘启峻　南方医科大学第一临床医学院
　　　　　刘晓汶　广东医科大学
　　　　　刘健菲　南方医科大学第一临床医学院
　　　　　刘梓轩　南方医科大学第一临床医学院
　　　　　李爱萍　南方医科大学第十附属医院（东莞市人民医院）
　　　　　肖卫民　南方医科大学第十附属医院（东莞市人民医院）
　　　　　陈绮婷　广东医科大学
　　　　　林伟丰　南方医科大学第十附属医院（东莞市人民医院）
　　　　　周宝玉　南方医科大学第一临床医学院

审译者名单（译者）

胡伟东　南方医科大学第十附属医院（东莞市人民医院）
钟伙花　南方医科大学第十附属医院（东莞市人民医院）
钟洪芬　南方医科大学第十附属医院（东莞市人民医院）
姚敏怡　南方医科大学第十附属医院（东莞市人民医院）
袁一棉　广东医科大学
袁淑兰　南方医科大学第十附属医院（东莞市人民医院）
袁锡球　南方医科大学第十附属医院（东莞市人民医院）
倪卓新　南方医科大学第十附属医院（东莞市人民医院）
黄龙龙　南方医科大学第十附属医院（东莞市人民医院）
梁灼源　南方医科大学第十附属医院（东莞市人民医院）
詹云浩　南方医科大学第十附属医院（东莞市人民医院）

主审简介

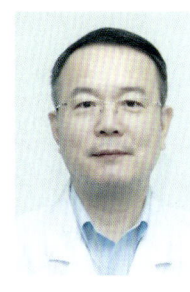

陈晓春 教授，博士研究生导师，福建医科大学附属协和医院神经内科主任医师。中国医师协会常务理事、神经内科医师分会候任会长、中华医学会神经病学分会痴呆与认知障碍学组组长。

长期从事神经退行性疾病的基础研究与临床诊疗工作，重点聚焦阿尔茨海默病、帕金森病的发病机制及防治策略，先后承担了科技创新2030-"脑科学与类脑研究计划"重大项目、国家科技支撑计划、国家自然科学基金等20多项国家级研究课题，在 *Molecular Neurodegeneration*、*Biological Psychiatry*、*Aging Cell* 等 SCI 源学术期刊发表高质量论文 100 余篇，主持完成的科研成果曾获教育部高等学校科学研究优秀成果奖——自然科学奖一等奖。

主审简介

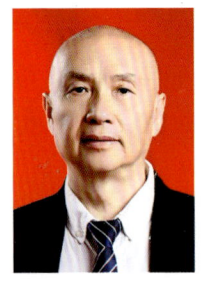

罗跃嘉 二级教授，博士研究生导师，现为北京师范大学心理学部聘任教授。曾任北京师范大学心理学部部长、深圳大学脑疾病与认知科学研究中心创始主任、北京师范大学脑与认知科学研究院创始院长、北京师范大学认知神经科学与学习国家重点实验室首任主任、中国科学院心理健康重点实验室创始主任等。现当选为中国心理学会候任理事长，欧洲自然科学院外籍院士、国际心理科学学会（APS）会士等，以及国家自然科学基金委员会、科技部、教育部、中组部、国家卫健委、国家科学技术奖励工作办公室评审专家。先后获国家杰出青年基金，首批"新世纪百千万人才工程"国家级人选，国务院特殊津贴获得者，中科院"百人计划"入选者等。20多年来主要从事情绪与认知的基础与临床应用研究，主持国家社科基金重大项目1项、国家自然科学基金重点项目2项、国际合作重点项目1项，以及国家重点基础研究发展计划（973计划）项目2项、国家科技支撑计划1项、教育部创新团队发展计划等20余项。发表学术论文560篇，其中SCI/SSCI论文276篇、《心理学报》论文近50篇；出版中英文专著、译著8部；获省部级科技奖15项（其中一等奖2项、二等奖6项）；培养博士后、博士研究生、硕士研究生150人。在推动中国认知神经科学的发展、参与中国心理学科和重点实验室建设以及脑电/ERP技术的研究与应用等方面，具有广泛学术影响力。

主译简介

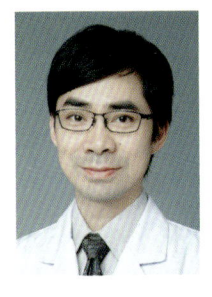

陈仰昆 教授，主任医师，博士研究生导师、博士后合作导师。

南方医科大学第十附属医院（东莞市人民医院）神经内科学科主任，暨南大学博士研究生导师，南方医科大学博士后合作导师，东莞市神经内科专业质量控制中心主任，中国人民政治协商会议第十四届东莞市委员会委员。1996—2003年在中山医科大学（现中山大学中山医学院）七年制本硕连读，获临床医学学士及神经病学硕士学位。2007—2010年在香港中文大学医学院内科科学部（神经病学）攻读博士学位。2018—2019年在英国伦敦国王学院圣托马斯医院进修卒中医学。先后获得"广东省杰出青年医学人才""东莞名医""东莞市医学领军人才"及"第八届东莞市优秀科技工作者"等称号。目前担任中华医学会神经病学分会神经康复学组委员、中国研究型医院学会脑小血管病分会常委、广东省医院协会神经内科专委会副主任委员、东莞市医学会神经病学分会主任委员、广东省医学会脑血管病分会常委及神经病学分会常委等学术职务。擅长脑血管病、帕金森病、认知障碍的诊疗。致力于推动东莞市卒中绿色通道及卒中中心建设；开设东莞首个帕金森病专病门诊及在东莞市率先进行DBS程控治疗。连续多年担任中国卒中学会培训中心全国培训讲师。创建东莞市重点实验室"智能脑影像及脑功能实验室"。研究领域包括卒中后认知及精神障碍、脑血流与代谢、脑小血管病及帕金森病的临床及影像学研究；脑卒中静脉影像、卒中后认知与精神障碍研究居于国内先进水平。主持省部级课题2项（含省级重点项目1项）及市厅级课题5项。共发表SCI论文73篇（其中第一或通讯作者32篇），最高影响因子10.1，H指数23。其中缺血性卒中谵妄、卒中后疲劳的研究被引用次数均超过50次，2篇SCI论文被国际指南引用。参与制定3项省级指南及标准。担任SCI期刊 *BMC Neurology* 编委、SCI期刊 *Frontiers in Neurology* 专刊客座副主编及SCI期刊 *Stroke and Vascular Neurology* 审委会委员。

主译序言

由澳大利亚西悉尼大学艾哈迈德·A. 穆斯塔法（Ahmed A. Moustafa）教授主编的著作《阿尔茨海默病：生物标志物、大数据及治疗学解析》（*Alzheimer's Disease: Understanding Biomarkers, Big Data, and Therapy*）是一部视角新颖、紧扣前沿的著作。我们认真阅读原著后，深受启发，故组织团队翻译出版，以介绍给国内的同行。

本书与一般的阿尔茨海默病的专著不同，其鲜明的特点是选用专题综述的形式来呈现，具有相当的深度。例如，本书关于阿尔茨海默病合并抑郁及焦虑的进展、瞳孔分析与认知障碍、深度学习在痴呆研究中的应用，以及阿尔茨海默病的创新治疗方法等，都是前沿和新颖的研究领域。本书中关于阿尔茨海默病对丘脑的影响，以及如何利用 ADNI 数据库进行研究的相关内容，对于神经内科医生及研究者，也会有不少的启发。

感谢翻译团队及编辑老师的辛勤工作，使本译著得以顺利出版。衷心感谢本领域国内著名学者、福建医科大学附属协和医院陈晓春教授及北京师范大学罗跃嘉教授对本译著审校工作的支持，以及对翻译团队的宝贵建议。

本译著的出版，将有助于我国认知障碍领域的研究者及临床医师开阔视野，从更全面的角度去理解阿尔茨海默病，并进一步探索前沿诊治方法。

最后，限于我们的能力，译著中可能存在翻译不够准确和不流畅之处，敬请读者谅解及指正。

2025 年 1 月 8 日

原著主编介绍

艾哈迈德·A. 穆斯塔法（Ahmed A. Moustafa）

澳大利亚新南威尔士州西悉尼大学心理学院

MARCS脑与行为研究所

南非约翰内斯堡大学健康科学学院人体解剖学与生理学系

贡献者名单

艾德·阿博·哈姆扎（Eid Abo Hamza）

埃及，坦塔，坦塔大学心理健康系教育学院；巴林，阿拉伯海湾大学研究生院

哈尼·阿拉什瓦尔（Hany Alashwal）

澳大利亚，新南威尔士，悉尼，西悉尼大学MARCS脑与行为研究所；阿拉伯联合酋长国，阿拉伯联合酋长国大学信息技术学院

菲比·贝利（Phoebo Bailey）

澳大利亚，新南威尔士，悉尼，西悉尼大学MARCS脑与行为研究所；澳大利亚，新南威尔士，悉尼，西悉尼大学心理学院

莉莉·比尔森（Lily Bilson）

澳大利亚，新南威尔士，悉尼，西悉尼大学心理学院

穆罕默德·哈吉（Mohamad El Haj）

法国，南特，昂热大学卢瓦尔省心理实验室（LPPL-EA 4638）；法国，图尔孔，图尔孔医院老年病科；法国，巴黎，法国大学

柔德拉·加里多（Sandra Garrido）

澳大利亚，新南威尔士，悉尼，西悉尼大学心理学院

希玛·阿德尔·海卡尔（Shimaa Adel Heikal）

埃及，新开罗，美国大学（开罗）科学与工程学院生物技术项目

艾哈迈德·希拉勒（Ahmed Helal）

埃及，坦塔大学心理健康系教育学院

瓦法·贾鲁迪（Wafa Jaroudi）

澳大利亚，新南威尔士，悉尼，西悉尼大学MARCS脑与行为研究所；澳大利亚，新南威尔士，悉尼，西悉尼大学心理学院

拉苏·卡尔基（Rasu Karki）

澳大利亚，新南威尔士，悉尼，西悉尼大学心理学院

阿布德拉博·苏莱星（Abdrabo Soliman）

卡塔尔，多哈，卡塔尔大学文理学院社会科学系

达斯汀·范德哈尔（Dustin van der Haar）

南非，约翰内斯堡大学计算机科学与软件工程学院

塞缪尔·洪伦（Samuel L. Warren）

澳大利亚，新南威尔士，悉尼，西悉尼大学心理学院心理学科

献 辞

致过去十年来所有在我工作研究中遇到过的阿尔茨海默病患者，您的付出和努力使这项研究成为可能。

目 录

第一部分 老年痴呆症中的心理健康

第一章 阿尔茨海默病中抑郁症的测量方法 ··················· 3

- 第一节 引言 ··················· 3
- 第二节 AD 中的抑郁症评估工具 ··················· 7
- 第三节 讨论和结论 ··················· 22

第二章 痴呆中抑郁症的本质：一项系统回顾 ··················· 31

- 第一节 引言：痴呆中抑郁症的诊断、患病率和影响 ··················· 31
- 第二节 方法 ··················· 33
- 第三节 抑郁症是导致老年痴呆症的一个危险因素 ··················· 33
- 第四节 痴呆中抑郁症的亚型 ··················· 36
- 第五节 抑郁与自知力 ··················· 38
- 第六节 痴呆亚型中的抑郁症：与自知力的关系 ··················· 39
- 第七节 结论及未来工作 ··················· 41

第三章 痴呆症患者的压力和焦虑 ··················· 51

- 第一节 痴呆症背景 ··················· 51
- 第二节 痴呆症患者的心理健康 ··················· 52
- 第三节 焦虑与痴呆症 ··················· 54
- 第四节 压力与痴呆症 ··················· 58
- 第五节 结论 ··················· 60

第二部分　痴呆研究的前沿主题

第四章　瞳孔中的阿尔茨海默病：瞳孔测量作为阿尔茨海默病认知过程的生物学标志物 ……………………………………………………………… 73

第一节　引言 ……………………………………………………………… 73
第二节　方法 ……………………………………………………………… 75
第三节　讨论 ……………………………………………………………… 76

第五章　维生素 D 缺乏与认知及神经的相关性：聚焦健康老龄化与阿尔茨海默病 ……………………………………………………………… 82

第一节　引言 ……………………………………………………………… 82
第二节　关于认知功能与维生素 D 水平的动物实验 …………………… 86
第三节　健康老龄化、痴呆及阿尔茨海默病 …………………………… 88
第四节　结论 ……………………………………………………………… 93
第五节　展望 ……………………………………………………………… 93

第六章　阿尔茨海默病对丘脑的影响 ……………………………………… 102

第一节　引言 ……………………………………………………………… 102
第二节　阿尔茨海默病对丘脑的影响 …………………………………… 103
第三节　丘脑与脑部其他部分之间的联系 ……………………………… 105
第四节　前额叶 - 纹状体环和内侧前额皮质 …………………………… 107
第五节　讨论 ……………………………………………………………… 109
第六节　未来的工作 ……………………………………………………… 111
第七节　结论 ……………………………………………………………… 111

第七章　利用大数据方法去理解阿尔茨海默病 …………………………… 117

第一节　引言 ……………………………………………………………… 117
第二节　什么是阿尔茨海默病 …………………………………………… 118

第三节	大数据方法	121
第四节	大数据分析	124
第五节	举例：阿尔茨海默病神经影像计划	128
第六节	结论	131

第八章 阿尔茨海默病的深度学习方法概况 142

第一节	引言	142
第二节	传统阿尔茨海默病CAD方法的趋势	143
第三节	深度学习情境下的阿尔茨海默病	147
第四节	使用深度学习的优势	155
第五节	使用深度学习的局限性	157
第六节	结论	157

第三部分 痴呆的治疗

第九章 阿尔茨海默病伴抑郁的治疗 169

第一节	引言	169
第二节	治疗	169
第三节	结论	175

第十章 用于音乐干预治疗的负面情绪易感性痴呆量表的开发 183

第一节	引言	183
第二节	方法	185
第三节	结果	187
第四节	讨论	189

第十一章 运用音乐改善痴呆人群的精神健康 196

| 第一节 | 引言 | 196 |

第二节　音乐疗法 ·· 196
　　第三节　非治疗师主导的音乐干预 ···························· 199
　　第四节　音乐疗法和干预措施作用机制的理论 ·············· 202
　　第五节　结论和未来的研究 ···································· 202

第十二章　多奈哌齐治疗阿尔茨海默病的疗效 ················ **207**
　　第一节　引言 ··· 207
　　第二节　多奈哌齐在阿尔茨海默病中的作用 ················· 208
　　第三节　多奈哌齐的联合治疗 ································· 213
　　第四节　结论 ··· 215

第一部分
老年痴呆症中的心理健康

第一章 阿尔茨海默病中抑郁症的测量方法

Ahmed A. Moustafa，Wafa Jaroudi，Ahmed Helal，Lily Bilson，Mohamad El Haj 编

翁汉育，林伟丰 译

陈仰昆 校

第一节 引言

抑郁症对痴呆及阿尔茨海默病（Alzheimer's disease，AD）患者产生了很大影响。一些研究报告显示，20%~60%的AD患者被诊断患有抑郁症[1]。由于症状重叠、交流不畅以及患者缺乏自知力，鉴别痴呆中的抑郁障碍困难重重[2,3]。抑郁和痴呆的相似症状包括睡眠障碍、饮食行为改变、主动性和兴趣减退（冷漠）、精神运动性激越、注意力不集中、焦虑和悲伤。而没有抑郁症的痴呆患者，往往不会出现常见的抑郁表现。例如，持续的悲伤、显著的晨间情绪恶化、无价值感或过度的内疚感、反复思考死亡以及自杀意念或行为。

尽管悲伤情绪是阿尔茨海默病中最常见的神经精神症状，但对于如何诊断AD中的抑郁症并没有普遍共识。美国国家心理健康研究所（National Institute of Mental Health，NIMH）提出了阿尔茨海默病中抑郁症的临时诊断标准（Provisional Diagnostic Criteria for Depression in Alzheimer's Disease，PDC-dAD）。然而，该标准尚未在科学研究及临床实践中得到严格验证。在制定诊断标准和监测AD变化时，常使用量表来辅助临床医生减少其中的不确定性。目前，用于测评痴呆患者抑郁程度的量表有以下几种（表1-1）。

表 1-1　现有常用的 AD 抑郁量表

量表	相关症状	说明	相关研究
贝克抑郁量表	悲伤；沮丧；失败感；满意度水平；内疚感；失望；惩罚感；自责；自杀；哭泣；易怒；兴趣；决策；外表；努力；睡眠；疲劳；食欲；体重；担心；性欲	—	[4-6]
《精神障碍诊断与统计手册第 4 版》标准	—	—	[7,8]
康奈尔痴呆抑郁量表	情绪（焦虑、悲伤、反应、易怒）；行为（激越、迟钝、身体不适、失去兴趣）；身体（食欲下降、体重减轻、精力不足）；循环功能（情绪日变化、入睡困难、睡眠中多次醒来、晨间早醒）；意念障碍（自杀、低自尊、悲观、情绪一致错觉）	评分系统：根据访谈前 1 周出现的症状和体征进行评分。如果症状是由身体残疾或疾病引起的，则不应给予评分	[9-13]
老年痴呆症情绪评估量表	运动活动；睡眠（失眠和白天嗜睡）；欲增加）；心身不适；精力；抑郁（易怒、烦躁）；享受反应；情绪反应；自尊；内疚感；绝望/无助；自杀想法；言语；每日情绪变化（早晚和严重程度）；偏执症状；其他精神病症状；表达性沟通能力；接受性认知能力；食欲（食欲下降和食欲增加、焦虑、抑郁外观）认知洞察力	—	[10]
老年抑郁量表	生活的满足感；放弃的活动/兴趣；生活的空虚；无聊；好的精神；害怕坏事情的发生；幸福；无助；待在家里/外出的偏好；记忆问题；无价值；精力；情况是无望的；生活与其他生活相比	—	—
汉密尔顿抑郁量表	情绪低落；内疚；自杀；失眠（最初、中间、延迟）；工作和兴趣；迟钝或激越；焦虑（精神、躯体）；躯体症状（胃肠道）；生殖器症状；疑病症（痴迷地认为他们的疾病未确诊）；体重减轻；洞察力；日变化；人格解体和意识障碍；偏执的症状；痴迷症状	—	[9]

续表

量表	相关症状	说明	相关研究
医院焦虑与抑郁量表	紧张;愉快;恐惧;微笑;担心;高兴;放松;关注外表;紧张?-逃逸?心神不宁;战斗(逃逸)-紧张?;物质享受	量表说明:你在过去的1周里一直的感觉如何	[9]
蒙哥马利-阿斯伯格抑郁量表	明显的悲伤;报告的悲伤;内心紧张;睡眠减少;食欲减退;注意力不集中;倦怠;无应感觉;悲观的想法;自杀的想法	Sheehan[9]评论说,该量表在干预研究中常用,这意味着它可能用于比较痴呆患者干预前和干预后的抑郁	[9,12,13]
老年患者护士观察量表	外貌;娱乐活动;悲伤;夜间躁动不安;对周围环境感兴趣;整洁;控制排便;记忆;购物能力;无价值;业余爱好活动(包括着装);重复语言;悲伤/哭泣/流泪;卫生不净整洁;爱好活动、在熟悉环境中定向;逃跑;记住名字;尽其所能帮助他人;在熟悉环境中定向;交谈中爱争吵易怒;攻击性(言语/身体);尿失禁;快乐;与朋友/家人联系;个体身份混乱;爱好活动(聚会);友好、积极;固执的行为	量表说明:基于护士的观察——患者在过去2周内的表现如何?护士被要求在过去2周内观察患者,反应是主观的,他们的关系类型和与患者的接触可能仍然会潜在地影响他们的反应	[13]
患者健康问卷	失去快乐、沮丧、低落、绝望、睡眠问题、疲劳、失败或肉疚感、注意力问题、缓慢语言、运动功能、食欲变化、不安;自杀或自残的想法	使用量表进行治疗和监测:一个需要治疗或改变治疗方案的抑郁症诊断、至少需要在过去2周内关于简易精神状态检查中的提问、被认为前两个问题中至少一个是肯定回答。举例说明:在过去的2周内,你有多久被以下问题困扰	[14,15]
NIMH AD 患者抑郁症的临时诊断标准	—	—	[7,8,16]

续表

量表	相关症状	说明	相关研究
剑桥大学老年人精神障碍测试	—	—	[8,17,18]
神经精神病学目录	—	—	[8,19]
ICD-10	—	—	[8,20]
痴呆情绪评估量表	—	—	[10]
阿尔茨海默病情绪量表	—	—	[21]
ZUNG氏抑郁症自评量表	悲伤；早晨感觉最好；哭泣；晚上难以入睡；食欲；性欲；减肥；便秘；心跳加快；疲劳；头脑清醒；做事困难/容易；不安；决策；有用的和需要的；生活很充实吗？自杀的想法；活动的享受	测量说明：在过去的几天里，你有多少上述感觉或行为	[22-24]

注：贝克抑郁量表（Beck's Depression Inventory, BDI）；康奈尔痴呆抑郁量表（Cornell Scale for Depression in Dementia, CSDD）；老年抑郁量表（Geriatric Depression Scale, GDS）；汉密尔顿抑郁量表（Hamilton Depression Scale, HAM-D）；医院焦虑与抑郁量表（Hospital Anxiety and Depression Scale, HADS）；蒙哥马利-阿斯伯格抑郁量表（Montgomery-Asberg Depression Scale, MADRS）；老年患者护士观察量表（Nurses Observations Scale for Geriatric Patients, NOSGR）；患者健康问卷（Patient Health Questionnaire, PHQ-9）；痴呆情绪评估量表（Dementia Mood Assessment Scale, DMAS）剑桥大学老年人精神障碍测试（Cambridge Examination for Mental Disorder of the Elderly, CAMDEX）；《精神障碍诊断与统计手册 第4版》（Diagnostic and Statistical Manual of Mental Disorders Version 4, DSM-Ⅳ）

第二节　AD 中的抑郁症评估工具

许多研究在评估痴呆患者的抑郁症时使用了几种抑郁量表[25,26]，然而，很少有人将这些量表进行比较和评估，以确定哪种量表能更好地识别痴呆患者的抑郁症，或者它们是否测量了不同或相似的抑郁症及痴呆变量。因此，2013 年，Knapskog 等[27]评估了 AD 患者在 CSDD 和 MADRS 量表中的得分，以比较对抑郁症的评估，并调查这些量表之间的相关性以及与患者年龄、性别、认知障碍水平和照顾者负担水平之间的关系。Knapskog 等[27]的研究共涉及 520 例患者，这些患者是从记忆门诊招募的，他们患有痴呆、轻度认知障碍（Mild Cognitive Impairment，MCI）或主观认知障碍。该研究对患者参与研究的适宜性进行了检测，包括痴呆诊断以及医生之间就以下评估结果达成共识：神经心理学检查 [使用简易精神状态检查表（Mini-Mental State Examination，MMSE）和画钟实验进行测量]、体格检查（通过血液样本和与患者或护理人员的访谈来评估，并记录所做观察）、形态学检查（使用 CT 或 MRI 脑部扫描、单光子发射 CT 和脊髓液测试进行测量），以及国际疾病分类统计学（International Statistical Classification of Diseases，ICD）评估。为了区分和评估受试者是否患有痴呆症、轻度认知障碍或主观认知障碍，我们使用日常生活能力（Activities of Daily Living，ADL）测量或让家庭医生将患者转诊至记忆门诊的方式来评估损害情况，从而使医生对患者的记忆问题有所了解。为了更具体地评估患者在参与研究前 1 个月内的抑郁情况，经过培训的护士们单独完成了 CSDD 问卷调查，而检查患者的医生则独立完成了 MADRS 问卷调查。该评估措施的完成是基于 2 次不同的面谈测试，使用了 2 个访谈者信息来源。在评估患者的照顾者负担水平时，护士根据照顾者提供的信息，使用 0（"完全没有"）到 4（"非常高"）的评分标准来完成相对压力量表。此外，我们采用斯皮尔曼相关系数和主成分分析来评估 CSDD 量表与 MADRS 量表之间的相关性。对 CSDD 和 MADRS 测量之间的相关性进行比较，轻度认知障碍和主观认知障碍患者之间的相关性较差，而痴呆患者之间的相关性更差。Knapskog 等[27]认为，痴呆患者在不同量表之间存在最弱相关性，这种相关性是由于他们受损的记忆与轻度认知障碍和主观认知障碍个体相比较所导致的。他们指出，与轻度认知障碍和主观认知障碍患者相比，受损的记忆可能导致痴呆患者较少报告抑郁症状。在评估影响抑郁测量之间相关性的患者特征变量时，统计分析总体上未显示出认知功能受损是影响 CSDD 和 MADRS 之间关系的因素。然而，患者的神经心理学检查使用 MMSE（得分为 26~28 分）与抑郁量表之间存在相关性，而画钟实验结果与 CSDD 或 MADRS 量表无相关性。此外，照顾者负担评估与 CSDD 和 MADRS 之间无相关性。从这项研究可以得出，CSDD 和 MADRS 作为评测痴呆患者抑郁症的 2 个量表，其相关性较差。此外，作者建议对于存在记忆问题的患者，应该同时使用患者和照顾者来评估其抑郁情况。因为随着患者记忆恶化（如在痴呆受试者样本中观察到），由其记忆问题导致报告的抑郁症状减少。

Sheehan[9] 对认知、功能、行为、生活质量（Quality of Life，QOL）、痴呆的抑郁症、照顾者负担以及整体痴呆严重程度等领域的量表进行了综述。Sheehan[9] 还讨论了量表作为评测痴呆症和抑郁症的准确且有效指标所需的重要特征。对于量表来说，具有面向效度（患者、家属和临床医生都认为问题是相关且重要的）、结构效度（实验是否真正测量到假设）、同时效度（与其他良好的测量工具相比表现良好）以及可靠性（互评和测试-再测试）非常重要。尽管有许多用于测量痴呆症患者抑郁症的工具，但 Sheehan[9] 认为，CSDD 是量化这些人群抑郁症状的金标准。其他抑郁量表，如 GDS、MADRS 和 HADS，在患有中度至重度痴呆的患者中被认为不够准确。Sheehan[9] 认为，这可能是因为这些患者难以理解这些量表中的问题。对 HAM-D 也进行了审查，但据报道该量表过于冗长，不适合用于痴呆患者。因此，该综述的结果强调，选择最准确的量表对于阐明痴呆症患者的干预效果至关重要。

Thorpe[10] 在痴呆症患者中诊断抑郁症时，确定了两个量表：DMAS 和 CSDD。Thorpe[10] 还详细介绍了收集一个谨慎的临床评估时需要考虑的必要领域，包括症状史、家族史和实验室调查。详细的症状史包括以下内容：对症状进行详细描述，包括其时间进程和发展情况，以及与其他干扰因素（如环境压力、疼痛、营养不良、其他医学条件和最近的药物变化）的关联。还需要特别关注在痴呆症中较少见的抑郁症状，如绝望、内疚表达、自卑感和自残念头。Thorpe[10]还指出，前额叶皮质相关的功能障碍，如缺乏抑制力、固执和主动性减退，更表明是强烈的额叶痴呆而不是抑郁症。建议了解家族情绪障碍史、个人抑郁症既往史和以前对治疗的反应，这些信息被认为是重要的。在直接面谈测试环境中，应密切关注患者情绪低落和无法对刺激做出反应的情况、绝望感、自责表达、无价值感以及自残念头。Thorpe[10]还建议对血液学、甲状腺功能、电解质、维生素B_{12}以及药物水平进行实验室检查，因为它们都有引起情绪症状（如抑郁）的倾向，尤其是在患有痴呆的患者中。

据 Kirkham 等[28]估计，20%~30% 的 AD 患者会发展成重度抑郁障碍（Major Depressive Disorder，MDD）。与没有痴呆的人群相比，痴呆患者仅需表现出 3 个症状而非 5 个即可被诊断为抑郁症。第一个症状必须是情绪低落或对活动失去兴趣。剩下的症状可能包括以下任何一种：体重或食欲明显改变，失眠或嗜睡，精神运动性激越或迟滞、疲劳、自卑感或内疚感，难以集中注意力以及反复出现死亡或自杀的念头。未经治疗的痴呆抑郁症与死亡率增加、认知衰退加速、入住养老院提前和生活质量降低有关。Kirkham 等[28]研究的首要目标是确定抑郁评定量表作为痴呆患者抑郁症筛查工具的准确性，并比较它们的诊断准确性。其次要目标是研究可能影响抑郁评定量表准确性的因素，包括用于诊断痴呆抑郁症的参考标准（《精神障碍诊断与统计手册》）、痴呆中抑郁症的基线患病率、年龄、性别、痴呆类型、研究环境和所在国家。参与该研究的对象是被诊断为阿尔茨海默病、血管性痴呆（Vascular Dementia，VaD）、血管性和阿尔茨海默病混合型痴呆以及路易体痴呆（Dementia with Lewy Bodies，DLB）的患者。指标测试包括几种通用抑郁量表，以及专门针对老年痴呆中抑郁情况的量表。

Portugal Mda 等[12]在 95 例 65 岁及以上的痴呆患者中评估了 MADRS 和 CSDD 的有效性。他们还尝试使用这 2 种评估工具，寻找最适合识别痴呆患者抑郁症的敏感性和特异性指标所对应的截断点。敏感性是指如果一个人患有该疾病，测试结果为阳性的概率；而特异性则是指测试结果为阴性且未患有该疾病的概率。GDS 和 NOSGER 在识别老年人抑郁症方面，尤其是对于患有痴呆的老年人来说，截断点并不一致，使它们变得不可靠。MADRS 和 CSDD 被认为是有用的，因为它们与金标准工具达成了令人满意的一致性，无论痴呆患者抑郁症严重程度如何都可用于诊断[13]。然而，MADRS 是一种基于观察者的评分量表，而 CSDD 是一种基于知情人的评分量表。这使得作者考虑到观察者（临床医生）和知情人（照顾者）在症状关注方面可能存在的差异。受试者根据 DSM-Ⅳ 标准进行了痴呆评估，并使用 DSM-Ⅳ、国际疾病分类第 10 版（International Classification of Disease，ICD-10）标准以及 PDC-dAD 进行抑郁诊断。痴呆和其严重程度是通过巴西适应版的临床痴呆评分（Clinical Dementia Rating，CDR）、MMSE 和神经精神量表（Neuropsychiatric Inventory，NPI）进行评估的。此外，所有患者都接受了巴西版本的 MADRS 抑郁筛查，并由相应的照顾者完成了改编版 CSDD 问卷调查。研究结果显示，MADRS 评分为 10 分和 CSDD 评分为 13 分是识别抑郁障碍的最佳截断点。该研究的结果与之前的研究不一致。几项研究报告称，在老年痴呆患者中，抑郁症的 CSDD 截断点为 5~8[11,29-31]。作者提出了几种可能性，包括拉丁美洲人口的文化差异以及照顾者可能提供虚假信息以迫使患者入院。作者得出结论，在与他们相似的样本中，MADRS 和 CSDD 都应被视为筛查工具，而不是诊断措施。

Starkstein 等[7]进行的一项研究的主要目标是验证一套诊断标准，以诊断 AD 患者的抑郁症。该研究招募的受试者包括 971 例患有轻度、中度或重度认知障碍的 AD 患者。所有受试者于 1993 年 1 月至 2002 年 10 月，在阿根廷布宜诺斯艾利斯市一个三级医疗中心的老年痴呆门诊接受了治疗。初始精神科检查使用 DSM-Ⅳ 结构化临床访谈（Structured Clinical Interview for DSM-Ⅳ，SCID）进行。根据 DSM-Ⅳ 定义（"悲伤情绪几乎每天大部分时间都存在，并持续超过 2 周"）对受试者的悲伤情绪进行了评定。其他应用检测包括 MMSE、CDR、HAM-D、汉密尔顿焦虑量表（Hamilton Anxiety Rating Scale，HAM-A）、冷漠量表和易怒性量表。采用潜在类别分析，一个聚类过程，来确定 AD 患者的潜在结构，并根据他们的 SCID 回答以及其他精神病学工具对其进行分类。通过潜在类别分析产生的最佳拟合模型是一个三类模型，其组别由他们的精神症状特征定义。第三类，占受试者的 21%，展示了对 9 个 DSM-Ⅳ 主要抑郁症标准的高频率。第二类占样本的 39%，抑郁症状的频率更广泛，范围从 4%~55%，相当于轻度抑郁。第一类占受试者的 40%，显示出非常低频率的抑郁症状。9 个 DSM-Ⅳ 主要抑郁症标准在不同组别之间存在显著差异。当与无抑郁情绪群体相比较时，96% 的第三类受试者符合未经修改的 DSM-Ⅳ 主要抑郁症标准。该研究还发现，焦虑和冷漠是 AD 患者抑郁症的重要预测因素，而易怒性则不是。最后，发现轻度抑郁的患者比没有抑郁的患者更容易出现冷漠情绪。这表明，AD 中的轻度抑郁可能是一个多样化的状况，包括真正抑郁的患者和那些没有抑郁但有倦怠感的患者。此外，还发现了更严重的抑郁与更晚期痴呆阶段之间存在显著关联。通过将美国国家精神卫生研究所 - 痴呆抑郁症（NIMH-dAD）的诊断与 DSM-Ⅳ 进行比较发现，受试者中有 38% 符合修改后的 NIMH-dAD 标准，而使用 DSM-Ⅳ 标准则为 27%。Starkstein 等[7]认为，根据 NIMH-dAD，抑郁症的发生频率可能被低估，因为他们在整个样本中使用了 DSM-Ⅳ 标准的时间标准来评估症状的频率。DSM-Ⅳ 的时间标准比 NIMH-dAD 更严格。作者得出结论，他们的研究验证了 DSM-Ⅳ 对于 AD 中重度抑郁症的诊断标准，并认为 DSM-Ⅳ 提供了最佳数量的症状来诊断重度抑郁症。

Vilalta-Franch 等[8]认为，与年轻患者相比，老年抑郁症患者的表现方式有所不同。老年患者常常否认自己感到悲伤，而是报告缺乏情感或失去了对活动的兴趣和快乐。本研究旨在通过横断面研究，比较特定的诊断标准与其他较一般的标准，确定 AD 患者抑郁发生率的差异。它还旨在根据使用的每个诊断标准确定患有抑郁症和无抑郁症患者的临床特征。本研究的数据来源于 491 例可能患有 AD 的患者，他们在 1998 年 5 月至 2003 年 5 月间完成了前一项研究——阿尔茨海默病型痴呆和护理负担演变（Evolution of Dementia of the Alzheimertype and Caregiver burden，EDAC）的基线访问。EDAC 是一项自然观察性研究，历时 24 个月。在基线访问中使用了 CAMDEX 和 NPI。CAMDEX 是一种标准化的、结构化的面谈测试和检查工具，可用于晚年常见心理障碍，特别是痴呆症的诊断。

它包括对患者的访谈、认知检查、与亲属或照顾者的访谈以及多个量表[布莱斯特痴呆评分量表（Blessed Dementia Rating Scale，BDRS）、缺血评分、MMSE]。CAMDEX 根据 DSM-Ⅳ 和 ICD-10 标准提供临床诊断，包括主要和次要的精神疾病诊断、对痴呆程度的临床估计、对抑郁症状严重程度的临床估计（CAMDEX 抑郁诊断量表）以及其他医学诊断。NPI 是一种用于评估患者行为和心理症状的量表，由看护人员或家属填写。该研究使用 ICD-10 和 DSM-Ⅳ 来诊断重度抑郁发作，使用 CAMDEX 标准来诊断抑郁症，使用 PDC-dAD 以及在 NPI 抑郁量表中对筛查问题"患者是否看起来悲伤或沮丧？他是否说自己感到悲伤或沮丧"作出积极回应。这相当于对抑郁症的五种概念化，按照诊断严格程度递增的顺序。研究结果发现，根据每个标准，AD 患者的抑郁症患病率如下：ICD-10 为 4.9%，CAMDEX 为 9.8%，DSM-Ⅳ 为 13.4%，PDC-dAC 为 27.4%，NPI 抑郁量表为 43.7%。按照 kappa 指数测量，分类系统之间的一致性百分比低至中等。没有任何一对标准达到 50% 的一致率。缺乏自信心或低自尊以及易怒是导致诊断不一致的主要因素。总之，本研究结果表明，抑郁在阿尔茨海默病中的患病率存在显著差异，这取决于所采用的诊断标准。各种测量方法之间的一致性较低，并且使用特定的抑郁诊断标准会增加患病率。

关于痴呆患者中抑郁症患病率的报告差异很大，最有可能的原因是认知障碍的严重程度不同，以及用于检测抑郁症的量表范围广泛[13]。由于抑郁症和痴呆症的症状相似，区分两者可能会很困难。然而，根据 Lyketsos 和 Olin[32] 的报道，痴呆中抑郁症的治疗是成功的。Muller-Thomsen 等[13] 使用 4 种不同的抑郁量表评估了与 AD 阶段相关联的抑郁发生率。次要目标是通过计算内部一致性和它们之间的相关性来测试每个量表的有效性。受试者是根据美国国立神经、语言交流障碍和卒中研究-阿尔茨海默病及相关疾病协会（National Institute of Neurological and Communicative Disorders and Stroke and the Alzheimer's Disease and Related Disorders Association，NINCDS-ADRDA）的标准，诊断为可能患有阿尔茨海默病的 316 例患者。这些患者于 1995 年至 2001 年间，在汉堡大学医院精神科记忆门诊部就诊，认知损伤严重程度使用 MMSE 进行确定。受试者分为两组——轻度痴呆组（MMSE 得分 18~30 分）和中度至重度痴呆组（MMSE 得分 0~17 分）。使用以下 4 个量表评估抑郁症：GDS——自评量表、MADRS——由神经心理学家评定的量表、NOSGER——照顾者评定的量表和 CSDD——医生评定的量表。根据 GDS 的数据，当使用 6 作为检测抑郁症的截断点时，AD 患者中抑郁症的患病率约为 35%。Muller-Thomsen 等[13]发现在中度至重度 AD 组中内部一致性明显下降。这说明，认知衰退程度可能会影响 GDS 结果。Muller-Thomsen 等[13]得出结论称，在 AD 中，特别是在后期阶段，GDS 不适用于检测抑郁症。这支持 Burke 等[33]以及 Zarb[34]之前的发现。与其他量表相比，由照顾者评定的 NOSGER 情绪量表报告了明显更高的抑郁率。然而，在中度至重度 AD 组中抑郁率较轻度 AD 组更高（68% vs. 53%），与其他量表一致。作者提出 3 种可能来解释 NOSGER 情绪量表报告的患病率较高的原因：首先，可能是照顾者将自己的个人负担投射出来，从而影响了他们的回答。其次，量表的截断点太低。最后，正如 Muller-Thomsen 等[13]所提到的，使用 NOSGER 的子量表是没有意义的。NOSGER 情绪量表的内部一致性是所有评估的量表中最差的，与其他量表结果之间存在较差的相关性。MADRS 和 CSDD 都将约 40% 的中度至重度 AD 患者分类为抑郁症，并且将轻度 AD 组中约 30% 的患者也归类为抑郁症。这 2 个量表在内部一致性方面均良好，并观察到 2 种评估之间有显著正相关性。作者们认为，这可能是由于这两个量表中某些项目相似导致的。总结起来，一个始终如一的发现是，在中度至重度 AD 组中抑郁症更为普遍，而在轻度 AD 组中则较少见。MADRS 和 CSDD 被推荐作为检测抑郁症和描述门诊 AD 患者的抑郁症状的有用工具。

汉密尔顿抑郁量表（Hamilton Rating Scale for Depression，HRSD）是一种常用的临床和研究工具。Naarding 等[35]评估了是否应该对包括卒中、AD 和帕金森病在内的各种神经系统疾病应用特定于疾病的截断点。作者们比较了 HAM-D 与 DSM-Ⅳ MDD 标准的同时效度。AD 组包括 274 例根据 DSM-Ⅳ 和 NINCDS-ADRDA 标准诊断为痴呆的患者。根据 DSM-Ⅳ 标准，HAM-D 被用作诊断 MDD 的症状检查量表。还使用 MMSE 评估了 239 例患者的认知状态。AD 组中 MDD

的患病率为22.6%。为了确定HAM-D是否可以用作预测性测试,在量表的中间范围内计算了不同截断点的阳性预测值(PPV)和阴性预测值(NPV)。在AD组中,高阳性预测值的最佳截断点为13/14,阴性预测值的最佳截断点为6/7。Naarding等[35]认为,在HAM-D中测量到的心理运动和自主神经症状在理论上可能与DSM对MDD的标准重合,从而使得AD患者的MDD诊断更加困难。然而,HAM-D与DSM-Ⅳ对于MDD标准之间存在较高的同时效度,因此这种重合不应引起临床关注。总之,该量表要实现最佳性能,则需要使用特定于疾病的截断点进行筛查、诊断和二分化。

以前认为,AD患者的抑郁症状与老年人正常认知状态下的抑郁症状有所不同[36]。人们曾认为AD患者更容易出现动机性症状和妄想,且较少出现抑郁的核心症状。如悲伤、睡眠障碍和食欲减退[37,38]。然而,更近期的研究并未证实这些发现,相反地,有报告称抑郁症的典型症状尤其是悲伤也存在于痴呆患者中[39-41]。这场争议的结果是,该领域的临床专家们提出了一个新的阿尔茨海默病抑郁症诊断标准:PDC-dAD。实施新标准的少数研究发现,使用该标准报告的AD患者抑郁症的患病率要高于使用DSM或ICD标准时所报告的。尽管关于老年痴呆患者常用抑郁测量工具(如HRSD)的研究较多[25],但也有其他专门针对阿尔茨海默病型老年痴呆患者使用的量表,如PDC-dAD[16]。Engedal等[36]旨在进一步研究PDC-dAD的实用性,并比较该量表与DSM-Ⅳ-TR和ICD-10标准中抑郁症状在同一名AD患者中的差异。具体来说,使用PDC-dAD测量方法识别症状的结果还与PDC-dAD对痴呆抑郁的诊断以及使用重性抑郁标准的《精神障碍诊断与统计手册第4版文本修订版》(Diagnostic and Statistical Manual of Mental Disorders Version 4,DSM-Ⅳ-TR)和ICD-10测量进行比较,以评估其在鉴定和诊断阿尔茨海默病患者抑郁方面的有效性。该研究包括112例阿尔茨海默病患者,其中55例来自养老院,57例来自老年精神科医院。根据ICD-10标准对阿尔茨海默病进行了诊断。由经过培训的护士使用CSDD对患者进行抑郁评估。使用身体自我维护量表进行ADL评估。通过MMSE和CDR量表评估认知功能和痴呆阶段。在CSDD被使用后1周内,经验丰富的老年精神科医生(对CSDD

结果不知情）根据 PDC-dAD 标准、ICD-10 研究标准以及 DSM-Ⅳ-TR（重性抑郁）标准记录存在的抑郁症状。正如预期的那样，PDC-dAD 标准比 DSM 和 ICD 标准识别到了更多的抑郁症患者。具体而言，结果报告了 AD 中抑郁症的患病率在以下水平：PCD-dAD——53.6%；ICD-10——47.3%；DSM-Ⅳ-TR——34.8%。PDC-dAD 标准在 Hosmer-Lemeshow 拟合度检验中表现不佳，使得该模型的有效性不如 ICD-10 和 DSM-Ⅳ-TR。这与其他研究[8,42]的发现一致。其原因被认为是诊断只需要 3 个症状，并且这些症状并非需要每天大部分时间都存在。PDC-dAD 还评估了妄想，在大多数患者有中度至重度阿尔茨海默病的情况下，妄想可能更加频繁地出现。3 个标准之间的一致性很高。使用 DSM 和 ICD 标准观察到的症状模式与没有痴呆的抑郁患者相似。抑郁症患者与非抑郁症患者相比，最显著的 6 个症状是焦虑、悲伤、多种身体不适、自杀意念、悲观情绪和低自尊。妄想和激越在 ICD 和 PDC-dAD 的诊断中是重要因素，但对于 DSM 来说并不重要。总之，AD 患者中抑郁症最突出和显著的症状与老年人中未患痴呆的核心抑郁症状相同，并且使用 PDC-dAD 标准诊断出的抑郁症患者比使用 DSM 或 ICD 标准更多。

为了探索使用 NIMH-dAD 的能力，Teng 等[42]使用 NIMH-dAD 测量痴呆抑郁症，并将其与使用其他测量标准诊断抑郁症的结果进行比较，评估抑郁症患者的缓解程度。他们从进行抑郁症描述性纵向研究的 AD 研究中心招募了 101 例符合 DSM-Ⅳ 标准的重度或轻度抑郁症患者。该研究对受试者在基线和 3 个月后的 2 个时间点进行评估，评估使用了多种量表来测量抑郁，如 NIMH-dAD、DSM-Ⅳ、CSDD 和 NPI-Q（问卷版本）。所使用的 DSM-Ⅳ 标准是主要或次要抑郁症，这也得到了使用 DSM-Ⅳ 轴 Ⅰ 障碍结构化临床访谈的支持。其他支持信息收集的来源，以支持某些措施（如 NIMH-dAD）的诊断，是与受试者及其照顾者进行访谈后临床医生的印象。在 3 个月后对这些评估和量表进行测量，可以评估受试者是否缓解。Teng 等[42]发现，与其他抑郁症测量工具相比，NIMH-dAD 测量方法在识别患有抑郁症的阿尔茨海默病患者方面更为有效。因此，建议使用 NIMH-dAD 量表来更好地区分抑郁症状。尽管 NIMH-dAD 量表在识别和区分患者的抑郁症状方面比其他测量工具更为有效，但其与 DSM-Ⅳ 在诊断轻度和重度抑郁症方面非常接近，因为它们具有非常相似的特征。例如，只需要存在少数抑郁症状（对于 NIMH-dAD 是 3 个，对于 DSM-Ⅳ 是 5 个）以及较不严格的时间要求来符合抑郁标准。NIMH-dAD 中派生自 DSM-Ⅳ 的 3 个症状包括心理运动改变、乏力以及罪恶感/无价值感。除了这 3 个症状外，DSM-Ⅳ 还包括社交孤立/退缩和易怒等其他症状。虽然谨慎并且认真对待个体的抑郁症状有其优势，但也可能存在低特异性的缺点，即在实际上没有抑郁症的情况下被诊断为抑郁症。该研究在 3 个月后随访时受试者的缓解率达到 51% 支持了这种解释。其他抑郁症测量指标中也发现了类似的缓解率，并且被认为是受试者接受抑郁症治疗所致，这可能是该研究结果的混杂或促成因素。总之，考虑与抑郁症相关的症状非常重要，因为尽管这些症状可能并不出现或反映在所有患有痴呆的患者身上[42]，但患者所经历的抑郁症状存在差异，而且更具体的诊断而不是过度诊断患者的抑郁似乎很重要，尤其是在随后需要进行治疗或药物干预的情况下。

为了评估抑郁症测量方法在痴呆患者中的有效性，Gilley 和 Wilson[13] 使用 GDS 和 HRSD 来诊断重度抑郁症。该研究还通过两组受试者，即认知受损的 AD 患者组和认知完好的对照组，以评估 GDS 对认知障碍的影响。总体而言，共有 715 例 AD 患者组成了认知受损组，93 名受试者组成了认知完好组。参与研究的所有受试者都接受了抑郁和认知功能的评估。使用 GDS 测量受试者过去 1 周内的情感/心境状态，并结合对过去 4 周中最常与受试者保持联系的 1 个知情人（家庭成员）进行访谈作为标准测量指标以评估抑郁情况。在评估受试者的抑郁状态时，使用 DSM-Ⅲ 结构化临床访谈（SCID）进行 MDD 诊断，其中 SCID 和 HRSD 也被纳入到访谈中以评估抑郁程度。为了探究认知障碍是否会影响 GDS 结果，对受试者进行的测量包括：MMSE——用于评估全面认知障碍水平；韦氏记忆量表-修订版的逻辑记忆和图形记忆子测试——用于评估记忆能力；多语种失语症检查（视觉命名量表和受控口头词汇联想量表）的子测试——用于评估语言功能。为了进一步评估认知障碍对 GDS 测量的影响，进行统计分析（例如，逻辑回归、乘积矩相关）。Gilley 和 Wilson[43] 研究的结果显示，在与认知完好组相比较时，AD 患者组的 GDS 测量得分与 SCID 和 HRSD 标准之间相关性较差。此外，在 AD 患者组中，他们的认知水平确实会影响 GDS 得分，这降低了在 AD 患者群体中使用 GDS 测量工具的有效性。解释这些发现时，可以提出一个观点：在 AD 患者中使用 GDS 测量工具可能导致高假阴性率，即 AD 患者可能存在抑郁症（或抑郁症状），但其测量得分却表明他们没有抑郁症。不同于其他研究[9]，如果建议在轻度阶段痴呆的使用中验证 GDS，可以得出应该进行更多的研究来调查 GDS 在轻度痴呆患者（如 CSDD）中有效性的结论[44]。

Korner 等[44]研究了抑郁测量工具在老年人和痴呆患者中的应用。该研究涉及对 145 名 65 岁或以上的老年受试者进行 GDS、CSDD 和 HDRS 的评估（其中 73 名抑郁，36 名抑郁和痴呆，36 名非抑郁，其中 11 人仅有痴呆）。对于患有痴呆的受试者，未指定其严重程度。Korner 等[44]还特别回顾了 GDS 和 CSDD 的敏感性和特异性以及 CSDD 的观察者间可靠性。这项研究采用了评估受试者抑郁和痴呆的方法，使用了 ICD 和临床整体印象测量。在与受试者进行面谈时使用 GDS、CDSS 和 HDRS，进一步探索和衡量受试者群体中的抑郁情况；而在探索受试者认知障碍时，则使用了 MMSE。研究结果表明，GDS、CSDD 和 HDRS 是评估抑郁症的良好指标。然而，尽管 CSDD 和 GDS 与 HDRS 量表密切相关，但在认知障碍或智力受损的受试者群体以及非认知障碍的受试者群体中，CSDD 比 GDS 更适合评估抑郁症。从量表内容来看，CSDD 和 HDRS 这两个测量工具之间存在着强烈的关系，其中有 4 个测量项目评估了抑郁症状（具体包括情绪、兴趣减退、精力低下和自杀意念），以及与抑郁相关的一些睡眠和精神病性症状。解释这些发现与评估痴呆患者抑郁症有效性的关系时，可以认为 GDS 不适合痴呆患者，而 CSDD 与 HDRS 在筛查抑郁症时对于痴呆患者的适用性和合适性也存在竞争问题。然而，其他研究表明，当涉及在痴呆患者中测量抑郁症时，HDRS 并非有效，这与抑郁症的症状有关。例如，无法保持对话能力，因为该量表需要 20~30 分钟才能完成[9]。因此，CSDD 被认为是最有效和适用于测量痴呆患者抑郁症的量表。根据量表长度适用于痴呆症患者的想法，Korner 等[44]还建议，量表的长度是测量工具有效性的重要特征，特别是在可能患有痴呆的老年人中。建议在痴呆和非痴呆的老年人群中，为了达到高敏感性和特异性水平，抑郁测量工具的长度应为4个项目。

Vida 等[45]比较了 CSDD 和 HDRS 2 种测量工具在检测 AD 患者抑郁症方面的有效性，并使用非参数统计分析受试者工作特征曲线（Receiver Operating Characteristic，ROC）来评估这些量表的适用性，包括特异性和敏感性。同时，该研究还评估了 CSDD 和 HDRS 量表与主要抑郁症的研究诊断标准（Research Diagnostic Criteria，RDC）之间的相关性。共有 10 名受试者参加了该项研究，并进行了一次访谈（连同他们的看护人员）以收集有关人口统计学、社会和医学信息的数据。此外，对受试者的认知和抑郁情绪状态使用多个测量工具进行评估：GDS、MMSE、HDRS 和 CSDD。在测量评估后，受试者进行了另一次访谈，研究人员使用 RDC 来测试（和评估）抑郁症的主要程度，从轻度到中度。研究结果显示，CSDD 和 HDRS 与 RDC 之间存在中度到高度的相关性。尽管 RDC 与两个量表之间都存在良好的关系，但 CSDD 与 RDC 的相关性略高于 HDRS，这表明在测量 AD 患者的抑郁程度方面，CSDD 与 RDC 之间存在更强的关联。此外，在特异性和敏感性分析中，CSDD 和 HDRS 都被证明是区分轻度至中度 AD 患者是否符合抑郁症诊断标准的有效措施。这种区分很重要，因为在早期痴呆阶段未能诊断出抑郁可能会导致绝望和自杀意念等严重后果[46,47]。因此，CSDD 可能比 HDRS 在识别痴呆患者的抑郁症方面更有效，这与其他文献[44]一致。该文献认为，CSDD 具有良好的内容效度和功能性，因为它是一种可以更易用于注意力不集中的痴呆患者身上的简化量表。因此，很显然 CSDD 比 HDRS 更有效，因其具备了在测量抑郁症时所需求的特点，并且这些特点被强调为理想特质，如敏感性和特异性。

Lam 等[48]评估了 GDS、更简短的抑郁评估量表（Even Briefer Assessment Scale for Depression，EBAS DEP）、单一问题以及 CSDD 在测量和诊断痴呆患者抑郁症方面的有效性。该研究涉及 88 例 60 岁或以上的老年痴呆患者（66 例无抑郁症；22 例有抑郁症）。受试者根据痴呆严重程度分为轻度和中至重度 2 组，以比较量表在不同痴呆严重程度阶段诊断抑郁的效果。研究中使用了 4 个量表来评估受试者的抑郁情况，这些量表由一位在招募时期对受试者是否患有抑郁症不知情的研究心理学家进行评定。所有的量表回答都是从最了解他们 ADL 并且和他们保持联系最为密切以及掌握信息最多的看护人那里获得的。然而，单一问题只能直接提问患者。采用卡方检验和曼 - 惠特尼 U 检验等统计分析方法，衡量量表的有效性以及性别、年龄和痴呆严重程度对抑郁与非抑郁痴呆受试者群体之间的影响，并确定单一问题是否能够诊断抑郁。另外，使用 ROC 曲线来比较 GDS、EBAS DEP 和 Cornell 量表的有效性，用于评估措施的敏感性和特异性。此外，还使用交叉表（另一种统计方法）对单一问题措施的特异性和敏感性进行了评估。该研究的结果表明，随着痴呆症在认知领域的恶化，抑郁症的诊断变得更加困难，需要选择更具体和短小的量表，以适应晚期痴呆患者注意力不集中的问题[9,25,44]。因此建议在中度至重度痴呆阶段，抑郁的截断点应该更高。此外，单一问卷的使用似乎比其他量表（GDS、EBAS DEP、CSDD 和单一问题）在诊断抑郁症方面力度更强，尤其是在晚期痴呆阶段。在选择最合适的测量方法后，CSDD 对于患有痴呆的受试者诊断抑郁症也是次有效的。正因为如此，Lam 等[48]建议，在选择一种用于诊断痴呆患者抑郁症的工具时，应首先使用单一问题量表，必要时再使用 CSDD，因为 CSDD 在诊断抑郁症方面敏感性和特异性最高，即使考虑到痴呆严重程度阶段。

尽管用于评估抑郁症的量表有许多，但它们往往更倾向于衡量抑郁症的严重程度，而不是确定个体是否真正患有抑郁症。还有不同的量表应该优先用于认知衰退（痴呆）患者和没有认知衰退的其他人。也就是说，MADRS 适用于测量认知正常的老年人的抑郁情况，而 CSDD 适用于既有痴呆又具备正常认知能力的老年人[49]。因此，本研究的目的是评估 MADRS 在识别 DSM-Ⅳ 诊断为抑郁症的认知正常个体中的有效性，并将其与 CSDD 进行比较。参与该研究的有 104 名 65 岁以上且没有痴呆迹象的受试者（101 名女性，39 名男性），他们接受了 MMSE 认知评估。此外，抑郁症的评估包括作为 MADRS 及其量表的一部分参与访谈，以及接受访谈的照顾者和患者作为 CSDD 测量的一部分。除了使用 MADRS 和 CSDD 两种量表来衡量抑郁程度之外，所有受试者均根据 DSM-Ⅳ

诊断出抑郁症，而只有70名受试者根据ICD-10被诊断出抑郁症。研究结果表明，MADRS适用于非痴呆人群的抑郁诊断，并具有良好的敏感性和特异性。与DSM-Ⅳ相比，ICD-10在抑郁诊断方面较为宽松（对重度抑郁的标准而言）。更具体地比较ICD-10与MADRS，当不将这些测量结果与DSM-Ⅳ进行比较时，ICD-10在识别抑郁症方面更准确。这些发现可能与MADRS在识别痴呆患者的抑郁症方面不如ICD-10有效有关，而且相比于DSM-Ⅳ，ICD-10在识别和诊断抑郁症方面也具有较宽松的标准。此外，在涉及CSDD时，相对而言，建议使用MADRS作为老年非痴呆受试者的测量方法。因此，可以得出结论，MADRS不仅是对非痴呆患者的抑郁更有用的测量指标，而且在区分受试者是否患有抑郁症方面比CSDD更有效。

Muller-Thomsen等[13]使用4种不同的抑郁量表，即GDS、MADRS、CSDD和NOSGER，探讨了阿尔茨海默病各阶段中抑郁的存在情况。该研究涉及对316例可能患有AD的患者进行探索，根据MMSE的测量结果将其分为两组：轻度AD和中度至重度AD，以评估认知障碍是否影响抑郁程度的测量。以下量表由个别专业人士（如医生、神经心理学家）或照顾者来评估受试者的抑郁情况：GDS、MADRS、CSDD和NOSGER，除非认知能力太差无法完成量表项目。通过SPSS进行统计分析，总体结果表明，与轻度AD组（26.8%）相比，中度到重度AD组受试者中的抑郁症较少（15.7%）。关于使用4个独立量表对两组人群进行抑郁症诊断，根据GDS测量结果发现35%的受试者被认定为抑郁。作者指出，在中度至重度AD组内，受试者自我诊断抑郁的内部一致性较低，这意味着在评估后期AD患者的抑郁时，GDS可能不是一个有效工具。此外，与其他3个量表相比，使用NOSGER情绪量表，受试者的抑郁症识别率相当高，尤其是在中度至重度AD患者群体中。然而，这样的发现被认为受到照顾者负担等其他因素的影响，包括内部一致性不足，在研究中与其他感兴趣的量表相比较差。在中度至重度AD组的受试者中，MADRS和CSDD发现40%的人有抑郁症，在轻度AD组中有30%的人有抑郁症。这些结果表明内部一致性足够，并存在正相关关系。总的来说，抑郁症在中度到重度组中被检测出更多，这表明阿尔茨海默病的神经进展可能会影响作者所提到的抑郁症状的出现或发展。总之，进一步可以提出的观点是，在研究 AD 疾病进展路径中检测抑郁时，MADRS 和 CSDD 似乎是 4 个量表中最合适的。这得到了量表内部一致性和相关性的支持。尽管这两种量表都被认为能很好地检测抑郁症，但一些使用者更喜欢其中一种，原因是 CSDD 更容易使用，其项目的措辞相对主观，而 MADRS 的项目则更客观、更容易理解和应用于患者[50]。此外，另一项研究发现，MADRS 和 CSDD 作为有效检测痴呆患者抑郁的指标也具有良好的内部一致性，并且能够很好地区分抑郁与非抑郁的痴呆受试者[50]。

Vilalta-Franch 等[8]将痴呆患者的抑郁症状与抑郁测量指标的特定症状特征联系起来，在 491 例可能患有阿尔茨海默病的患者中使用不同抑郁量表来调查诊断抑郁症的患病率。在研究的基线阶段，受试者完成了 CAMDEX 和 NPI 以进行临床诊断痴呆，并使用剑桥认知测验、MMSE 和 BDRS 等量表对认知和功能进行评估，同时还使用 NPI 评定疾病的行为和神经心理症状。为了评估抑郁症，患者完成了以下测量：ICD-10、DSM-Ⅳ（用于主要抑郁发作的诊断）、CAMDEX（抑郁症）、PDC-dAD 以及 NPI 抑郁亚量表（筛查问题的积极回应）。研究结果确实显示不同量表在检测抑郁症方面存在差异。ICD-10 将人群中的 4.9% 诊断为抑郁，PDC-dAD 为 27.4%，DSM-Ⅳ 为 13.4%，CAMDEX 为 9.8%，NPI 抑郁亚量表则高达 43.7%，这可能是由于看护者过分强调患者症状严重程度而导致结果被高估。通过比较量表检测到的患病率，发现 PDC-dAD 更具体地识别了 ICD-10、CAMDEX 和 DSM-Ⅳ 在诊断痴呆患者抑郁症时未考虑的症状。研究结果发现，与其他在研究中使用的量表相比，PDC-dAD 量表在识别患有痴呆的抑郁症患者方面最为有效。具体而言，在 DSM-Ⅳ、CAMDEX 和 NPI 之间存在较低的一致性水平时，该量表与其他量表之间达成了最高程度的一致性。此外，NPI 在检测抑郁症方面也存在 15% 的假阴性率，即当实际上患者确实有抑郁症时，该量表会将其判断为无抑郁症。

第三节 讨论和结论

总之，通过综述表明，抑郁症在老年人、轻度认知障碍患者和痴呆症患者的几个领域（包括心理和生理方面）都有广泛的影响。更为重要的是，痴呆和抑郁之间的关系是双向的。例如，既往有抑郁史会增加患 AD 的机会，而痴呆症状（认知衰退、执行功能障碍和其他认知障碍）也会影响情绪并导致 AD 的抑郁出现。值得注意的是，治疗 AD 患者的抑郁症（或患有轻度认知障碍和主观认知障碍的个体）也能改善认知能力下降。另外，也有其他关于抑郁症和痴呆症之间关系的综述（表 1-2，也见于文献[44,51-53]），这里我们也试图关注用于评估痴呆患者抑郁的几种方法，以解释文献中相互矛盾的结论。

阿尔茨海默病中抑郁症的患病率因研究而异，一些研究报告的发病率为 20%~80%。这些差异背后的原因之一是使用了许多不同的量表来测量抑郁（见表 1-1）。其中一些量表包括 BDI、CSDD、GDS、HAM-D、HADS、MADRS、NOSGER 患者健康问卷、NIMH PDC-dAD、CAMDEX、NPI、ICD-10、DMAS 阿尔茨海默病情绪量表、Zung 氏抑郁自评量表等。而这些量表大多测量抑郁症的不同方面，因此导致了准确估计 AD 患者抑郁发病率的差异。

自知力（对自己症状的认识）和抑郁症之间的关系并不直接，因为一些研究报告了相悖的发现，即自知力良好的痴呆症患者有更多的抑郁症状。意识到自己的症状可能会让人对自己的病情感到难过，从而导致抑郁。此外，有研究调查了患者症状的严重程度与其照顾者的健康状况之间的关系，发现痴呆症状越严重，其照顾者的 QOL 就越低。然而，今后的研究应该扩大调查抑郁（患者或他们的照顾者）在他们之间的相互影响。

表 1-2　既往关于痴呆与抑郁症关系的代表性综述

量表/领域	内容
Sheehan[9] 回顾对痴呆症严重程度的测试，并协助提示性治疗设施	
康奈尔大学的患者和护理人员量表	优点：已被验证用于有或无痴呆症的患者，并被一些人认为是诊断痴呆症患者抑郁症状的金标准 作者：患者和护理人员都可以回答问题；如果患者不能回答而护理人员可以，这非常有用
蒙哥马利-阿斯伯格抑郁量表	评估心理症状 优点：过去对轻度痴呆症的作用有限 作者：很适用于干预研究。我们认为，通过（假设的）比较抑郁（先前的干预）和当前的抑郁（干预后），即历史和当前的抑郁，来评估干预的有效性是有用的
汉密尔顿抑郁量表	优点：最常用于抑郁症评估 问题和面谈测试 缺点：不太可能用于痴呆症患者 作者：不太可能用于痴呆症患者。由于痴呆症的症状包括难以跟上或跟踪对话，我们认为管理这个量表可能会很困难，因为它包括一个需要 20~30 分钟的半结构化访谈
老年抑郁量表	优点：最常用的老年人抑郁情绪评估方法 自我评价或由评估人评定 在老年人的护理机构可靠 缺点：对变化敏感。验证为轻度痴呆，但不是中度至重度痴呆——由于难以理解问题，完成率较低。考虑到利弊，我们认为它可能仅适用于轻度痴呆
医院焦虑与抑郁量表	优点：针对住院患者的抑郁和焦虑症筛查试验。易于使用，并能准确地检测出抑郁症 缺点：对于有显著认知障碍的老年患者，几乎没有实际应用，因为对项目的反应是主观的 我们认为，与其他量表相比，该量表不适合用于已过轻度期的痴呆症患者，因为对他们的症状了解有限或没有了解可能会影响他们对项目的反应
Kirkham 等 [28] 探讨了抑郁评定量表诊断 AD 痴呆、血管性痴呆和路易体痴呆抑郁的准确性	
康奈尔痴呆抑郁量表	专门针对痴呆症患者的抑郁 作者：≥9 筛选为阳性
痴呆情绪评估量表	护理人员的报告是基于临床医生的面谈。包含情绪和认知评估
老年患者护士观察量表	护理人员报告 作者：≥10 提示抑郁症

续表

量表/领域	内容
老年抑郁量表	自我报告 ≥6、≥8 或 ≥9 预示着抑郁症的存在
汉密尔顿抑郁量表	临床医生的访谈 ≥8 被认为是抑郁症的阳性反应
蒙哥马利-阿斯伯格抑郁量表	临床医生的访谈 ≥13 筛查为阳性
贝克抑郁量表	自我报告 ≥13 筛查为阳性
患者健康问卷	自我报告 ≥8~11 提示抑郁
Thorpe[10] 讨论了抑郁症和痴呆症的症状	
认知和功能下降	过度关注缺陷。对症状缺乏关注或否认 作者：很难对痴呆症中的抑郁症做出明确的诊断，尤其是在晚期患者中
情绪	大多数情况下，悲伤和刺激/支持并没有多大帮助。大部分正常。这取决于具体情况和波动。如果情绪低落，支持就会有帮助
兴趣和主动性	几个月来失去兴趣和快乐，包括感到悲伤、内疚、自残、绝望。长时间的冷漠，但并不涉及悲伤
饮食行为和减肥方法	几周内食欲的变化，导致了体重的增加或减少。经过几个月到几年的时间，体重逐渐下降。由于活动减少，药物治疗导致身高增长
睡眠	长达数月至数年睡眠周期紊乱导致大脑发生变化。晚上醒来，白天睡觉 在几周内，睡眠时间增加或减少
精神运动性激越	发生在几周内，往往发生在白天，在早上更糟。包括虚无主义的陈述（例如，生活是毫无意义的）或过度的内疚 发生在几个月或几年内，容易在一天结束后因疾病进展更糟。患者开始从他们早期的生活经历中寻找人或地方
精神运动性阻滞	发生在严重的抑郁症中，持续数周 发生在轻度至中度痴呆症中，更多发生在后期。可与帕金森病（面部掩蔽，运动功能迟缓）/皮克病相似

续表

量表/领域	内容
精力	低能量和有疲劳的症状 正常能量，但由于缓慢的执行功能导致的活动减少
有罪感/无价值感	在严重抑郁症中很常见。包括情绪低落，以及食欲和睡眠方面的变化 当对仍有疾病洞察力的患者施加压力时，内疚/无价值的陈述是很常见的
注意力和思考	注意力不集中，优柔寡断，害怕犯错 像思维这样的事情在疾病的后期阶段都会受到影响

参考文献

1. Reichman, W. E., & Coyne, A. C. (1995). Depressive symptoms in Alzheimer's disease and multi-infarct dementia. Journal of Geriatric Psychiatry and Neurology, 8(2), 96-99. Available from https://doi.org/10.1177/089198879500800203.

2. Burke, A. D., Goldfarb, D., Bollam, P., & Khokher, S. (2019). Diagnosing and treating depression in patients with Alzheimer's disease. Neurology Therapy, 8(2), 325-350. Available from https://doi.org/10.1007/s40120-019-00148-5.

3. Dias, N. S., Barbosa, I. G., Kuang, W., & Teixeira, A. L. (2020). Depressive disorders in the elderly and dementia: An update. Dementia & Neuropsychologia, 14(1), 1-6. Available from https://doi.org/10.1590/1980-57642020dn14-010001.

4. Chiu, I., Piguet, O., Diehl-Schmid, J., Riedl, L., Beck, J., Leyhe, T., & Sollberger, M. (2018). Facial emotion recognition performance differentiates between behavioral variant frontotemporal dementia and major depressive disorder. The Journal of Clinical Psychiatry, 79(1). Available from https://doi.org/10.4088/JCP.16m11342.

5. O'Shea, D. M., Dotson, V. M., Woods, A. J., Porges, E. C., Williamson, J. B., O'Shea, A., & Cohen, R. (2018). Depressive symptom dimensions and their association with hippocampal and entorhinal cortex volumes in community dwelling older adults. Frontiers in Aging Neuroscience, 10, 40. Available from https://doi.org/10.3389/fnagi.2018.00040.

6. Zlatar, Z. Z., Muniz, M., Galasko, D., & Salmon, D. P. (2017). Subjective cognitive decline correlates with depression symptoms and not with concurrent objective

cognition in a clinic-based sample of older adults. The Journals of Gerontology. Series B, Psychological Sciences and Social Sciences. Available from https://doi.org/10.1093/geronb/gbw207.

7. Starkstein, S. E., Dragovic, M., Jorge, R., Brockman, S., & Robinson, R. G. (2011). Diagnostic criteria for depression in Alzheimer disease: A study of symptom patterns using latent class analysis. The American Journal of Geriatric Psychiatry: Official Journal of the American Association for Geriatric Psychiatry, 19(6), 551-558. Available from https://doi.org/10.1097/JGP.0b013e3181ec897f.

8. Vilalta-Franch, J., Garre-Olmo, J., Lopez-Pousa, S., Turon-Estrada, A., LozanoGallego, M., Hernandez-Ferrandiz, M., & Feijoo-Lorza, R. (2006). Comparison of different clinical diagnostic criteria for depression in Alzheimer disease. The American Journal of Geriatric Psychiatry: Official Journal of the American Association for Geriatric Psychiatry, 14(7), 589-597. Available from https://doi.org/10.1097/01.JGP.0000209396.15788.9d.

9. Sheehan, B. (2012). Assessment scales in dementia. Therapeutic Advances in Neurological Disorders, 5(6), 349-358. Available from https://doi.org/10.1177/1756285612455733.

10. Thorpe, L. (2009). Depression vs. Dementia: How Do We Assess? The Canadian Review of Alzheimer's Disease and Other Dementias, 12(3), 17-21.

11. Barca, M. L., Selbaek, G., Laks, J., & Engedal, K. (2008). The pattern of depressive symptoms and factor analysis of the Cornell Scale among patients in Norwegian nursing homes. International Journal of Geriatric Psychiatry, 23(10), 1058-1065. Available from https://doi.org/10.1002/gps.2033.

12. Portugal Mda, G., Coutinho, E. S., Almeida, C., Barca, M. L., Knapskog, A. B., Engedal, K., & Laks, J. (2012). Validation of Montgomery-Asberg Rating Scale and Cornell Scale for Depression in Dementia in Brazilian elderly patients. International Psychogeriatrics / IPA, 24(8), 1291-1298. Available from https://doi.org/10.1017/S1041610211002250.

13. Muller-Thomsen, T., Arlt, S., Mann, U., Mass, R., & Ganzer, S. (2005). Detecting depression in Alzheimer's disease: Evaluation of four different scales. Archives of Clinical Neuropsychology: The Official Journal of the National Academy of Neuropsychologists, 20(2), 271-276. Available from https://doi.org/10.1016/j.acn.2004.03.010.

14. Kroenke, K., Spitzer, R. L., & Williams, J. B. (2003). The Patient Health Questionnaire-2: Validity of a two-item depression screener. Medical Care, 41(11), 1284-1292. Available from https://doi.org/10.1097/01.MLR.0000093487.78664.3C.

15. Kroenke, K., Spitzer, R. L., Williams, J. B., & Lowe, B. (2010). The Patient Health Questionnaire Somatic, Anxiety, and Depressive Symptom Scales: A systematic review.

General Hospital Psychiatry, 32(4), 345-359. Available from https://doi.org/10.1016/j.genhosppsych.2010.03.006.

16. Sepehry, A. A., Lee, P. E., Hsiung, G. R., Beattie, B. L., Feldman, H. H., & Jacova, C. (2017). The 2002 NIMH Provisional Diagnostic Criteria for Depression of Alzheimer's Disease (PDC-dAD): Gauging their validity over a decade later. Journal of Alzheimer's Disease: JAD, 58(2), 449-462. Available from https://doi.org/10.3233/JAD-161061.

17. Ball, S. L., Holland, A. J., Huppert, F. A., Treppner, P., Watson, P., & Hon, J. (2004). The modified CAMDEX informant interview is a valid and reliable tool for use in the diagnosis of dementia in adults with Down's syndrome. Journal of Intellectual Disability Research: JIDR, 48(Pt 6), 611-620. Available from https://doi.org/10.1111/j.1365-2788.2004.00630.x.

18. Martinelli, J. E., Cecato, J. F., Bartholomeu, D., & Montiel, J. M. (2014). Comparison of the diagnostic accuracy of neuropsychological tests in differentiating Alzheimer's disease from mild cognitive impairment: Can the Montreal Cognitive Assessment be better than the Cambridge Cognitive Examination? Dementia and Geriatric Cognitive Disorders Extra, 4(2), 113-121. Available from https://doi.org/10.1159/000360279.

19. Connor, D. J., Sabbagh, M. N., & Cummings, J. L. (2008). Comment on administration and scoring of the Neuropsychiatric Inventory in clinical trials. Alzheimer's & Dementia: The Journal of the Alzheimer's Association, 4(6), 390-394. Available from https://doi.org/10.1016/j.jalz.2008.09.002.

20. Wang, J., Li, W., Yue, L., Hong, B., An, N., Li, G., & Xiao, S. (2018). The study of White Matter Hyperintensity (WMH) and factors related to geriatric late-onset depression. Shanghai Archives of Psychiatry, 30(1), 12-19. Available from https://doi.org/10.11919/j.issn.1002-0829.217038.

21. Robert, P., Ferris, S., Gauthier, S., Ihl, R., Winblad, B., & Tennigkeit, F. (2010). Review of Alzheimer's disease scales: Is there a need for a new multi-domain scale for therapy evaluation in medical practice? Alzheimer's Research & Therapy, 2(4), 24. Available from https://doi.org/10.1186/alzrt48.

22. Gottlieb, G. L., Gur, R. E., & Gur, R. C. (1988). Reliability of psychiatric scales in patients with dementia of the Alzheimer type. The American Journal of Psychiatry, 145(7), 857-860. Available from https://doi.org/10.1176/ajp.145.7.857.

23. Zung, W. W. (1965). A self-rating depression scale. Archives of General Psychiatry, 12, 63-70.

24. Zung, W. W., Richards, C. B., & Short, M. J. (1965). Self-rating depression scale in an outpatient clinic. Further validation of the SDS. Archives of General Psychiatry, 13(6), 508-515.

25. Brodaty, H., & Luscombe, G. (1996). Depression in persons with dementia. International Psychogeriatrics/IPA, 8(4), 609622.
26. Teresi, J., Abrams, R., Holmes, D., Ramirez, M., & Eimicke, J. (2001). Prevalence of depression and depression recognition in nursing homes. Social Psychiatry and Psychiatric Epidemiology, 36(12), 613-620.
27. Knapskog, A. B., Barca, M. L., & Engedal, K. (2013). A comparison of the Cornell Scale for Depression in Dementia and the Montgomery-Aasberg Depression Rating Scale in a memory clinic population. Dementia and Geriatric Cognitive Disorders, 35(5-6), 256-265. Available from https://doi.org/10.1159/000348345.
28. Kirkham, J. G., Takwoingi, Y., Quinn, T. J., Rapoport, M., Lanctôt, K. L., Maxwell, C.J., & Seitz, D. P. (2016). Depression rating scales for detection of major depression in people with dementia (Protocol). Cochrane Database of Systematic Reviews, 8.
29. Alexopoulos, G. S., Abrams, R. C., Young, R. C., & Shamoian, C. A. (1988). Cornell Scale for Depression in Dementia. Biological Psychiatry, 23(3), 271-284.
30. Barca, M. L., Engedal, K., Laks, J., & Selbaek, G. (2010). A 12 months follow-up study of depression among nursing-home patients in Norway. Journal of Affective Disorders, 120(13), 141-148. Available from https://doi.org/10.1016/j.jad.2009.04.028.
31. Schreiner, A. S., Hayakawa, H., Morimoto, T., & Kakuma, T. (2003). Screening for late life depression: cut-off scores for the Geriatric Depression Scale and the Cornell Scale for Depression in Dementia among Japanese subjects. International Journal of Geriatric Psychiatry, 18(6), 498-505. Available from https://doi.org/10.1002/gps.880.
32. Lyketsos, C. G., & Olin, J. (2002). Depression in Alzheimer's disease: Overview and treatment. Biological Psychiatry, 52(3), 243-252.
33. Burke, W. J., Roccaforte, W. H., & Wengel, S. P. (1991). The short form of the GeriatricDepression Scale: A comparison with the 30-item form. Journal of Geriatric Psychiatry and Neurology, 4(3), 173-178.
34. Zarb, J. (1996). Correlates of depression in cognitively impaired hospitalized elderly referred for neuropsychological assessment. Journal of Clinical and Experimental Neuropsychology, 18(5), 713-723. Available from https://doi. org/10.1080/01688639608408294.
35. Naarding, P., Leentjens, A. F., van Kooten, F., & Verhey, F. R. (2002). Disease-specific properties of the Rating Scale for Depression in patients with stroke, Alzheimer's dementia, and Parkinson's disease. The Journal of Neuropsychiatry and Clinical Neurosciences, 14(3), 329-334. Available from https://doi.org/10.1176/jnp.14.3.329.
36. Engedal, K., Barca, M. L., Laks, J., & Selbaek, G. (2011). Depression in Alzheimer's disease: Specificity of depressive symptoms using three different clinical criteria. International Journal of Geriatric Psychiatry, 26(9), 944-951. Available from https://doi.

org/10.1002/gps.2631.
37. Olin, J. T., Katz, I. R., Meyers, B. S., Schneider, L. S., & Lebowitz, B. D. (2002). Provisional diagnostic criteria for depression of Alzheimer disease: Rationale and background. The American Journal of Geriatric Psychiatry: Official Journal of the American Association for Geriatric Psychiatry, 10(2), 129-141.
38. Olin, J. T., Schneider, L. S., Katz, I. R., Meyers, B. S., Alexopoulos, G. S., Breitner, J. C., & Lebowitz, B. D. (2002). Provisional diagnostic criteria for depression of Alzheimer disease. The American Journal of Geriatric Psychiatry: Official Journal of the American Association for Geriatric Psychiatry, 10(2), 125-128.
39. Ballard, C., Neill, D., O'Brien, J., McKeith, I. G., Ince, P., & Perry, R. (2000). Anxiety, depression and psychosis in vascular dementia: Prevalence and associations. Journal of Affective Disorders, 59(2), 97-106.
40. Chemerinski, E., Petracca, G., Sabe, L., Kremer, J., & Starkstein, S. E. (2001). The specificity of depressive symptoms in patients with Alzheimer's disease. The American Journal of Psychiatry, 158(1), 68-72. Available from https://doi.org/10.1176/appi.ajp.158.1.68.
41. Starkstein, S. E., Mizrahi, R., & Garau, L. (2005). Specificity of symptoms of depression in Alzheimer disease: A longitudinal analysis. The American Journal of Geriatric Psychiatry: Official Journal of the American Association for Geriatric Psychiatry, 13(9), 802-807. Available from https://doi.org/10.1176/appi.ajgp.13.9.802.
42. Teng, E., Ringman, J. M., Ross, L. K., Mulnard, R. A., Dick, M. B., & Bartzokis, G. (2008). Diagnosing depression in Alzheimer disease with the national institute of mental health provisional criteria, Alzheimer's Disease Research Centers of California Depression in Alzheimer's Disease, IThe American Journal of Geriatric Psychiatry: Official Journal of the American Association for Geriatric Psychiatry, 16(6), 469-477. Available from https://doi.org/10.1097/JGP.0b013e318165dbae.
43. Gilley, D. W., & Wilson, R. S. (1997). Criterion-related validity of the Geriatric Depression Scale in Alzheimer's disease. Journal of Clinical and Experimental Neuropsychology, 19(4), 489-499. Available from https://doi.org/10.1080/01688639708403739.
44. Korner, A., Lauritzen, L., Abelskov, K., Gulmann, N., Marie Brodersen, A., Wedervang Jensen, T., & Marie Kjeldgaard, K. (2006). The Geriatric Depression Scale and the Cornell Scale for Depression in Dementia. A validity study. Nordic Journal of Psychiatry, 60(5), 360-364. Available from https://doi.org/10.1080/08039480600937066.
45. Vida, S., Des Rosiers, P., Carrier, L., & Gauthier, S. (1994). Depression in Alzheimer'sdisease: Receiver operating characteristic analysis of the Cornell Scale for Depression in Dementia and the Hamilton Depression Scale. Journal of Geriatric Psychiatry

and Neurology, 7(3), 159-162. Available from https://doi.org/10.1177/089198879400700306.

46. Harwood, D. G., & Sultzer, D. L. (2002). "Life is not worth living": Hopelessness in Alzheimer's disease. Journal of Geriatric Psychiatry and Neurology, 15(1), 38-43. Available from https://doi.org/10.1177/089198870201500108.

47. Sabodash, V., Mendez, M. F., Fong, S., & Hsiao, J. J. (2013). Suicidal behavior in dementia: A special risk in semantic dementia. American Journal of Alzheimer's Disease and Other Dementias, 28(6), 592-599. Available from https://doi.org/10.1177/1533317513494447.

48. Lam, C. K., Lim, P. P., Low, B. L., Ng, L. L., Chiam, P. C., & Sahadevan, S. (2004). Depression in dementia: A comparative and validation study of four brief scales in the elderly Chinese. International Journal of Geriatric Psychiatry, 19(5), 422-428. Available from https://doi.org/10.1002/gps.1098.

49. Engedal, K., Kvaal, K., Korsnes, M., Barca, M. L., Borza, T., Selbaek, G., & Aakhus, E. (2012). The validity of the Montgomery-Aasberg Depression Rating Scale as a screening tool for depression in later life. Journal of Affective Disorders, 141(2-3), 227-232. Available from https://doi.org/10.1016/j.jad.2012.02.042.

50. Leontjevas, R., van Hooren, S., & Mulders, A. (2009). The Montgomery-Asberg Depression Rating Scale and the Cornell Scale for Depression in Dementia: A validation study with patients exhibiting early-onset dementia. The American Journal of Geriatric Psychiatry: Official Journal of the American Association for Geriatric Psychiatry, 17(1), 56-64. Available from https://doi.org/10.1097/JGP.0b013e31818b4111.

51. Monastero, R., Mangialasche, F., Camarda, C., Ercolani, S., & Camarda, R. (2009). A systematic review of neuropsychiatric symptoms in mild cognitive impairment. Journal of Alzheimer's Disease: JAD, 18(1), 11-30. Available from https://doi.org/10.3233/JAD-2009-1120.

52. Novais, F., & Starkstein, S. (2015). Phenomenology of depression in Alzheimer's disease. Journal of Alzheimer's Disease: JAD, 47(4), 845-855. Available from https://doi.org/10.3233/JAD-148004.

53. Wragg, R. E., & Jeste, D. V. (1989). Overview of depression and psychosis in Alzheimer's disease. The American Journal of Psychiatry, 146(5), 577-587. Available from https://doi.org/10.1176/ajp.146.5.577.

第二章 痴呆中抑郁症的本质：一项系统回顾

Ahmed A. Moustafa，Phoebe Bailey，Wafa Jaroudi，Lily Bilson，Mohamad El Haj，Eid Abo hamza 编

黄龙龙，钟洪芬 译

陈仰昆 校

第一节 引言：痴呆中抑郁症的诊断、患病率和影响

抑郁症与各种类型的痴呆共病[1-3]。据报道，抑郁症是老年人中最严重的心理健康问题之一，也是痴呆患者的常见症状[4]。在大多数阿尔茨海默病（AD）患者中，抑郁症状表现为轻度至中度，严重的抑郁症状并不普遍。5%~30%的阿尔茨海默病患者可能被诊断为重度抑郁发作[5]。痴呆患者的抑郁症状包括淡漠、运动迟缓、心境恶劣，或者轻微、不典型的抑郁症状[6]。一些研究表明，不到10%的阿尔茨海默病患者的抑郁表现为先前存在的抑郁症的复发[7]。然而，对于大多数阿尔茨海默病患者，抑郁症的症状为首次出现。

研究痴呆中的抑郁症很重要，因为它对患者生活的某些方面有负面影响。例如，研究表明，抑郁可以增加痴呆患者海马的斑块和缠结[8]。阿尔茨海默病患者的抑郁也可以同时合并淡漠[9]和焦虑[10]。Benoit等[11]评估了可能患有阿尔茨海默病个体中淡漠和抑郁的作用：参与者进行了痴呆患者的抑郁标准及神经精神量表（NPI）评估，734名轻度AD参与者中，41.8%被发现存在淡漠合并或不合并抑郁，47.8%被发现抑郁合并或不合并淡漠。特别是关于抑郁症的问题，15.4%的参与者存在抑郁，然而仅有9.4%的参与者存在淡漠，提示了抑郁是轻度阿尔茨海默病的常见症状。抑郁相关的主要症状是疲劳和精力丧失以及社交场合及活动的积极情绪或愉悦感的降低和焦虑不安等其他症状[11]。Benoit等[11]的研究表明，抑郁是痴呆患者常见的感受，如果没有干预或没有有效干预，可

影响整体健康状况,并对生活方式产生负面影响。

此外,一些研究表明抑郁的痴呆患者更容易跌倒[12,13]。抑郁的阿尔茨海默病患者可导致更大的孤立感、更高的发病率,以及行为问题,如身体和言语的攻击[14,15]。抑郁同样影响有痴呆风险的老年人、轻度认知障碍(MCI)和阿尔茨海默病患者的生活质量[16],尽管有些研究未发现抑郁对生活质量的影响[17]。

据报道,阿尔茨海默病患者抑郁症的患病率有很大差异,这些差异很大程度归因于诊断标准的不统一[18,19]。一些研究讨论,大多数评估结果只使用抑郁评估量表或主观判断而不是标准化的诊断标准和临床访谈[20,21]。阿尔茨海默病患者抑郁的研究差异,不仅在于发病率的评估,还包括临床相关性及治疗反应等方面。

在一个研究中,通过对 279 例未分型的痴呆临终患者和 24 名非临终健康对照者的评估来完成抑郁的诊断、患病率和治疗问题[14]。所有参与者在其生命的最后 6 个月均居住在慢性护理机构。对情绪障碍、抑郁症状、服药情况和痴呆的严重程度等数据进行回顾。包括国际疾病分类 -9(ICD-9)抑郁障碍编码确定的抑郁症临床诊断。痴呆患者中重度抑郁的患病率为 29%,而非痴呆对照组为 42%。同时,痴呆患者的抑郁往往被漏诊,而且相对于对照组,严重痴呆症患者的抑郁症的认知度明显较低。Evers 等[14]的研究也发现,两组参与者抑郁的治疗均不足。然而,他们能够评估抑郁筛查计划对痴呆症患者抑郁诊断和治疗的影响。筛查计划包括护理人员在入院时及每季度对居民进行筛查,筛查内容包括孤僻和消极行为、悲伤情绪、参与活动能力的缺乏,以及睡眠及食欲的改变,有这些症状的参与者会被转诊到精神病医生处进行评估。结果提示,当将纳入筛查计划的患者与未纳入筛查计划的患者进行比较时,抑郁症状的记录有所改善。

Novais 和 Starkstein[22]的综述表明,在关于阿尔茨海默病合并抑郁症方面,评估的频率、主要临床相关性和治疗的反应上,均有显著的差异。这种差异,可部分地解释为方法学上的局限性所致:缺乏特异的诊断标准、依赖于照顾者或患者提供的信息。阿尔茨海默病患者抑郁症诊断的最主要的困难是抑郁的症状和痴呆患者认知减退的症状存在潜在的重叠，包括失眠、兴趣丧失、精神运动迟滞和注意力缺失，同时还包括食欲差、体重下降和自卑。Novais 和 Starkstein[22]建议，尽管事实上许多标准未被证实有效，但阿尔茨海默病患者抑郁症的诊断，需基于精神病学诊断的系统性精神状态检查。

下面将讨论几个关于抑郁症和痴呆关系的话题，包括抑郁症是发展为痴呆的一个危险因素、痴呆患者的抑郁症亚型，以及不同痴呆类型其抑郁症状的表现是怎样的。

第二节 方法

在此研究中，我们提供了一个关于抑郁症和痴呆症之间的关系的叙述性综述。我们的检索策略包括了来自两组词中的两个关键词的组合。第一组包括抑郁、消极情绪或抑郁的症状；第二组包括痴呆、阿尔茨海默病、血管性痴呆、词义性痴呆和 MCI。我们已经在 PubMed、PsychoInfo 和谷歌上检索了之前的研究。此外，我们还仔细检查了每一篇论文，以确保研究的目标是研究痴呆症中的抑郁症。没有涉及这一主题的研究被排除在外。

第三节 抑郁症是导致老年痴呆症的一个危险因素

抑郁症和痴呆症存在两个潜在的因果影响方向：从抑郁症到痴呆症（例如，抑郁症可增加痴呆的患病率）和从痴呆症到抑郁症（痴呆症的症状可导致抑郁症的发展）[23]。现有的研究大多集中在抑郁症到痴呆症方面[7,24]。而关于后一观点的讨论，请看 Barnes 等[25]、Fischer 等[26]、Moustafa 等[27]、Moustafa 等[28]、Russell-Williams 等[29]、Zeki Al Hazzouri 等[30] 相关文献。

有证据表明，抑郁症是痴呆症的早期前驱期，所以抑郁症可发展为痴呆症[31]，抑郁症也被确定为 MCI 或由 MCI 进展为阿尔茨海默病的潜在危险因素[32-35]。事实上，抑郁症已经被证明可以调节 MCI 和痴呆症之间的联系[36-42]。一些研究表明，抑郁症的出现至少可以使发展为阿尔茨海默病的可能性增加1倍[43-48]。即使是教育程度高的患者，抑郁也会导致晚年的记忆衰退[43]。

值得注意的是，抑郁症在个体一生中发生的时间与发展为痴呆症的风险有关。Li等[49]通过一项纵向研究，探讨了早期和晚期抑郁症与痴呆症风险之间的关系。对3410名参与者进行了实验室检测、神经影像检查、使用《精神障碍诊断与统计手册第4版》（DSM-Ⅳ）进行的痴呆症测试，以及使用流行病学研究中心抑郁量表（Center for Epidemiological Studies Depression，CES-D）对抑郁症进行测量。结果表明，当抑郁症发生在晚年时，会增加痴呆的风险。在50岁及以上的个体中发生的抑郁症会增加患痴呆的风险，但在50岁之前发生的抑郁症并不会增加患痴呆的风险。提示抑郁症是痴呆症发展的一个危险因素[49]。

另一个影响痴呆症发展的因素是抑郁症状发生频率。Dotson等[50]研究了抑郁发作的次数是否与患痴呆症的风险有关。与Li等[49]研究类似，Dotson等[50]进行了一项为期约24年的纵向研究，涉及1239名参与者。在整个研究过程中，使用临床痴呆评分（CDR）、痴呆问卷和《诊断和统计手册第3版修订版》（Diagnostic and Statistical Manual Version 3 Revised，DSM-Ⅲ-R）来测量痴呆的进展和严重程度。抑郁也使用CES-D进行了测量。结果显示，87%的参与者当经历过一次抑郁发作时表现出痴呆的风险增加，同时，经历过两次抑郁发作的参与者患痴呆症的风险甚至是2倍。此外，研究结果还强调，每发作1次抑郁，个体患痴呆症的风险就会增加14%[50]。这些发现强调了行为和认知干预的必要性，以管理抑郁症的症状和经历，因为抑郁可能对痴呆症的发展和经历产生不利影响[49-52]。

Harwood等[51]招募了243例AD患者，以探讨AD患者的抑郁史与当前抑郁之间是否存在关系。目前的抑郁是使用康奈尔量表进行测量的，而患者和照料人员的访谈也评估了抑郁和情绪障碍的病史（例如，自杀意念、精神病院住院治疗）。结果显示，有抑郁和情绪障碍史的AD患者中，目前有抑郁的患者明显多于无抑郁史的患者。因此，有人认为，有抑郁病史增加了AD患者发生情绪障碍的可能性，包括抑郁[53]。

为了探讨 AD 患者抑郁的发生及临床特征，Zubenko 等[52]招募了可能的 AD 患者和认知正常个体的对照组。通过回顾医学和行为障碍史，以及通过体格检查、神经影像和神经心理评估，对认知状态和功能进行了一些评估。例如，简易精神状态检查（MMSE）和临床痴呆评定量表（Clinical Dementia Rating Scale，CDRS）。重度抑郁症的评估采用痴呆患者抑郁临床评估（Clinical Assessment of Depression in Dementia，CADD），这是一种诊断访谈，包含汉密尔顿抑郁量表（HDRS）和 NPI 量表中与痴呆患者神经精神经历相关的部分，如幻觉和抑郁症状。总的来说，研究发现，与没有抑郁的患者相比，经历重度抑郁发作的 AD 患者在被诊断为可能的 AD 时往往更年轻。此外，CADD 结果显示，与无重度抑郁发作的 AD 患者相比，伴有重度抑郁症的 AD 患者的 HDRS 评分更高，且有更多的妄想和幻觉。这一发现的解释是重度抑郁症可能是痴呆症的早期迹象。此外，AD 患者先前抑郁的发生率（44.9%）高于认知正常的参与者（28.5%）。在 AD 组中，18.5% 的患者在诊断前经历过抑郁发作，提示抑郁增加了 AD 发展的风险和 AD 后抑郁复发的发生率（34.6%）。

上述研究表明，抑郁症可以先于痴呆症的发展。这些研究表明，抑郁症可以影响海马的功能，进而导致痴呆症的发展[7,54,55]。然而，一些研究表明，虽然抑郁在 AD 患者中可能先于认知能力下降和记忆问题出现，但抑郁并不一定是 AD 发展的危险因素[56-58]。也就是说，抑郁症有可能发生在痴呆症发展之前，而不会引起 AD。未来的动物研究可能能够提供一些关于抑郁症和痴呆症之间的因果关系的信息。此外，如前所述，也有证据表明了从痴呆到抑郁的途径。痴呆症患者可能会因其疾病而发展为抑郁症。此外，痴呆中抑郁症的患病率因痴呆的类型、使用的工具和诊断性的定义不同而有很大不同。无论潜在的途径如何，痴呆症和抑郁症的共病都会导致功能缺陷、行为问题、养老院安置、照顾者压力[59]和死亡率的增加。

第四节 痴呆中抑郁症的亚型

抑郁症有不同类型：重度抑郁症、轻度抑郁症以及心境恶劣。重度抑郁症是指根据DSM-5对抑郁症的正式定义，而轻度抑郁症是抑郁症的一种亚临床形式，定义为有2~4种抑郁症状，包括抑郁情绪或失去兴趣[60]。心境恶劣被定义为轻度痴呆，但通常持续时间更长[61]。

轻度和重度抑郁发作（按DSM-Ⅳ标准，经神经心理检查确定）的患病率通过对109例AD门诊患者评估来确定[62]。所有参与者都符合可能发生AD的标准。患者的平均年龄为74.4岁[标准差（SD）7.9]；79%是女性，84%住在自己或家人的家中。17%的参与者在AD发病前有抑郁症病史。所有参与者都采用康奈尔痴呆抑郁量表（CSDD）、精神老年依赖评定量表（身体依赖和行为障碍分量表）和一般医疗健康评分。参与者根据他们的CSDD分数被分为三组：重度抑郁发作（22%的参与者）、轻度抑郁发作（27%的参与者），以及"剩余的患者"。重度抑郁发作与日常生活能力（ADL）的严重损害、严重的非情绪行为障碍和频繁的走神有关。轻度抑郁发作与中度至重度非情绪行为障碍和频繁走神相关。这些发现支持了Teri和Wagner[6]的研究发现，即AD患者的重度抑郁症与更严重的行为障碍相关。

Migliorelli等[63]对103例符合可能的AD临床标准的患者进行了抑郁的患病率、危险因素和相关性检查。采用结构化的精神病学访谈来评估这些患者是否存在认知障碍、日常生活能力缺陷、社会功能障碍和嗅觉失认症。至少对2例患者的一级亲属进行结构化的精神病学评估。我们使用了以下精神病学工具：DSM-Ⅲ-R的结构化临床访谈（SCID）、DSM-Ⅲ-R人格障碍的结构化临床访谈（SCID-Ⅱ）、现状调查、家族史研究诊断标准、HDRS、汉密尔顿焦虑量表（HAM-A）、痴呆病觉缺失问卷、功能独立性测量和社会关系调查表。并进行MMSE以及广泛的神经心理检查，包括视觉感知、听觉注意、意识形态运动异常、抽象推理和其他神经机制。结果显示，51%的患者患有抑郁症（28%为心境恶劣，23%为重度抑郁症）。其中，重度抑郁症或心境恶劣的患者大多数为女性，而重度抑郁症患者的正规教育年限明显较少。一半的重度抑郁症患者在痴呆发作之前就有抑郁症发作。而86%的心境恶劣患者在痴呆发作后就出现了抑郁症，与重度抑郁症患者形成鲜明的对比。另一个重要的发现是，心境恶劣患者与重度抑郁症患者和健康对照组相比，出现失认症更少（即更好地意识到他们的认知和行为问题）。Migliorelli 等[63]认为，心境恶劣可能与他们察觉到其进展性认知能力下降有关。有趣的是，只有6例患者（53例患有心境恶劣或重度抑郁症）正在服用抗抑郁药物。重度抑郁症患者的HDRS评分明显高于心境恶劣或非抑郁患者，而心境恶劣患者的HDRS评分明显高于非抑郁患者。Migliorelli 等[63]还根据DSM-Ⅲ-R标准对轻度、中度和重度痴呆阶段的心境恶劣和重度抑郁症的患病率进行了研究。他们发现，心境恶劣在轻度痴呆患者中更为普遍，而重度抑郁症在整个进展阶段也同样普遍。

Chemerinski 等[64]调查了AD患者中"隐性抑郁症"的患病率——这个术语用来描述符合DSM-Ⅳ标准的重度或轻度抑郁，而没有抑郁情绪和兴趣丧失的患者（即他们符合DSM的4个或以上标准的重度或轻度抑郁，而没有必要的抑郁情绪或兴趣丧失的初始症状）。共有233例AD患者、47例抑郁症/无痴呆患者和20例健康对照者，其中AD患者随后被分为2组：非抑郁的AD患者和抑郁的AD患者。使用了以下评估量表：SCID、MMSE、HDRS、HAM-A、CDRS和冷漠量表。AD患者由照顾者在HDRS的"抑郁情绪"项目中评分大于2分者被标记为"抑郁情绪"（$n=92$）。那些在这个项目上评分为0的人则标记为"没有抑郁情绪"（$n=62$）。抑郁的AD患者在焦虑、冷漠和帕金森病样症状方面的得分明显高于非抑郁的AD患者。抑郁的AD患者在以下HDRS项目上的得分明显高于非抑郁的AD患者：内疚、自杀、中度失眠、晚期失眠、兴趣丧失、精神运动发育迟缓、躁动、担忧、焦虑、精力丧失、性欲减退、疑病症和体重减轻。在食欲不振方面没有显著差异。相对于患有AD的抑郁患者，非AD的抑郁患者在自杀、食欲不振和体重减轻等HDRS项目方面的得分明显更高。然而，AD患者的精神运动发育迟缓得分明显高于非AD患者。此外，96%的AD抑郁患者（根据他们的照顾者在HDRS的"抑郁情绪"标准上的得分大于2分）符合DSM-Ⅳ

重度（61%）或轻度（35%）抑郁的标准。只有2%符合隐性重度抑郁症的条件，而18%符合隐性轻度抑郁症的标准。抑郁情绪与大范围抑郁症状之间的显著相关性表明，抑郁症的情感性和自主神经症状在AD患者中都是常见的。此外，这些症状似乎是情感障碍特有的，而不是慢性神经系统疾病的异常表现。

总的来说，一些研究表明，痴呆症患者有不同类型的抑郁症：重度抑郁症、轻度抑郁症和心境恶劣。这些类型的抑郁症对痴呆和记忆力下降的临床方面有不同的影响。此外，相较于青年或中年，痴呆的发展被发现与晚年抑郁症更相关[65]。因此，建议临床医生在考虑不同类型的抑郁症的影响时，也需考虑发生在早期还是晚期的抑郁对患者健康的影响。

第五节 抑郁与自知力

一些研究报道了痴呆患者的自知力和抑郁之间的关系。有研究探索了人格特征、认知功能和个体患AD风险之间的关系[66]。结果表明，抑郁症和意识的症状与认知功能的发展和恶化有关，因此，越是意识到自己的疾病（即自知力越强），则抑郁程度越严重。抑郁症更多发生在对自己疾病有认知的人身上，这一观点得到了文献的支持。研究发现，与疾病自知力受损的人相比，疾病自知力完整的痴呆症患者的抑郁症状出现得更频繁、更强烈[67]。研究中，MMSE评分较高的参与者在HDRS上的评分较低，反之亦然[67]。结果表明，随着认知障碍的发生、进展，抑郁程度逐渐达到顶峰，然后随着认知和疾病自知力的恶化抑郁程度反而逐渐下降。

为了支持抑郁症和疾病自知力之间存在关系的观点，Harwood和Sultzer[68]探讨了AD患者是否经历绝望、情绪障碍以及精神和行为症状，这些是抑郁症的关键特征。研究人员调查了这些关于疾病自知力的感觉的存在。91例AD参与者的样本完成了HDRS，以测量抑郁和绝望。他们还完成了神经行为评定量表来测量精神和行为情绪障碍以及自知力，并完成了MMSE来测量认知。结果表明，大多数参与者都有绝望和其他消极的想法，以及情绪障碍的心理症状。这些参与者倾向于了解他们的疾病。基于这些发现，可以说抑郁症影响痴呆早期的个体，因为绝望的感觉可以导致自杀意念[68,69]。这些发现强调了疾病自知力和情绪障碍之间的关系。更具体地说，在早期痴呆期间，当个体意识到他们的疾病以及他们的认知和功能恶化时，他们会经受更多的情绪障碍并出现抑郁症状。

第六节　痴呆亚型中的抑郁症：与自知力的关系

抑郁症的严重程度因MCI、AD、血管性痴呆以及疾病严重程度（如轻度痴呆 *vs.* 严重痴呆）而异。虽然有些人认为，随着痴呆症状的恶化，抑郁症的严重程度可能会增加，但事实并非如此。有研究显示，抑郁症在轻度痴呆中比在重度痴呆中更常见，这可能是因为人们对疾病有更深刻的认识[70]。按照这一思路，Barca等（2008年）[70]报告称，由于心理和生物风险因素（在研究中未指明）所致，轻度痴呆 [临床痴呆评分（CDR）1 分] 和重度痴呆（CDR 3 分）患者的抑郁症状发生率高于未患痴呆的患者或中度痴呆（CDR 2 分）患者。

一项研究调查了270例MCI患者和402例AD患者的显著抑郁症状患病率[71]。使用CSDD评估抑郁症状。行为评估由患者和他们的照顾者在2周内使用以下量表完成：MFS（Middelheim Frontality Score），阿尔茨海默病行为病理学评定量表（behavior-AD），科恩-曼斯菲尔德焦虑量表和CSDD。结果表明，抑郁症状在AD患者（25%）中高于MCI患者（16%）。有抑郁症状的AD患者与有抑郁症状的MCI患者相比，表现出更严重的额叶症状、行为症状和激越行为。有抑郁症状的MCI患者额叶症状的严重程度（使用MFS量表）也高于无抑郁症状的MCI患者。此外，有抑郁症状的AD患者的额叶症状严重程度高于无抑郁症状的AD患者。相比于没有抑郁症的患者，有抑郁症的AD患者中躁动不安、情绪控制受损、欣快感和情绪迟钝、去抑制、自发性和刻板行为更为普遍。阿尔茨海默病行为病理学评定量表显示，有抑郁症状的AD患者中，74%表现为中度至重度行为症状。

有研究招募了1002例患者，其中329例为痴呆症患者（214例AD患者；

62例血管性痴呆；44例病因不明的痴呆；4例额颞叶痴呆；3例酒精相关性痴呆；2例创伤后应激障碍相关痴呆）[9]。对参与者当前的心理、认知和行为状况史进行评估。评估包括痴呆严重程度和使用CDR、NPI的精神和行为评估，考虑幻觉和抑郁等体验。结果表明，冷漠行为障碍在痴呆患者中最为常见，其次是抑郁/攻击行为障碍。血管性痴呆患者抑郁的发生率高于AD患者，而AD患者妄想的发生率高于血管性痴呆患者。Lyketsos等[9]发现，抑郁和幻觉在严重痴呆症中减少，这可能与疾病后期缺乏意识（或自知力）有关。然而，也有可能是意识的缺乏阻止了严重痴呆患者表达他们的情绪状态。因此，未来的工作应该尝试评估轻度和重度痴呆患者抑郁的生物标志物。

在另一项研究中，对AD（$n=111$）和语义性痴呆（$n=25$）患者的自杀行为与抑郁和自知力的关系进行了比较[69]。使用神经精神症状调查表收集参与者自杀意念和抑郁的历史和现状信息，以及相关的家族史信息。使用MMSE和简易波士顿命名测试评估认知功能。用加州大学洛杉矶分校的洞察力访谈来测量自知力，其涉及患者对其疾病/残疾的意识以及他们如何表达它（如是否关心或否认）。结果发现，语义性痴呆患者大多有抑郁和自杀行为史，部分患者在疾病早期就有抑郁发作。此外，还发现语义性痴呆患者比AD患者有更多的抑郁和自杀意念（2例语义性痴呆患者死于自杀）。作者认为，语义性痴呆患者对他们的疾病有更多的意识（也就是说，有更多的自知力），并认为这种痴呆更令人担忧，因其导致患者抑郁和绝望的想法增加。

与AD患者相比，血管性痴呆患者更容易出现抑郁症[9]，这两种类型的痴呆在自知力和人格变化水平上也可能存在差异。利用CT扫描对AD和血管性痴呆患者的神经病理学进行评估。使用GDS和简短痴呆量表评估痴呆的严重程度[72]。HDRS被用来评估抑郁症，在一次涉及患者和照顾者的访谈中，用一个4分评分量表确定患者的病史和对疾病的了解之间的差异。研究发现，与AD患者相比，抑郁症在血管性痴呆患者中更为常见。这与Lyketsos等[9]的观点一致，他们认为血管性痴呆表现影响与情绪相关的大脑区域，而AD病理则影响与认知相关的大脑区域。然而，Verhey等[72]发现，尽管患者组间的自知力没有显著差异，但两种疾病的轻度期患者与晚期患者相比，抑郁水平相似。这表明对痴呆症的意识（即自知力）可能与抑郁症无关。

与上述研究不同，一项研究调查了不同亚型痴呆症中的不同亚型抑郁症。有研究在 6440 例痴呆患者（2947 例 AD、725 例血管性痴呆和 2768 例未指明的痴呆）中调查了重度抑郁障碍、复发、心境恶劣障碍、抑郁性精神病和适应障碍的患病率[73]。使用综合医疗信息服务数据库确定抑郁症的亚型，并根据 ICD-9 诊断标准对痴呆症的亚型进行分类。在所有痴呆患者中抑郁障碍的患病率为 27%。血管性痴呆组报告的每种抑郁症的患病率均显著高于 AD 和未指明的痴呆组。此外，与 AD 组相比，未指明的痴呆组患者的抑郁障碍患病率显著较高。与 78 岁及以上患者相比，60~64 岁患者的抑郁症患病率较低（分别为 27.94% 和 26.2%），并且这些差异在痴呆亚组之间持续存在。抑郁性精神病的患病率较低，各组之间具有可比性。血管性痴呆组的心境恶劣障碍和适应障碍伴抑郁症状的发生率明显高于 AD 患者，但与未指明的痴呆患者相比则无显著差异。

AD 和未指明的痴呆组之间的心境恶劣障碍没有显著差异；然而，AD 组与未指明的痴呆组在适应障碍方面存在显著差异。在 AD 患者中，心境恶劣的患病率为 2%，在未指明的痴呆患者中为 3%，在血管性痴呆患者中为 4%。总之，这项研究表明，抑郁障碍在血管性痴呆患者中比 AD 和未指明的痴呆患者中更为普遍。重性抑郁障碍、抑郁障碍和伴有抑郁特征的适应障碍在血管性痴呆中更为常见；然而，在未指明的痴呆和血管性痴呆患者中，心境恶劣的患病率相似。

综上所述，与 AD 相比，抑郁症在血管性痴呆和语义性痴呆中更为常见。此外，痴呆患者的抑郁症患病率可能与他们的自知力水平（即对疾病的认识）有关。然而，还需要进一步的研究来阐明痴呆和抑郁症之间的关系。

第七节　结论及未来工作

综述表明，抑郁症和痴呆之间的关系是复杂的。关于抑郁症在痴呆中的流行程度有许多相互矛盾的结果。这与几种用于测量抑郁的量表有关，也与照顾者或临床医生对患者的评估有关。未来的工作应该尝试整合并提供一种统一的痴呆抑郁症的测量方法。此外，虽然有几项研究发现抑郁症先于痴呆症的发展，但尚不清楚抑郁症是否确实会导致痴呆症。这是因为大多数研究都是不可控的（这在人类临床研究中很难做到）。然而，动物研究可能会提供一些信息，以确定抑郁症是否会导致痴呆的发展。此外，自知力可能与痴呆患者的抑郁经历有关，因此，具有完整自知力的痴呆患者更有可能报告抑郁症状。未来的工作应该提供与自知力不相关的痴呆抑郁症的生物标志物。综述显示，痴呆中有几种抑郁症亚型，抑郁症状的严重程度取决于痴呆类型，因为抑郁症在血管性痴呆和语义性痴呆患者中比在 AD 患者中更普遍。然而，未来的工作应该解释抑郁症在痴呆中流行的神经机制，以及其在血管性痴呆和语义性痴呆中比在 AD 中更常见的原因。

参考文献

1. Amore, M., Tagariello, P., Laterza, C., & Savoia, E. M. (2007). Subtypes of depression in dementia. Archives of Gerontology and Geriatrics, 44(Suppl 1), 23-33. Available from https://doi.org/10.1016/j.archger.2007.01.004.
2. Baruch, N., Burgess, J., Pillai, M., & Allan, C. L. (2019). Treatment for depression comorbid with dementia. Evidence-based Mental Health, 22(4), 167-171. Available from https://doi.org/10.1136/ebmental-2019-300113.
3. Kuring, J. K., Mathias, J. L., & Ward, L. (2018). Prevalence of depression, anxiety and PTSD in people with dementia: A systematic review and meta-analysis. Neuropsychology Review, 28(4), 393-416. Available from https://doi.org/10.1007/s11065-018-9396-2.
4. Australian Bureau of Statistics (2015). National Health Survey: First results (no. 4364.0.55.001). Retrieved from http://www.abs.gov.au/ausstats/abs@.nsf/Lookup/by %20Subject/4364.0.55.001B2014-15BMain%20FeaturesBMental%20and%20behavioural%20conditionsB32.
5. Reichman, W. E., & Coyne, A. C. (1995). Depressive symptoms in Alzheimer's disease and multi-infarct dementia. Journal of Geriatric Psychiatry and Neurology, 8(2), 96-99.

Available from https://doi.org/10.1177/089198879500800203.

6. Teri, L., & Wagner, A. (1992). Alzheimer's disease and depression. Journal of Consulting and Clinical Psychology, 60(3), 379-391.

7. Jaroudi, W., Garami, J., Garrido, S., Hornberger, M., Keri, S., & Moustafa, A. A. (2017). Factors underlying cognitive decline in old age and Alzheimer's disease: The role of the hippocampus. Reviews in the Neurosciences, 28(7), 705-714. Available from https://doiorg/10.1515/revneuro-2016-0086.

8. Rapp, M. A., Schnaider-Beeri, M., Grossman, H. T., Sano, M., Perl, D. P., Purohit, D. P., & Haroutunian, V. (2006). Increased hippocampal plaques and tangles in patients with Alzheimer disease with a lifetime history of major depression. Archives of General Psychiatry, 63(2), 161-167. Available from https://doi.org/10.1001/ archpsyc.63.2.161.

9. Lyketsos, C. G., Steinberg, M., Tschanz, J. T., Norton, M. C., Steffens, D. C., & Breitner, J. C. (2000). Mental and behavioral disturbances in dementia: Findings from the cache county study on memory in aging. The American Journal of Psychiatry, 157(5), 708-714. Available from https://doi.org/10.1176/appi.ajp.157.5.708.

10. Porter, V. R., Buxton, W. G., Fairbanks, L. A., Strickland, T., O'Connor, S. M., Rosenberg-Thompson, S., & Cummings, J. L. (2003). Frequency and characteristics of anxiety among patients with Alzheimer's disease and related dementias. The Journal of Neuropsychiatry and Clinical Neurosciences, 15(2), 180-186. Available from https://doi.org/10.1176/jnp.15.2.180.

11. Benoit, M., Berrut, G., Doussaint, J., Bakchine, S., Bonin-Guillaume, S., Fremont, P., & Robert, P. (2012). Apathy and depression in mild Alzheimer's disease: A crosssectional study using diagnostic criteria. Journal of Alzheimer's Disease: JAD, 31(2), 325-334. Available from https://doi.org/10.3233/JAD-2012-112003.

12. Gostynski, M., Ajdacic-Gross, V., Heusser-Gretler, R., Gutzwiller, F., Michel, J. P., & Herrmann, F. (2001). [Dementia, depression and activity of daily living as risk factors for falls in elderly patients]. Sozial-und Praventivmedizin, 46(2), 123.

13. Shua-Haim, J. R., Haim, T., Shi, Y., Kuo, Y. H., & Smith, J. M. (2001). Depression among Alzheimer's caregivers: Identifying risk factors. American Journal of Alzheimer's Disease and Other Dementias, 16(6), 353-359. Available from https://doi.org/10.1177/153331750101600611.

14. Evers, M. M., Samuels, S. C., Lantz, M., Khan, K., Brickman, A. M., & Marin, D. B.(2002). The prevalence, diagnosis and treatment of depression in dementia patients in chronic care facilities in the last six months of life. International Journal of Geriatric Psychiatry, 17(5), 464-472. Available from https://doi.org/10.1002/gps.634.

15. Menon, A. S., Gruber-Baldini, A. L., Hebel, J. R., Kaup, B., Loreck, D., Itkin

Zimmerman, S., & Magaziner, J. (2001). Relationship between aggressive behaviors and depression among nursing home residents with dementia. International Journal of Geriatric Psychiatry, 16(2), 139-146.

16. Winter, Y., Korchounov, A., Zhukova, T. V., & Bertschi, N. E. (2011). Depression in elderly patients with Alzheimer dementia or vascular dementia and its influence on their quality of life. Journal of Neurosciences in Rural Practice, 2(1), 27-32. Available from https://doi.org/10.4103/0976-3147.80087.

17. Nikmat, A. W., Hawthorne, G., & Al-Mashoor, S. H. (2011). Quality of life in dementia patients: Nursing home versus home care. International Psychogeriatrics/IPA, 23(10), 1692-1700. Available from https://doi.org/10.1017/S1041610211001050.

18. Teng, E., Ringman, J. M., Ross, L. K., Mulnard, R. A., Dick, M. B., & Bartzokis, G. (2008). Diagnosing depression in Alzheimer disease with the national institute of mental health provisional criteria, Alzheimer's Disease Research Centers of California Depression in Alzheimer's Disease, I.The American Journal of Geriatric Psychiatry: Official Journal of the American Association for Geriatric Psychiatry, 16(6), 469-477. Available from https://doi.org/10.1097/JGP.0b013e318165dbae.

19. Vilalta-Franch, J., Garre-Olmo, J., Lopez-Pousa, S., Turon-Estrada, A., LozanoGallego, M., Hernandez-Ferrandiz, M., & Feijoo-Lorza, R. (2006). Comparison of different clinical diagnostic criteria for depression in Alzheimer disease. The American Journal of Geriatric Psychiatry: Official Journal of the American Association for Geriatric Psychiatry, 14 (7), 589-597. Available from https://doi.org/10.1097/01.JGP.0000209396.15788.9d.

20. Byers, A. L., & Yaffe, K. (2011). Depression and risk of developing dementia. Nature Reviews Neurology, 7(6), 323-331. Available from https://doi.org/10.1038/nrneurol.2011.60.

21. Wragg, R. E., & Jeste, D. V. (1989). Overview of depression and psychosis in Alzheimer's disease. The American Journal of Psychiatry, 146(5), 577-587. Available from https://doi.org/10.1176/ajp.146.5.577.

22. Novais, F., & Starkstein, S. (2015). Phenomenology of depression in Alzheimer's disease. Journal of Alzheimer's Disease: JAD, 47(4), 845-855. Available from https://doi.org/10.3233/JAD-148004.

23. Thorpe, L. (2009). Depression vs. dementia: How do we assess? The Canadian Review of Alzheimer's Disease and Other Dementias, 12(3), 17-21.

24. Herbert, J., & Lucassen, P. J. (2016). Depression as a risk factor for Alzheimer's disease: Genes, steroids, cytokines and neurogenesis-What do we need to know? Frontiers in Neuroendocrinology, 41, 153-171. Available from https://doi.org/10.1016/

j.yfrne.2015.12.001.

25. Barnes, D. E., Yaffe, K., Byers, A. L., McCormick, M., Schaefer, C., & Whitmer, R. A. (2012). Midlife vs late-life depressive symptoms and risk of dementia: Differential effects for Alzheimer disease and vascular dementia. Archives of General Psychiatry, 69(5), 493-498. Available from https://doi.org/10.1001/archgenpsychiatry.2011.1481.

26. Fischer, A., Dourado, M. C. N., Laks, J., Landeira-Fernandez, J., Morris, R. G., & Mograbi, D. C. (2019). Modelling the impact of functionality, cognition, and mood state on awareness in people with Alzheimer's disease. International Psychogeriatrics/IPA, 1-11. Available from https://doi.org/10.1017/S1041610219001467.

27. Moustafa, A. A., Crouse, J. J., Herzallah, M. M., Salama, M., Mohamed, W., Misiak, B., & Mattock, K. (2019). Depression following major life transitions in women: A review and theory. Psychological Reports. Available from https://doi.org/10.1177/0033294119872209, 33294119872209.

28. Moustafa, A. A., Tindle, R., Frydecka, D., & Misiak, B. (2017). Impulsivity and its relationship with anxiety, depression and stress. Comprehensive Psychiatry, 74, 173-179. Available from https://doi.org/10.1016/j.comppsych.2017.01.013.

29. Russell-Williams, J., Jaroudi, W., Perich, T., Hoscheidt, S., El Haj, M., & Moustafa, A. A. (2018). Mindfulness and meditation: Treating cognitive impairment and reducing stress in dementia. Reviews in the Neurosciences, 29(7), 791-804. Available from https://doi.org/10.1515/revneuro-2017-0066.

30. Zeki Al Hazzouri, A., Vittinghoff, E., Byers, A., Covinsky, K., Blazer, D., Diem, S., & Yaffe, K. (2014). Long-term cumulative depressive symptom burden and risk of cognitive decline and dementia among very old women. The Journals of Gerontology. Series A, Biological Sciences and Medical Sciences, 69(5), 595-601. Available from https://doi.org/10.1093/gerona/glt139.

31. Muliyala, K. P., & Varghese, M. (2010). The complex relationship between depression and dementia. Annals of Indian Academy of Neurology, 13(Suppl 2), S69 S73. Available from https://doi.org/10.4103/0972-2327.74248.

32. Lebedeva, A. K., Westman, E., Borza, T., Beyer, M. K., Engedal, K., Aarsland, D., & Haberg, A. K. (2017). MRI-based classification models in prediction of mild cognitive impairment and dementia in late-life depression. Frontiers in Aging Neuroscience, 9, 13. Available from https://doi.org/10.3389/fnagi.2017.00013.

33. Lee, G. J., Lu, P. H., Hua, X., Lee, S., Wu, S., Nguyen, K., & Alzheimer's Disease Neuroimaging, I. (2012). Depressive symptoms in mild cognitive impairment predict greater atrophy in Alzheimer's disease-related regions. Biological Psychiatry, 71(9), 814-821. Available from https://doi.org/10.1016/j.biopsych.2011.12.024.

34. Mah, L., Binns, M. A., Steffens, D. C., & Alzheimer's Disease Neuroimaging, I. (2015). Anxiety symptoms in amnestic mild cognitive impairment are associated with mediatemporal atrophy and predict conversion to Alzheimer disease. The American Journal of Geriatric Psychiatry: Official Journal of the American Association for Geriatric Psychiatry, 23 (5), 466-476. Available from https://doi.org/10.1016/j.jagp.2014.10.005.

35. Monastero, R., Mangialasche, F., Camarda, C., Ercolani, S., & Camarda, R. (2009). A systematic review of neuropsychiatric symptoms in mild cognitive impairment. Journal of Alzheimer's Disease: JAD, 18(1), 11-30. Available from https://doi.org/10.3233/JAD-2009-1120.

36. Devanand, D. P., Sano, M., Tang, M. X., Taylor, S., Gurland, B. J., Wilder, D., & Mayeux, R. (1996). Depressed mood and the incidence of Alzheimer's disease in the elderly living in the community. Archives of General Psychiatry, 53(2), 175-182.

37. Gabryelewicz, T., Styczynska, M., Luczywek, E., Barczak, A., Pfeffer, A., Androsiuk, W., & Barcikowska, M. (2007). The rate of conversion of mild cognitive impairment to dementia: Predictive role of depression. International Journal of Geriatric Psychiatry, 22(6), 563-567. Available from https://doi.org/10.1002/gps.1716.

38. Li, Y. S., Meyer, J. S., & Thornby, J. (2001a). Longitudinal follow-up of depressive symptoms among normal versus cognitively impaired elderly. International Journal of Geriatric Psychiatry, 16(7), 718-727.

39. Li, Y., Meyer, J. S., & Thornby, J. (2001b). Depressive symptoms among cognitively normal versus cognitively impaired elderly subjects. International Journal of Geriatric Psychiatry, 16(5), 455-461.

40. Simard, M., van Reekum, R., & Cohen, T. (2000). A review of the cognitive and behaioral symptoms in dementia with Lewy bodies. The Journal of Neuropsychiatry and Clinical Neurosciences, 12(4), 425-450. Available from https://doi.org/10.1176/jnp.12.4.425.

41. Teng, E., Lu, P. H., & Cummings, J. L. (2007). Neuropsychiatric symptoms are associated with progression from mild cognitive impairment to Alzheimer's disease. Dementia and Geriatric Cognitive Disorders, 24(4), 253-259. Available from https://doi.org/10.1159/000107100.

42. Vloeberghs, R., Opmeer, E. M., De Deyn, P. P., Engelborghs, S., & De Roeck, E. E. (2018). [Apathy, depression and cognitive functioning in patients with MCI and dementia]. Tijdschrift Voor Gerontologie en Geriatrie, 49(3), 95-102. Available from https://doi.org/10.1007/s12439-018-0248-6.

43. Geerlings, M. I., Schoevers, R. A., Beekman, A. T., Jonker, C., Deeg, D. J., Schmand,

B., & Van Tilburg, W. (2000). Depression and risk of cognitive decline and Alzheimer's disease. Results of two prospective community-based studies in the Netherlands. The British Journal of Psychiatry: The Journal of Mental Science, 176, 568-575.

44. Jorm, A. F. (2001). History of depression as a risk factor for dementia: An updated review. The Australian and New Zealand Journal of Psychiatry, 35(6), 776-781. Available from https://doi.org/10.1046/j.1440-1614.2001.00967.x.

45. Modrego, P. J., & Ferrandez, J. (2004). Depression in patients with mild cognitive impairment increases the risk of developing dementia of Alzheimer type: A prospective cohort study. Archives of Neurology, 61(8), 1290-1293. Available from https://doi.org/10.1001/archneur.61.8.1290.

46. Ownby, R. L., Crocco, E., Acevedo, A., John, V., & Loewenstein, D. (2006). Depression and risk for Alzheimer disease: Systematic review, meta-analysis, and metaregression analysis. Archives of General Psychiatry, 63(5), 530-538. Available from https://doi.org/10.1001/archpsyc.63.5.530.

47. Palmer, K., Berger, A. K., Monastero, R., Winblad, B., Backman, L., & Fratiglioni, L. (2007). Predictors of progression from mild cognitive impairment to Alzheimer disease. Neurology, 68(19), 1596-1602. Available from https://doi.org/10.1212/01.wnl.0000260968.92345.3f.

48. Palmer, K., Di Iulio, F., Varsi, A. E., Gianni, W., Sancesario, G., Caltagirone, C., & Spalletta, G. (2010). Neuropsychiatric predictors of progression from amnestic-mild cognitive impairment to Alzheimer's disease: The role of depression and apathy. Journal of Alzheimer's Disease: JAD, 20(1), 175-183. Available from https://doi.org/10.3233/JAD-2010-1352.

49. Li, G., Wang, L. Y., Shofer, J. B., Thompson, M. L., Peskind, E. R., McCormick, W., & Larson, E. B. (2011). Temporal relationship between depression and dementia: Findings from a large community-based 15-year follow-up study. Archives of General Psychiatry, 68(9), 970-977. Available from https://doi.org/10.1001/archgenpsychiatry.2011.86.

50. Dotson, V. M., Beydoun, M. A., & Zonderman, A. B. (2010). Recurrent depressive symptoms and the incidence of dementia and mild cognitive impairment. Neurology, 75(1), 27-34. Available from https://doi.org/10.1212/WNL.0b013e3181e62124.

51. Harwood, D. G., Barker, W. W., Ownby, R. L., & Duara, R. (1999). Association between premorbid history of depression and current depression in Alzheimer's disease. Journal of Geriatric Psychiatry and Neurology, 12(2), 72-75. Available from https://doi.org/10.1177/089198879901200206.

52. Zubenko, G. S., Zubenko, W. N., McPherson, S., Spoor, E., Marin, D. B., Farlow, M. R., & Sunderland, T. (2003). A collaborative study of the emergence and clinical featuresof

the major depressive syndrome of Alzheimer's disease. The American Journal of Psychiatry, 160(5), 857-866. Available from https://doi.org/10.1176/appi.ajp.160.5.857.

53. Zubenko, G. S. (1996). Clinicopathologic and neurochemical correlates of major depression and psychosis in primary dementia. International Psychogeriatrics/IPA, 8(Suppl 3), 219-223, discussion 269-272.

54. Chung, J. K., Plitman, E., Nakajima, S., Chakravarty, M. M., Caravaggio, F., Takeuchi, H., & Graff-Guerrero, A. (2016). Depressive symptoms and small hippocampal volume accelerate the progression to dementia from mild cognitive impairment. Journal of Alzheimer's Disease: JAD, 49(3), 743-754. Available from https://doi.org/10.3233/JAD-150679.

55. Steffens, D. C., Payne, M. E., Greenberg, D. L., Byrum, C. E., Welsh-Bohmer, K. A., Wagner, H. R., & MacFall, J. R. (2002). Hippocampal volume and incident dementia in geriatric depression. The American Journal of Geriatric Psychiatry: Official Journal of the American Association for Geriatric Psychiatry, 10(1), 62-71.

56. Bennett, S., & Thomas, A. J. (2014). Depression and dementia: Cause, consequence or coincidence? Maturitas, 79(2), 184-190. Available from https://doi.org/10.1016/j.maturitas.2014.05.009.

57. Chen, P., Ganguli, M., Mulsant, B. H., & DeKosky, S. T. (1999). The temporal relationship between depressive symptoms and dementia: A community-based prospective study. Archives of General Psychiatry, 56(3), 261-266.

58. Chen, R., Hu, Z., Wei, L., Qin, X., & Copeland, J. R. (2009). Is the relationship between syndromes of depression and dementia temporal? The MRC-ALPHA and Hefei-China studies. Psychological Medicine, 39(3), 425-430. Available from https://doi.org/10.1017/S0033291708003735.

59. Berger, G., Bernhardt, T., Weimer, E., Peters, J., Kratzsch, T., & Frolich, L. (2005). Longitudinal study on the relationship between symptomatology of dementia and levels of subjective burden and depression among family caregivers in memory clinic patients. Journal of Geriatric Psychiatry and Neurology, 18(3), 119-128. Available from https://doi.org/10.1177/0891988704273375.

60. Fils, J. M., Penick, E. C., Nickel, E. J., Othmer, E., Desouza, C., Gabrielli, W. F., & Hunter, E. E. (2010). Minor versus major depression: A comparative clinical study. Primary Care Companion to the Journal of Clinical Psychiatry, 12(1). Available from https://doi.org/10.4088/PCC.08m00752blu, PCC 08m00752.

61. Niculescu, A. B., 3rd, & Akiskal, H. S. (2001). Proposed endophenotypes of dysthymia: Evolutionary, clinical and pharmacogenomic considerations. Molecular Psychiatry, 6(4), 363-366. Available from https://doi.org/10.1038/sj.mp.4000906.

62. Lyketsos, C. G., Steele, C., Baker, L., Galik, E., Kopunek, S., Steinberg, M., & Warren, (1997). Major and minor depression in Alzheimer's disease: Prevalence and impact. The Journal of Neuropsychiatry and Clinical Neurosciences, 9(4), 556-561. Available from https://doi.org/10.1176/jnp.9.4.556.

63. Migliorelli, R., Teson, A., Sabe, L., Petracchi, M., Leiguarda, R., & Starkstein, S. E. (1995). Prevalence and correlates of dysthymia and major depression among patients with Alzheimer's disease. The American Journal of Psychiatry, 152(1), 37-44. Available from https://doi.org/10.1176/ajp.152.1.37.

64. Chemerinski, E., Petracca, G., Sabe, L., Kremer, J., & Starkstein, S. E. (2001). The specificity of depressive symptoms in patients with Alzheimer's disease. The American Journal of Psychiatry, 158(1), 68-72. Available from https://doi.org/10.1176/appi.ajp.158.1.68.

65. Singh-Manoux, A., Dugravot, A., Fournier, A., Abell, J., Ebmeier, K., Kivimaki, M., & Sabia, S. (2017). Trajectories of depressive symptoms before diagnosis of dementia: A 28-year follow-up study. JAMA Psychiatry, 74(7), 712-718. Available from https://doi.org/10.1001/jamapsychiatry.2017.0660.

66. Wilson, R. S., Schneider, J. A., Arnold, S. E., Bienias, J. L., & Bennett, D. A. (2007). Conscientiousness and the incidence of Alzheimer disease and mild cognitive impairment. Archives of General Psychiatry, 64(10), 1204-1212. Available from https://doi.org/10.1001/archpsyc.64.10.1204.

67. Brodaty, H., & Luscombe, G. (1996). Depression in persons with dementia. International Psychogeriatrics/IPA, 8(4), 609622.

68. Harwood, D. G., & Sultzer, D. L. (2002). "Life is not worth living" 130. : Hopelessness in Alzheimer's disease. Journal of Geriatric Psychiatry and Neurology, 15(1), 38-43. Available from https://doi.org/10.1177/089198870201500108.

69. Sabodash, V., Mendez, M. F., Fong, S., & Hsiao, J. J. (2013). Suicidal behavior in dementia: A special risk in semantic dementia. American Journal of Alzheimer's Disease and Other Dementias, 28(6), 592-599. Available from https://doi.org/10.1177/1533317513494447.

70. Barca, M. L., Selbaek, G., Laks, J., & Engedal, K. (2008). The pattern of depressive symptoms and factor analysis of the Cornell scale among patients in Norwegian nursing homes. International Journal of Geriatric Psychiatry, 23(10), 1058-1065. Available from https://doi.org/10.1002/gps.2033.

71. Van der Mussele, S., Bekelaar, K., Le Bastard, N., Vermeiren, Y., Saerens, J., Somers, N., & Engelborghs, S. (2013). Prevalence and associated behavioral symptoms of depression in mild cognitive impairment and dementia due to Alzheimer's diseaseInternational

Journal of Geriatric Psychiatry, 28(9), 947-958. Available from https://doi. org/10.1002/gps.3909.

72. Verhey, F. R., Ponds, R. W., Rozendaal, N., & Jolles, J. (1995). Depression, insight, and personality changes in Alzheimer's disease and vascular dementia. Journal of Geriatric Psychiatry and Neurology, 8(1), 23-27.

73. Castilla-Puentes, R. C., & Habeych, M. E. (2010). Subtypes of depression among patients with Alzheimer's disease and other dementias. Alzheimer's & Dementia: The Journal of the Alzheimer's Association, 6(1), 63-69. Available from https://doi.org/10.1016/j.jalz.2009.04.1232.

第三章 痴呆症患者的压力和焦虑

Ahmed A. Moustafa, Shimaa Adel Heikal, Wafa Jaroudi, Ahmed Helal 编
袁锡球,刘启峻,肖卫民 译
陈仰昆 校

第一节 痴呆症背景

痴呆症的发病率在全球范围内不断上升,预计到2050年将影响超过1.3亿人[1]。在澳大利亚,被诊断为痴呆症的人数也在增加[2]。痴呆症是一个综合征,包括各种影响记忆和认知能力、干扰职业和社会功能的疾病[3,4]。痴呆症是一种慢性和进展性疾病,由多种脑部疾病引起,患者的记忆力、认知能力和行为等出现退化,显著损害了个体的日常功能,世界卫生组织(World Health Organization,WHO)在2012年将痴呆症归类为公共卫生优先事项[5-7]。随着人口老龄化,痴呆症的患病率不断增加,在中老年人口比例高的国家尤为严重[7]。痴呆症是老年人残疾和丧失自理能力的主要原因之一,同时老龄化正在影响痴呆症的患病率,因此各国政府应积极制定行动计划来应对该病[8]。

2010年,全球大约有3560万人患有痴呆症,每年约有770万人被诊断为痴呆症患者[7]。到2050年预计被诊断出患有痴呆症的人数将增加3倍,超过1.52亿人[9]。2015年痴呆症护理的财务负担估计为8180亿美元,较低收入国家的人均费用较低;在高收入国家,人均费用估计为32 865美元,中上等收入国家为6827美元,中下等收入国家为3109美元,低收入国家为868美元[4,10]。尽管早发型痴呆症的病例数量有所增加,但该疾病通常与年龄相关[8,11]。年龄越大,发展成为痴呆的机会就越高[12]。

痴呆症是澳大利亚85岁以上人群的第二大死因[12,13]。据澳大利亚统计局报道,2015年有159 052例与痴呆症相关的死亡。研究表明,在9年内,将有

58.9万人被诊断出患有痴呆症，而这一数据将在39年内增加到超过100万人[2]。由于区分因年龄引起的整体认知功能自然下降与异常的神经认知损害之间的固有困难，研究表明大约有40%的痴呆症患者未被诊断出来，故这些数据可能还会增加[14]。统计数据显示，随着时间的推移，痴呆症的发病率在以惊人的速度增长，这凸显了对这个问题研究的重要性。了解痴呆症的症状对于有效制定干预措施以减轻疾病后果并提高患者生活质量至关重要。

认知能力的下降通常是老年患者报告的主要症状。然而，随着年龄的增长[15]，人们通常会出现一定程度的认知功能下降。当认知下降的症状进展到影响日常功能的程度时，痴呆症的诊断就会成为一个典型情况。正常认知与痴呆之间的中间阶段被称为轻度认知障碍（MCI）[15]。记忆力受损是发展成认知障碍最突出的线索之一，这之后会进展为痴呆。更具体地说，Holzer和Warshaw[16]认为，记忆的回忆能力下降是痴呆最早的迹象之一。其他症状包括从事重复行为和表现出判断力恶化，这可能对他们的日常生活活动（如驾驶或保持对话）产生重大影响[16,17]。

第二节 痴呆症患者的心理健康

心理健康问题包括焦虑和抑郁[18]。澳大利亚统计局指出，2014—2015年间，有210万人患有与抑郁和焦虑相关的心理健康问题。此外，心理困扰（即长期的压力感）在澳大利亚人口中也普遍存在[19]。根据现有的文献，痴呆症和心理健康之间存在一种联系，特别是与抑郁和焦虑，有时还涉及压力。同时，有必要探讨每种情绪状态是如何对痴呆症患者的生活产生影响的，特别是对他们的日常生活和生活质量的影响。这样的研究或许能启发我们找到能够改善当前心理健康和痴呆症日益严重趋势的思路和措施。

与痴呆症相关的许多心理健康问题会使人变得衰弱，影响个人的生活质量和完成日常生活所需的能力。阿尔茨海默病（AD）是最常见的痴呆症类型，占所有痴呆症病例的60%~80%[20]，了解其相关风险因素（如抑郁和焦虑）也有助于延缓痴呆症的发病[21]。例如，研究表明，焦虑症对痴呆症的进展有影响[22]。因此，研究心理健康问题在 AD 发病中的作用有重要意义[23,24]。

许多被诊断为痴呆症的患者都会出现抑郁、焦虑和压力等共病[25-27]。抑郁、焦虑和压力可能会导致认知功能损害和痴呆症的发展，并且是痴呆症患者常见的表现，特别是在疾病的轻度和中度阶段[28]。这 3 种负面情绪通常被忽视，并被认为是老年期和痴呆症患者的正常经历。抑郁被忽视或误诊为衰老或痴呆症的原因之一，部分在于情绪障碍症状与痴呆症之间存在相当大的重叠。

重要的是，痴呆症患者的认知能力有限，这使得识别和测量这些负面情绪状态更加困难[29-33]。痴呆症患者的记忆力、注意力和语言理解能力较差，这使得他们很难完成抑郁、焦虑和压力的测量。痴呆症患者的心理健康问题常常被住院护士和护理助理等忽视和低估[33]。情绪障碍的误诊和漏诊是需要解决的重要问题，因为抑郁等负面情绪会增加自杀的风险和发生率[34,35]。据我们所知，抑郁 - 焦虑 - 压力量表（Depression-Anxiety-Stress Scale，DASS-21）[36]是唯一能够测量抑郁、焦虑和压力的综合心理量表，但不能用于测试认知损害的个体，如患有痴呆症的个体。

除了压力、焦虑和抑郁之外，Van Der Linde 等[37]还发现冷漠是痴呆症的一个主要心理症状，其与抑郁和焦虑症重叠。两者都涉及对生活的不满或不幸感。据报道，在痴呆症的整个病程中，冷漠现象非常普遍且持续存在[38]；在额颞叶痴呆症（Frontotemporal Dementia，FTD）、原发性进行性失语症（Primary Progressive Aphasia，PPA）和年轻时发病的注意力缺失症病例中，冷漠现象的报告频率非常高[39]。

除了冷漠，Wilson 等[40]还确定孤独是导致抑郁、压力和 AD 疾病发展和糟糕经历的因素。此外，Wilson 等[40]进行了一项涉及认知健康的老年参与者的纵向研究。他们发现，孤独是导致抑郁、压力和 AD 的因素，并且使晚发性 AD 的风险增加了 2 倍。

Wilson 等[41]探讨了神经质的哪些方面与痴呆的发展有关。神经质是一种以倾向于感受负面情绪而著称的人格特质，涉及焦虑、担忧、恐惧、愤怒、沮丧、内疚和抑郁情绪等体验。在 785 名未患痴呆症的老年人中，神经质与痴呆症相关的两个方面通常是焦虑和压力。关于神经质与痴呆症的发展，研究发现，抑郁会对信息处理和信息保持等特定认知功能（如记忆）产生负面影响[41]。研究结果表明，抑郁、焦虑和压力会影响认知过程和疾病（痴呆症）的发生和进展，会加重记忆等认知功能的恶化[41]。最近的一项研究调查了人格特质是否与个体认知状态的差异有关。Zufferey 等[24]使用分层多元线性模型量化了人格特质与内侧颞叶认知损害之间的相互作用。结果发现，人格特质与认知状态，尤其是神经质与相关的焦虑、抑郁和压力之间存在明显的交互作用。

第三节 焦虑与痴呆症

痴呆症患者通常会出现焦虑症状。焦虑是痴呆和痛苦的常见症状，与生活质量下降和神经心理学表现恶化有关[42]。据估计，超过 25% 的痴呆症患者被诊断患有焦虑症[43]。焦虑症在痴呆症患者身上发生的概率是健康老人的 2~4 倍[44]。此外，痴呆症患者出现焦虑症状时常常需要安置到养老院，相应地增加了照顾者的负担[43,45]。因此，解决痴呆症患者的焦虑症状已成为未来疾病管理方案的重点。在下一节中，我们将讨论有关焦虑作为痴呆症风险因素的研究、焦虑在不同类型痴呆症中的发病率以及痴呆症早期和晚期的焦虑情况。

一、焦虑是痴呆症的一个危险因素

多项研究调查了焦虑如何影响健康人和痴呆症患者的记忆和痴呆症状。例如，Wilson 等[46]调查了老年人的焦虑与认知功能之间的关系。男性和女性所体验到的苦恼（包括焦虑和悲伤的症状）是不同的。女性参与者比男性经历更多的痛苦，这导致前者的认知能力下降更严重[46]。这一发现与焦虑和悲伤的经历会使整体认知能力下降的观点一致。

为了详细阐述痛苦、焦虑和悲伤之间的关系，Wilson 等[47,48]调查了持久的痛苦体验与 MCI 发展之间的关系。经过 12 年的数据收集，研究发现，持续的痛苦体验会影响情景记忆，并随着时间的推移患上 MCI 的机会增加。研究发现，苦恼和焦虑会导致早期认知能力下降。因此，有必要适当地监测和管理早期的症状，同时在老年人群中推广有效的干预措施。

在一项研究中，研究人员探讨了焦虑与老年男性（48~67 岁）痴呆的关联，发现焦虑是痴呆症发病的一个危险因素[49]。最近的系统综述和荟萃分析侧重于将焦虑作为痴呆症和认知能力下降的预测因素。结果表明，焦虑会增加认知障碍的风险，尤其是在老年人中[50]。

主观认知下降（subjective cognitive decline，SCD）是指自我认知能力的感知。Liew[51] 每年测量 SCD 参与者的焦虑症状，以探讨痴呆症或 MCI 的发生情况。SCD 和焦虑被证明是 MCI 和痴呆的危险因素，这两种症状同时出现的可能性最高[51]。此外，Norman 等[52] 研究了老年个体对罹患阿尔茨海默病的恐惧（Fear of Developing Alzheimer's Disease，FDAD），以了解其如何影响老年人的主观记忆的抱怨（Subjective Memory Complaints，SMC）。研究对象包括 65~93 岁的成年人，他们自我报告了抑郁、焦虑和记忆症状，研究人员对他们关于罹患 AD 的恐惧进行了评估。结论是焦虑与 FDAD 和主观记忆的抱怨有关。评估老年人的焦虑症状可能有助于确定那些有发展为冷漠和痛苦风险的人[52]。

因此，早期干预非常重要，因为能识别焦虑的经历，并侧重于缓解与之相关的症状，这反过来又能降低焦虑和认知障碍的可能性，从而改善痴呆症患者的生活质量。

二、焦虑症在不同类型痴呆症中的发病率

不同的研究更深入地调查了焦虑症在不同类型痴呆症中的发生情况。例如，Porter 等[53] 评估了不同类型痴呆症（如 AD、血管性痴呆、FTD）中焦虑症的患病率，并将其与健康对照组参与者的焦虑症患病率进行了比较。该研究收集了 191 例痴呆症患者和 40 名对照组患者的数据，使用神经精神量表（NPI）测量焦虑和行为障碍，使用简易精神状态检查量表（MMSE）测量认知能力下降，使用功能活动问卷测量日常生活活动能力，使用磁共振成像脑部扫描和血液测试测

量激素水平。

总体而言，痴呆症患者的焦虑程度高于对照组患者。在比较痴呆症类型时，VaD 和 FTD 的参与者比 AD 的参与者有更高的焦虑。值得注意的是，患有焦虑的 AD 参与者有早发痴呆，即在 65 岁之前发生的痴呆症[53]。这些研究结果表明，焦虑会增加患痴呆症的风险，并使痴呆症患者的生活中经历更严重的精神疲劳。

与 Ballard 等[54] 的观点一致，Porter 等[53] 发现 VaD 的患者比 AD 患者更容易出现焦虑症状。Ballard 等[54] 报告称，这是因为 VaD 和 AD 的病理学有所不同，比如它们的潜在发展及其影响。此外，Porter 等[53] 研究结果表明，焦虑与认知之间存在相关性。也就是说，焦虑会影响认知能力，并且最常发生在早发性痴呆症患者身上。因此，焦虑与痴呆症之间可能存在一种模式，即焦虑是痴呆症的一个危险因素，并在疾病的轻度阶段达到高峰。

与 Porter 等[53] 研究类似，Teri 等[55] 也探讨了焦虑症状的发生及其与抑郁症共病性的关系。为此，研究者分别使用 MMSE 和 Mattis 痴呆评定量表测量 523 例痴呆症患者的认知能力[55]。此外，还使用 Blessed Dementia 评定量表测量了参与者完成日常活动的能力。结果显示，70% 的参与者有一种或多种焦虑症状，最主要的症状是恐惧。参与者常见的其他行为症状包括漫无目的地走动和幻觉[55]。

最近，一项系统性综述报告显示，焦虑是 AD 和 VaD 的危险因素。Rasmussen 等[56] 报告称，焦虑和抑郁是 AD 和 FTD 患者的独立危险因素。焦虑和 FTD 之间有明显关联，而 AD 与抑郁的关联度更高[56]。此外，一项针对 AD 和路易体痴呆（DLB）患者的回顾性研究发现，在控制年龄、性别和认知状态后，DLB 患者中焦虑比 AD 患者更常见。症状在临床诊断前 4~5 年出现，以严重的惊恐发作为特征，需要医疗帮助。AD 患者较少出现焦虑，或至少从未需要过医疗帮助。因此，该研究建议，所有因焦虑和认知能力下降而入院的老年患者都应考虑 DLB[57]。

另外，对 AD 和 DLB 患者进行的一项为期 4 年的研究显示，焦虑与认知能力下降或疾病严重程度无明显关联。这表明，在最初被诊断为痴呆的患者中，焦虑并不是一个重要的因素[58]。另一项研究中，与不同类型痴呆症相关的神经精神症状在不同研究中各不相同。抑郁症在 AD 和 FTD 中非常普遍，而焦虑症在 FTD 中经常被报道[39]。

三、痴呆症早期与晚期的焦虑症

一些研究测量了焦虑与痴呆症的不同阶段之间的关系。例如，Seignourel 等[43]认为，焦虑最常影响痴呆症早期阶段的患者，因为患者保留对自己的疾病的了解。研究比较了处于认知能力衰退和 AD 不同阶段的患者的焦虑和抑郁模式，发现在认知能力衰退的早期阶段，患者会表现出诸多焦虑和抑郁症状，随着病情向诊断 AD 的发展，这些情绪症状会逐渐减少[25]。最初意识到衰退会加重患者的焦虑和抑郁症状，而随着病情的进展和认知的减弱，焦虑和冷漠的感觉就不那么明显。根据这些研究结果，最需要心理健康评估和帮助的是那些有认知损害并处于轻度至中度痴呆的患者。痴呆症早期阶段患者的认知水平从健康状态发展到受损状态，其心理健康方面受到的影响最大。

类似地，Piccininni 等[27]调查了 AD 患者中行为和心理症状的频率，以更好地了解这些症状在疾病进展中的严重程度。50 例 AD 患者和他们的照顾者参加了这项研究，研究内容包括对他们的心理健康、神经心理健康和神经影像学的评估。测试包括测量语言功能、记忆过程和完成日常任务的能力的量表。为了测量参与者妄想、焦虑、易怒和运动等行为和心理症状的严重程度，研究人员使用 NPI 对照顾者进行了访谈。结果包括 AD 参与者中报告最多的冷漠、异常运动活动（如起搏和强迫）、烦躁不安和焦虑增加，发生率为 46%~74%，这是非常频繁的[27]。此外，Piccininni 等[27]发现妄想、幻觉和异常运动活动的症状随着疾病进展而变得更加频繁和严重。另外，当患者意识到他们的能力下降时，也就是所谓的具有完整的疾病洞察力时，心理症状（如烦躁不安）在疾病的轻度阶段最频繁和严重[27]。焦虑症伴随着抑郁、焦虑和烦躁等情绪，通常发生在轻度痴呆症患者身上，这强调了评估和测量痴呆症患者负面情绪的重要性。

第四节 压力与痴呆症

除了焦虑，压力也是一种与痴呆症患者认知损害有关的情绪状态[59,60]。众所周知，压力是增加罹患认知损害的危险因素。Johansson 等[61] 探讨了压力经历与痴呆症发展之间的联系。在长达 35 年的时间里，通过定期完成由医生实施的心理压力测量来监测参与者的压力。此外，还使用神经精神病学检查和《精神障碍诊断与统计手册》对痴呆症患者进行筛查和评估。研究发现，持续的中年压力与罹患痴呆症的风险增加有关，而压力经历与早发性和晚发性痴呆症都有关联[61]。

对压力的生理反应会影响大脑，这可能会增加患痴呆症的风险[62,63]。压力对大脑的影响及其与痴呆症的联系尚未完全明确；但已提出了几种机制，包括长期压力引起的皮质醇水平升高会导致下丘脑 - 垂体 - 肾上腺轴调节失调，从而导致压力反应性增加[63]。在本节中，我们将讨论心理压力如何影响记忆和认知、痴呆症中的社会 - 心理压力、痴呆症中的创伤后应激障碍（Posttraumatic Stress Disorder，PTSD）、中年时期感知到的压力和痴呆、儿童时期的压力和痴呆，以及痴呆患者所经历的压力。

一、心理压力、轻度认知障碍和痴呆症

心理压力是罹患 MCI 和痴呆症的一个新兴的风险因素。许多研究都调查了心理压力与晚年认知能力下降之间的关系[40,61,64,65]。然而，压力与认知结果之间的确切关系仍不清楚。

Katz 等[66] 通过一项纵向研究调查了压力与认知的关系，特别是遗忘性轻度认知障碍（amnestic Mild Cognitive Impairment，aMCI）的发展。研究发现，压力是 aMCI 发展的一个决定因素。一个重要的发现是，患有 aMCI 和显著压力水平的女性参与者也表现出较高的抑郁评分。基于这些发现，感知压力量表测量中获得高压力评分的个体罹患 aMCI 的概率增加 2.5 倍。

工作压力、高要求和工作处理能力不足等社会心理问题已被证明会造成个

体压力[67,68]。研究表明，工作场所的社会心理压力是导致痴呆症的一个重要因素[69]。工作处理能力不足和工作压力大等因素被认为是痴呆症和AD的危险因素，而这些因素与其他已知因素无关[68]。

二、童年压力、中年压力和痴呆症

多项研究对童年时期的经历进行了调查，并将其与成年后的健康状况和疾病联系起来。遭受虐待或在社会经济劣势环境中成长与后来的精神障碍有关[70]。早期经历诸如丧失父母之类的压力事件会增加患痴呆症的风险[71-73]。此外，童年时期的压力还包括生活在孤儿院、被托管、经历危机或战争。童年时期承受的压力越大，患痴呆症的风险就越高，强调了童年时期的经历对日后生活的影响[74]。因此，应为遭受压力的儿童提供特殊支持，以保护他们免受在成年后可能发展成痴呆或AD的风险。

至于中年压力，一项长达35年的纵向研究发现，患痴呆症的女性在中年时表示经常承受着巨大且持续的压力[61]。一项长达27年的跟踪研究表明，在先前报告过精神压力的参与者中，痴呆的发病率增加了50%[75]。研究发现，年龄是一个重要因素，因为在中年期间经历压力的人比在成年后经历压力的人更可能发展为痴呆。

三、痴呆症患者的创伤后应激障碍

PTSD是一种常见的压力形式，指个人在经历战争或虐待等危及生命的事件后出现的严重临床障碍[76,77]。PTSD被认为是痴呆症发病的潜在风险因素[78-83]。Wang等[84]指出，患有PTSD的个体患痴呆症的风险增加了4倍。这些研究结果强调了长期的压力感受和体验对认知的负面影响，尤其是当压力类型涉及战争或虐待等创伤性经历时[85,86]。Katz等[66]认为，压力是痴呆症患者的一种经历，并可能增加罹患MCI的概率。这些研究结果表明，有必要采取干预措施来缓解压力，从而降低罹患MCI的风险。Yaffe等[87]支持"压力会导致发生认知问题"的观点，而这些认知问题可能会在后期发展为痴呆症。Yaffe等[87]调查了有无

PTSD 的退伍军人罹患痴呆症的情况。研究结果表明，有 PTSD 的退伍军人罹患痴呆症的风险比没有 PTSD 的退伍军人更高。他们的研究结果还表明，压力和 PTSD 会导致海马萎缩，而海马是记忆过程的重要区域。此外，压力和 PTSD 还会导致记忆和学习能力（如短期记忆）恶化或受损。经历过压力的人也具有更高的皮质醇水平，这是一种为应对压力而释放的化学物质。这些人的海马也会发生神经萎缩[88]。因此，压力的后果可能比增加患痴呆症的风险更具体，因为它明确地影响了海马的记忆功能。

Flatt 等[89]研究了男性和女性的 PTSD 及其与痴呆症的关系。报告称，与没有 PTSD 的人相比，患有 PTSD 的人更容易患痴呆症。此外，无论性别如何，遭受 PTSD 的个体都有患痴呆症的风险[89]。Flatt 等[89]研究还表明，患有 PTSD 和合并抑郁症的人患痴呆症的风险是普通人的 2 倍[76]。不仅是早期的 PTSD，迟发性 PTSD 也与痴呆有关。此外，Ball 等[78]还研究了痴呆症和 PTSD 患者攻击性行为增加的情况。结果表明，同时患有痴呆症和 PTSD 的患者更具攻击性，但还需要更多的研究来支持这一假设。

PTSD 患者的海马积小于正常健康人，这一发现进一步证实了压力导致认知障碍的观点。大脑扫描还显示，PTSD 患者的海马萎缩与细胞退化有关，导致记忆回忆能力受损[85,86]。皮质醇水平对突触可塑性以及海马树突的形态和结构可产生负面影响，进一步说明了压力与记忆受损的关系[90,91]。

这些结果表明，及早识别个体的创伤是有益的。尽早接受适当的心理干预，有助于保护 PTSD 患者免受罹患痴呆症和可能出现的认知能力下降的影响[92]。

第五节　结论

综述研究发现，焦虑在 VaD 中比在 AD 中更常见，其会影响记忆和认知能力，因此是痴呆发病的危险因素。和焦虑一样，压力也会增加罹患 MCI 和痴呆症的概率。研究还表明，童年和中年的压力都会增加患痴呆症的机会。最后，PTSD 与痴呆症之间有一定的联系。

对受痴呆症影响的认知和心理健康两方面进行干预，可能会对痴呆症患者产生双向的帮助。也就是说，改善认知功能的干预措施可以改善心理健康，同样，改善心理健康的干预措施也能改善认知功能。因此，在制定干预措施时，研究人员必须同时考虑到认知和心理健康因素，包括个人特质（如神经质）、以往的焦虑或压力经历以及现有的并发症（如抑郁症）。正确识别早期痴呆症患者的焦虑或压力症状对于个性化治疗和有效的心理护理是非常必要的，这也是减缓病情发展的一种手段。最后，公共卫生干预措施应以减少慢性压力为目标，为儿童期遭受压力和PTSD的患者提供适当的护理，并为痴呆症高危人群提供更好的社会整体环境。

参考文献

1. Martin Prince, A., Wimo, A., Guerchet, M., Gemma-Claire Ali, M., Wu, Y.-T., Prina, M., ... Xia, Z. (2015). World Alzheimer Report 2015, The Global Impact of Dementia: An analysis of prevalence, incidence, cost and trends. Retrieved from www.alz.co.uk/worldreport 2015 corrections.
2. Health Direct. (2018). Dementia Statistics. Retrieved from https://www.healthdirect.gov.au/dementia-statistics.
3. Gale, S. A., Acar, D., & Daffner, K. R. (2018). Dementia. American Journal of Medicine, 131(10), 1161-1169. Available from https://doi.org/10.1016/j.amjmed.2018.01.022, Elsevier Inc.
4. WHO. (2017). WHO|Global action plan on the public health response to dementia 2017-2025. WHO.
5. Baumgart, M., Snyder, H. M., Carrillo, M. C., Fazio, S., Kim, H., & Johns, H. (2015). Summary of the evidence on modifiable risk factors for cognitive decline and dementia: A population-based perspective. Alzheimer's & Dementia, 11(6), 718-726. Available from https://doi.org/10.1016/j.jalz.2015.05.016.
6. Ferri, C. P., Prince, M., Brayne, C., Brodaty, H., Fratiglioni, L., Ganguli, M., ... Scazufca, M. (2005). Global prevalence of dementia: A Delphi consensus study. Lancet, 366(9503), 2112-2117. Available from https://doi.org/10.1016/S0140-6736 (05)67889-0.
7. WHO. (2012). Dementia: a public health priority. Retrieved from https://apps. who.

int/iris/ bitstream/handle/10665/75263/9789241564458_eng.pdf;jsessionid = 91F60603FF109 08D2230F876DE20819C?sequence = 1.

8. Prince, M., Bryce, R., Albanese, E., Wimo, A., Ribeiro, W., & Ferri, C. P. (2013). The global prevalence of dementia: A systematic review and metaanalysis. Alzheimer's & Dementia, 9(1), 63-75. Available from https://doi.org/10.1016/j.jalz.2012.11.007, Elsevier Inc.

9. WHO. (2018). WHO|Towards a dementia plan: A WHO guide. WHO.

10. WHO. (2015). WHO|Thematic briefs for the First WHO Ministerial Conference on Global Action Against Dementia, March 16-17, 2015. WHO. Retrieved from https://www.who.int/mental_health/neurology/dementia/thematic_briefs_dementia/en/.

11. Prince, M. (2000). Methodological issues for population-based research into dementia in developing countries: A position paper from the 10/66 Dementia Research Group. International Journal of Geriatric Psychiatry, 15(1), 21-30, https://doi.org/10.1002/(SICI)1099-1166(200001)15:1 < 21::AID-GPS71 > 3.0.CO;2-5.

12. Australian Bureau of Statistics. (2015a). Causes of Death, Australia (no. 3303.0). Retrieved from http://www.abs.gov.au/ausstats/abs@.nsf/Lookup/by%20Subject/3303.0~2015~Main%20Features~Dementia~10002.

13. Waite, L. M., Broe, A., Grayson, D. A., & Creasey, H. (2001). The incidence of dementia in an Australian community population: The Sydney older persons study. International Journal of Geriatric Psychiatry, 16(7), 680-689. Available from https://doi.org/10.1002/gps.404.

14. Slavin, M. J., Brodaty, H., & Sachdev, P. S. (2013). Challenges of diagnosing dementia in the oldest old population. Journal of Gerontology, Series A: Biological Sciences and Medical Science, 68(9), 1103-1111. doi:10.1093/gerona/glt051.

15. Hugo, J., & Ganguli, M. (2014). Dementia and cognitive impairment. Epidemiology, diagnosis, and treatment. Clinics in Geriatric Medicine, 30(3), 421-442. Available fromhttps://doi.org/10.1016/j.cger.2014.04.001, W.B. Saunders.

16. Holzer, C., & Warshaw, G. (2000). Clues to early Alzheimer dementia in the outpatient setting. Archives of Family Medicine, 9(10), 1066, Retrieved from. Available from https://triggered.clockss.org/ServeContent?url=http://archfami.ama-assn.org%2Fcgi%2Freprint%2F9%2F10%2F1066.pdf.

17. Aretouli, E., & Brandt, J. (2010). Everyday functioning in mild cognitive impairment and its relationship with executive cognition. International Journal of Geriatric Psychiatry: A Journal of the Psychiatry of Late Life and Allied Sciences, 25(3), 224-233. Available from https://doi.org/10.1002/gps.2325.

18. Mental Health Foundation. (2016). The interface between dementia and mental health:

An evidence review policy paper 2016.

19. Australian Bureau of Statistics. (2015c). National Health Survey: First Results (no. 4364.0.55.001). Retrieved from http://www.abs.gov.au/ausstats/abs@.nsf/Lookup/by%20Subject/4364.0.55.001~2014-15~Main%20Features~Psychological%20distress~16.

20. Alzheimer's association. (2020). 2020 Alzheimer's disease facts and figures. Alzheimer's & Dementia, 16(3), 391-460. Available from https://doi.org/10.1002/alz.12068.

21. Santabárbara, J., Lipnicki, D. M., Bueno-Notivol, J., Olaya-Guzmán, B., Villagrasa, B., & López-Antón, R. (2020). Updating the evidence for an association between anxiety and risk of Alzheimer's disease: A meta-analysis of prospective cohort studies. Journal of Affective Disorders. Available from https://doi.org/10.1016/j.jad.2019.11.065, Elsevier B.V.

22. Becker, E., Orellana Rios, C. L., Lahmann, C., Rücker, G., Bauer, J., & Boeker, M. (2018). Anxiety as a risk factor of Alzheimer's disease and vascular dementia. British Journal of Psychiatry, 213(5), 654-660. Available from https://doi.org/10.1192/bjp.2018.173.

23. Terracciano, A., Iacono, D., O'Brien, R. J., Troncoso, J. C., An, Y., Sutin, A. R., ... Resnick, S. M. (2013). Personality and resilience to Alzheimer's disease neuropathology: A prospective autopsy study. Neurobiology of Aging, 34(4), 1045-1050. Available from https://doi.org/10.1016/j.neurobiolaging.2012.08.008.

24. Zufferey, V., Donati, A., Popp, J., Meuli, R., Rossier, J., Frackowiak, R., ... Kherif, F. (2017). Neuroticism, depression, and anxiety traits exacerbate the state of cognitive impairment and hippocampal vulnerability to Alzheimer's disease. Alzheimer's and Dementia: Diagnosis, Assessment and Disease Monitoring, 7, 107-114. Available from https://doi.org/10.1016/j.dadm.2017.05.002.

25. Bierman, E. J. M., Comijs, H. C., Jonker, C., & Beekman, A. T. F. (2007). Symptoms of anxiety and depression in the course of cognitive decline. Dementia and Geriatric Cognitive Disorders, 24(3), 213-219. Available from https://doi.org/10.1159/000107083.

26. Dementia Australia. (2015). Don't forget dementia on World Mental Health Day. Retrieved from https://www.dementia.org.au/media-releases/2015/dont-forgetdementiaon-world-mental-health-day.

27. Piccininni, M., Di Carlo, A., Baldereschi, M., Zaccara, G., & Inzitari, D. (2005). Behavioral and psychological symptoms in Alzheimer's disease: Frequency and relationship with duration and severity of the disease. Dementia and Geriatric Cognitive Disorders, 19(5-6), 276-281. Available from https://doi.org/10.1159/000084552.

28. Zubenko, G. S. (1996). Clinicopathologic and neurochemical correlates of major depression and psychosis in primary dementia. International Psychogeriatrics, 8(3), 219-223. Available from https://doi.org/10.1017/S1041610297003384.

29. Alzheimer's Association. (2018). Depression. Retrieved from https://www.alz.org/help-

30. Brodaty, H., & Luscombe, G. (1996). Depression in persons with dementia. International Psychogeriatrics, 8(4), 609-622. Available from https://doi.org/10.1017/S104161029600292X.

31. Forstl, H., Burns, A., Luthert, P., Cairns, N., Lantos, P., & Levy, R. (1992). Clinical and neuropathological correlates of depression in Alzheimer's disease. Psychological Medicine, 22(4), 877-884. Available from https://doi.org/10.1017/S0033291700038459.

32. Kim, E., & Rovner, B. W. (1994). Depression in dementia. Psychiatric Annals, 24(4), 173-177. Available from https://doi.org/10.3928/0048-5713-19940401-06.

33. Teresi, J., Abrams, R., Holmes, D., Ramirez, M., & Eimicke, J. (2001). Prevalence of depression and depression recognition in nursing homes. Social Psychiatry and Psychiatric Epidemiology, 36(12), 613-620. Available from https://doi.org/10.1007/s127-001-8202-7.

34. Harwood, D. G., & Sultzer, D. L. (2002). "Life is not worth living": Hopelessness in Alzheimer's disease. Journal of Geriatric Psychiatry and Neurology, 15(1), 38-43. Available from https://doi.org/10.1177/089198870201500108.

35. Sabodash, V., Mendex, M. F., Fong, S., & Hsiao, J. J. (2013). Suicidal behavior in dementia: A special risk in semantic dementia. American Journal of Alzheimer's Disease & Other Dementias, 28(6), 592-599. Available from https://doi.org/10.1177/1533317513494447.

36. Lovibond, S. H., & Lovibond, P. F. (1995). Manual for the Depression Anxiety & Stress Scales (2nd ed.). Sydney: Psychology Foundation.

37. Van Der Linde, R. M., Dening, T., Matthews, F. E., & Brayne, C. (2014). Grouping of behavioural and psychological symptoms of dementia. International Journal of Geriatric Psychiatry, 29(6), 562-568. Available from https://doi.org/10.1002/gps.4037.

38. van der Linde, R. M., Dening, T., Stephan, B. C. M., Prina, A. M., Evans, E., & Brayne, C. (2016). Longitudinal course of behavioural and psychological symptoms of dementia: Systematic review. British Journal of Psychiatry, 209(5), 366-377. Available from https://doi.org/10.1192/bjp.bp.114.148403.

39. Collins, J. D., Henley, S. M. D., & Suárez-González, A. (2020). A systematic review of the prevalence of depression, anxiety, and apathy in frontotemporal dementia, atypical and youngonset Alzheimer's disease, and inherited dementia. International Psychogeriatrics. Cambridge University Press. Available from https://doi.org/10.1017/

S1041610220001118.

40. Wilson, R. S., Krueger, K. R., Arnold, S. E., Schneider, J. A., Kelly, J. F., Barnes, L. L., ... Bennett, D. A. (2007). Loneliness and risk of Alzheimer disease. Archives of General Psychiatry, 64(2), 234-240. Available from https://doi.org/10.1001/archpsyc.64.2.234.

41. Wilson, R. S., Begeny, C. T., Boyle, P. A., Schneider, J. A., & Bennett, D. A. (2011). Vulnerability to stress, anxiety, and development of dementia in old age. The American Journal of Geriatric Psychiatry, 19(4), 327-334. Available from https://doi.org/10.1097/JGP.0b013e31820119da.

42. Hoe, J., Hancock, G., Livingston, G., & Orrell, M. (2006). Quality of life of people with dementia in residential care homes. British Journal of Psychiatry, 188(May), 460-464. Available from https://doi.org/10.1192/bjp.bp.104.007658.

43. Seignourel, P. J., Kunik, M. E., Snow, L., Wilson, N., & Stanley, M. (2008). Anxiety in dementia: A critical review. Clinical Psychology Review, 28(7), 1071-1082. Available from https://doi.org/10.1016/j.cpr.2008.02.008.

44. Chemerinski, E., Petracca, G., Manes, F., Leiguarda, R., & Starkstein, S. E. (1998). Prevalence and correlates of anxiety in Alzheimer's disease. Depression and Anxiety, 7(4), 166-170, 10.1002/(SICI)1520-6394(1998)7:4 < 166::AID-DA4 > 3.0.CO;2-8.

45. Gibbons, L., Teri, L., Logsdon, R., McCurry, S., Kukull, W., Bowen, J., ... Larson, E. (2002). Anxiety symptoms as predictors of nursing home placement in patients with Alzheimer's disease. Journal of Clinical Geropsychology, 8(4), 335-342. Available from https://doi.org/10.1023/A:1019635525375.

46. Wilson, R. S., Bennett, D. A., de Leon, C. F. M., Bienias, J. L., Morris, M. C., & Evans, D. A. (2005). Distress proneness and cognitive decline in a population of older persons. Psychoneuroendocrinology, 30(1), 11-17. Available from https://doi.org/10.1016/j.psyneuen.2004.04.005.

47. Wilson, R. S., Schneider, J. A., Arnold, S. E., Bienias, J. L., & Bennett, D. A. (2007). Conscientiousness and the incidence of Alzheimer disease and mild cognitive impairment. Archives of General Psychiatry, 64(10), 1204-1212. Available from https://doi.org/10.1001/archpsyc.64.10.1204.

48. Wilson, R. S., Schneider, J. A., Boyle, P. A., Arnold, S. E., Tang, Y., & Bennett, D. A. (2007). Chronic distress and incidence of mild cognitive impairment. Neurology, 68(24),2085-2092. Available from https://doi.org/10.1212/01.wnl.0000264930.97061.82.

49. Gallacher, J., Bayer, A., Fish, M., Pickering, J., Pedro, S., Dunstan, F., ... Ben-Shlomo, Y. (2009). Does anxiety affect risk of dementia? Findings from the Caerphilly Prospective Study. Psychosomatic Medicine, 71(6), 659-666. Available from https://doi.org/10.1097/

PSY.0b013e3181a6177c.

50. Gulpers, B., Ramakers, I., Hamel, R., Köhler, S., Oude Voshaar, R., & Verhey, F. (2016). Anxiety as a predictor for cognitive decline and dementia: A systematic review and meta-analysis. American Journal of Geriatric Psychiatry, 24(10), 823-842. Available from https://doi.org/10.1016/j.jagp.2016.05.015, Elsevier B.V.

51. Liew, T. M. (2020). Subjective cognitive decline, anxiety symptoms, and the risk of mild cognitive impairment and dementia. Alzheimer's Research and Therapy, 12(1), 107. Available from https://doi.org/10.1186/s13195-020-00673-8.

52. Norman, A. L., Woodard, J. L., Calamari, J. E., Gross, E. Z., Pontarelli, N., Socha, J., ... Armstrong, K. (2020). The fear of Alzheimer's disease: Mediating effects of anxiety on subjective memory complaints. Aging and Mental Health, 24(2), 308-314. Available from https://doi.org/10.1080/13607863.2018.1534081.

53. Porter, V. R., Buxton, W. G., Fairbanks, L. A., Strickland, T., O'Connor, S. M., Rosenberg-Thompson, S., & Cummings, J. L. (2003). Frequency and characteristics of anxiety among patients with Alzheimer's disease and related dementias. The Journal of Neuropsychiatry and Clinical Neurosciences, 15(2), 180-186. Available from https://doi.org/10.1176/jnp.15.2.180.

54. Ballard, C., Neill, D., O'brien, J., McKeith, I. G., Ince, P., & Perry, R. (2000). Anxiety, depression and psychosis in vascular dementia: Prevalence and associations. Journal of Affective Disorders, 59(2), 97-106. Available from https://doi.org/10.1016/S0165-0327(99)00057-9.

55. Teri, L., Ferretti, L. E., Gibbons, L. E., Logsdon, R. G., McCurry, S. M., Kukull, W. A., ... Larson, E. B. (1999). Anxiety in Alzheimer's disease: Prevalence and comorbidity. Journals of Gerontology Series A: Biomedical Sciences and Medical Sciences, 54(7), M348 M352. Available from https://doi.org/10.1093/gerona/54.7.M348.

56. Rasmussen, H., Rosness, T. A., Bosnes, O., Salvesen, Ø., Knutli, M., & Stordal, E. (2018). Anxiety and depression as risk factors in frontotemporal dementia and Alzheimer's disease: The HUNT study. Dementia and Geriatric Cognitive Disorders Extra, 8(3), 414-425. Available from https://doi.org/10.1159/000493973.

57. Segers, K., Benoit, F., Meyts, J., & Surquin, M. (2020). Anxiety symptoms are quantitatively and qualitatively different in dementia with Lewy bodies than in Alzheimer's disease in the years preceding clinical diagnosis. Psychogeriatrics, 20(3), 242-246. Available from https://doi.org/10.1111/psyg.12490.

58. Breitve, M. H., Hynninen, M. J., Brønnick, K., Chwiszczuk, L. J., Auestad, B. H., Aarsland, D., & Rongve, A. (2016). A longitudinal study of anxiety and cognitive decline in dementia with Lewy bodies and Alzheimer's disease. Alzheimer's Research

and Therapy, 8(1), 3. Available from https://doi.org/10.1186/s13195-016-0171-4.
59. Greenberg, M. S., Tanev, K., Marin, M.-F., & Pitman, R. K. (2014). Stress, PTSD, and dementia. Alzheimer's & Dementia, 10(3 Suppl.), S155-S165. Available from https://doi.org/10.1016/j.jalz.2014.04.008.
60. Mohlenhoff, B. S., O'Donovan, A., Weiner, M. W., & Neylan, T. C. (2017). Dementia risk in posttraumatic stress disorder: The relevance of sleep-related abnormalities in brain structure, amyloid, and inflammation. Current Psychiatry Reports, 19(11), 89.Current Medicine Group LLC 1. Available from https://doi.org/10.1007/s11920-017-0835-1.
61. Johansson, L., Guo, X., Waern, M., Östling, S. Ö., Gustafson, D., Bengtsson, C., & Skoog, I. (2010). Midlife psychological stress and risk of dementia: A 35-year longitudinal population study. Brain, 133(8), 2217-2224. Available from https://doi.org/10.1093/brain/awq116.
62. Islamoska, S., Hansen, Å. M., Ishtiak-Ahmed, K., Garde, A. H., Andersen, P.K., Garde, E., ... Nabe-Nielsen, K. (2020). Stress diagnoses in midlife and risk of dementia: A register-based follow-up study. Aging & Mental Health, 1-10. Available from https://doi.org/10.1080/13607863.2020.1742656.
63. Ouanes, S., & Popp, J. (2019). High cortisol and the risk of dementia and Alzheimer's disease: A review of the literature. Frontiers in Aging Neuroscience, 11. Available from https://doi.org/10.3389/fnagi.2019.00043.
64. Comijs, H. C., van den Kommer, T. N., Minnaar, R. W. M., Penninx, B. W. J. H., & Deeg, D. J. H. (2011). Accumulated and differential effects of life events on cognitive decline in older persons: Depending on depression, baseline cognition, or ApoE epsilon4 status? The Journals of Gerontology. Series B, Psychological Sciences and Social Sciences, 66(Suppl 1). Available from https://doi.org/10.1093/geronb/gbr019.
65. Tschanz, J. T., Pfister, R., Wanzek, J., Corcoran, C., Smith, K., Tschanz, B. T., ... Norton, M. C. (2013). Stressful life events and cognitive decline in late life: Moderation by education and age. The Cache County Study. International Journal of Geriatric Psychiatry, 28(8), 821-830. Available from https://doi.org/10.1002/gps.3888.
66. Katz, M. J., Derby, C. A., Wang, C., Sliwinski, M. J., Ezzati, A., Zimmerman, M. E., ... Lipton, R. B. (2016). Influence of perceived stress on incident amnestic mild cognitive impairment: Results from the Einstein Aging Study. Alzheimer Disease and Associated Disorders, 30(2), 93. Available from https://doi.org/10.1097/WAD.0000000000000125.
67. Karasek, R. A. (1979). Job demands, job decision latitude, and mental strain: Implications for job redesign. Administrative Science Quarterly, 24(2), 285. Available from https://doi.org/10.2307/2392498.

68. Wang, H.-X., Wahlberg, M., Karp, A., Winblad, B., & Fratiglioni, L. (2012). Psychosocial stress at work is associated with increased dementia risk in late life Alzheimer's & Dementia, 8(2), 114-120. Available from https://doi.org/10.1016/j.jalz.2011.03.001.
69. Seidler, A., Nienhaus, A., Bernhardt, T., Kauppinen, T., Elo, A. L., & Frölich, L. (2004). Psychosocial work factors and dementia. Occupational and Environmental Medicine, 61 (12), 962-971. Available from https://doi.org/10.1136/oem.2003.012153.
70. McCrory, C., Dooley, C., Layte, R., & Kenny, R. A. (2015). The lasting legacy of childhood adversity for disease risk in later life. Health Psychology, 34(7), 687-696. Available from https://doi.org/10.1037/hea0000147.
71. Conde-Sala, J. L., & Garre-Olmo, J. (2020). Early parental death and psychosocial risk factors for dementia: A case control study in Europe. International Journal of Geriatric Psychiatry, 35(9), 10511059. Available from https://doi.org/10.1002/gps.5328.
72. Norton, M. C., Østbye, T., Smith, K. R., Munger, R. G., & Tschanz, J. T. (2009). Early parental death and late-life dementia risk: Findings from the Cache County Study. Age and Ageing. Available from https://doi.org/10.1093/ageing/afp023.
73. Radford, K., Delbaere, K., Draper, B., Mack, H. A., Daylight, G., Cumming, R., ... Broe, G. A. (2017). Childhood stress and adversity is associated with late-life dementia in aboriginal Australians. American Journal of Geriatric Psychiatry, 25(10), 1097-1106. Available from https://doi.org/10.1016/j.jagp.2017.05.008.
74. Donley, G. A. R., Lönnroos, E., Tuomainen, T. P., & Kauhanen, J. (2018). Association of childhood stress with late-life dementia and Alzheimer's disease: The KIHD study. European Journal of Public Health, 28(6), 1069-1073. Available from https://doi.org/10.1093/eurpub/cky134.
75. Skogen, J. C., Bergh, S., Stewart, R., Knudsen, A. K., & Bjerkeset, O. (2015). Midlife mental distress and risk for dementia up to 27 years later: The Nord-Trøndelag Health Study (HUNT) in linkage with a dementia registry in Norway. BMC Geriatrics, 15(1). Available from https://doi.org/10.1186/s12877-015-0020-5.
76. Flatt, J. D., Gilsanz, P., Quesenberry, C. P., Albers, K. B., & Whitmer, R. A. (2018). Post-traumatic stress disorder and risk of dementia among members of a health care delivery system. Alzheimer's & Dementia, 14(1), 28-34. Available from https://doi.org/10.1016/j.jalz.2017.04.014.
77. Mawanda, F., Wallace, R. B., McCoy, K., & Abrams, T. E. (2017). PTSD, psychotropic medication use, and the risk of dementia among US veterans: A Retrospective cohort study. Journal of the American Geriatrics Society, 65(5), 1043-1050. Available from https://doi.org/10.1111/jgs.14756.

78. Ball, V. L., Hudson, S., Davila, J., Morgan, R., Walder, A., Graham, D. P., ... Kunik, M. E. (2009). Post-traumatic stress disorder and prediction of aggression in persons with dementia. International Journal of Geriatric Psychiatry, 24(11), 1285-1290. Available from https://doi.org/10.1002/gps.2258.

79. Bruneau, M., Desmarais, P., & Pokrzywko, K. (2020). Post-traumatic stress disorder mistaken for behavioural and psychological symptoms of dementia: Case series and recommendations of care. Psychogeriatrics, 20(5), 754759. Available from https://doi.org/10.1111/psyg.12549.

80. Günak, M. M., Billings, J., Carratu, E., Marchant, N. L., Favarato, G., & Orgeta, V. (2020). Post-traumatic stress disorder as a risk factor for dementia: Systematic review and meta-analysis. The British Journal of Psychiatry: The Journal of Mental Science, 217(5), 600-608. Available from https://doi.org/10.1192/bjp.2020.150.

81. Kuring, J. K., Mathias, J. L., & Ward, L. (2020). Risk of dementia in persons who have previously experienced clinically-significant depression, anxiety, or PTSD: A systematic review and meta-analysis. Journal of Affective Disorders, 274, 247-261. Available from https://doi.org/10.1016/j.jad.2020.05.020, Elsevier B.V.

82. Lawrence, K. A., Pachner, T. M., Long, M. M., Henderson, S., Schuman, D. L., & Plassman, B. L. (2020). Risk and protective factors of dementia among adults with posttraumatic stress disorder: A systematic review protocol. British Medical Journal Open, 10(6). Available from https://doi.org/10.1136/bmjopen-2019-035517, e035517.

83. Nilaweera, D., Freak-Poli, R., Ritchie, K., Chaudieu, I., Ancelin, M. L., & Ryan, J. (2020). The long-term consequences of trauma and posttraumatic stress disorder symptoms on later life cognitive function and dementia risk. Psychiatry Research, 294, 113506. Available from https://doi.org/10.1016/j.psychres.2020.113506.

84. Wang, T. Y., Wei, H. T., Liou, Y. J., Su, T. P., Bai, Y. M., Tsai, S. J., ... Chen, M. H. (2016). Risk for developing dementia among patients with posttraumatic stress disorder: A nationwide longitudinal study. Journal of Affective Disorders, 205, 306-310. Available from https://doi.org/10.1016/j.jad.2016.08.013.

85. Uddo, M., Vasterling, J. J., Brailey, K., & Sutker, P. B. (1993). Memory and attention in combat-related post-traumatic stress disorder (PTSD). Journal of Psychopathology and Behavioral Assessment, 15(1), 43-52. Available from https://doi.org/10.1007/BF00964322.

86. Weniger, G., Lange, C., Sachsse, U., & Irle, E. (2008). Amygdala and hippocampal volumes and cognition in adult survivors of childhood abuse with dissociative disorders. Acta Psychiatrica Scandinavica, 118(4), 281-290. Available from https://doi.org/10.1111/j.1600-0447.2008.01246.x.

87. Yaffe, K., Vittinghoff, E., Lindquist, K., Barnes, D., Covinsky, K. E., Neylan, T., ... Marmar, C. (2010). Post-traumatic stress disorder and risk of dementia among U.S. post-traumatic stress disorder and risk of dementia among U.S. veterans. Archives of General Psychiatry, 67(6), 608-613. Available from https://doi.org/10.1001/archgenpsychiatry.2010.61.
88. Duman, R. S. (2002). Pathophysiology of depression: the concept of synaptic plasticity. European Psychiatry, 17, 306-310. Available from https://doi.org/10.1016/S0924-9338(02)00654-5.
89. Flatt, J., Quesenberry, C. P., Liu, J. Y., Albers, K., & Whitmer, R. A. (2016). 01-02-03: Post-traumatic stress disorder and risk of dementia among men and women members of a healthcare delivery system. Alzheimer's & Dementia, 12. Available from https://doi.org/10.1016/j.jalz.2016.06.300, P174.
90. Kim, J. J., & Diamond, D. M. (2002). The stressed hippocampus, synaptic plasticity and lost memories. Nature Reviews. Neuroscience, 3(6), 453. Available from https://doi.org/10.1038/nrn849.
91. McEwen, B. S. (2000). The neurobiology of stress: From serendipity to clinical relevance. Brain Research, 886(1-2), 172-189. Available from https://doi.org/10.1016/S0006-8993(00)02950-4.
92. Martinez-Clavera, C., James, S., Bowditch, E., & Kuruvilla, T. (2017). Delayed-onset post-traumatic stress disorder symptoms in dementia. Progress in Neurology and Psychiatry, 21(3), 26-31. Available from https://doi.org/10.1002/pnp.477.

第二部分
痴呆研究的前沿主题

第四章 瞳孔中的阿尔茨海默病：瞳孔测量作为阿尔茨海默病认知过程的生物学标志物

Mohamad El Haj, Ahmed A. Moustafa 编
陈绮婷，周宝玉，陈仰昆 译
肖卫民 校

第一节 引言

阿尔茨海默病（AD）是一种神经退行性疾病，随着人口老龄化问题的加剧，已经成为一项重大的公共卫生问题。尽管人们为开发出有效的药物治疗做了许多努力，但目前仍无法治愈 AD。正因为缺乏有效的治疗方法，故 AD 管理的主要焦点之一是识别有 AD 风险的个体。这是为了预测疾病的发生，理想情况下，在神经功能明显下降之前，维持认知和功能能力。AD 可以由 2 个主要生物标志物来反映，分别是脑脊液（cerebral spinal fluid，CSF）中 β-淀粉蛋白（β-Amyloid，Aβ）和 tau 蛋白的存在，以及 MRI 上观察到的海马积的缩小。尽管这些生物标志物早已被广泛用于检测 AD，但仍然需要寻找更好的疾病标志物。这种标志物最好可以通过无创的方法（因为 CSF 检测需要医疗干预）或更经济的检测获得（因为 MRI 通常昂贵）。为了解决这个问题，我们研究瞳孔扩张是否能作为一种非侵入性和更经济的认知衰退标志。因此，我们提供一个案例研究来评估瞳孔扩张是否可以在患有 AD 的患者中反映认知努力，旨在揭示瞳孔扩张是否具有反映 AD 中认知过程的潜力。

基于大量的研究，我们展示了瞳孔直径如何反映非病理性人群中的认知努力。然而，在谈到这些文献之前，了解瞳孔的基本功能是有意义的。瞳孔直径通常在 1.5~9.0 mm 不等[1,2]。在自然光线条件下，瞳孔直径约为 3.0 mm[1,2]。瞳孔直径由

开大肌和括约肌控制：开大肌收缩使瞳孔扩大，括约肌收缩使瞳孔缩小[3,4]。开大肌和括约肌通过落入视网膜的光量来调节视野：亮光使瞳孔缩小，弱光使瞳孔扩大。这种对光反射通常发生在 200 ms 内。在 AD 患者中，也可以观察到瞳孔光反射的变化。一项研究表明，AD 患者在接受托吡卡胺治疗后瞳孔对光反射能力减弱[5]。这些变化可能与蓝斑核的变化有关，而蓝斑核是 AD 中 Aβ 的沉积部位[6]。因此，瞳孔活动可以反映 AD 中的神经病理学变化。正如下文所示，瞳孔活动反映了认知努力。

有大量的研究表明，在工作记忆任务中，尤其是在跨度任务中，瞳孔直径会随认知努力而增加。在跨度任务中，通常要求参与者按正向顺序（即前向跨度）或逆向顺序（即后向跨度）重复一串数字。研究表明，在数字跨度任务中，每多保留一个数字都会导致瞳孔直径增加，直到数字的长度超出工作记忆的容量为止，此时瞳孔直径开始趋于稳定甚至减小[7-11]。这些研究表明，瞳孔扩张可以作为认知努力的可靠和有效的心理生理标志。

研究也报告了认知努力对瞳孔扩张的影响。例如，已有研究表明，在处理复杂句子与简单句子时[12]，进行复杂与简单的视觉搜索时[13]，以及在执行功能任务时[14-18]，瞳孔直径是如何增加的。在记忆回溯过程中也可以观察到瞳孔扩张。一项研究调查了自传记忆（即个人生活事件的记忆）期间的瞳孔扩张，通过邀请参与者在眼动跟踪眼镜监测其瞳孔的情况下，回忆个人事件[19]。在控制变量下，参与者需要大声计数。分析结果表明，在自传式记忆期间，瞳孔较对照组大。这种扩张被归因于需要用于重构记忆的认知负荷。一项处理未来思维（即生成未来假设情景的能力）的研究也得出了类似的结论。一项研究记录了参与者在回忆过去个人信息和构建未来可能发生事件时的瞳孔直径[20]。结果表明，在构建未来时，瞳孔较大。这种较大的瞳孔归因于在构建未来时需要将可用信息重新组合成新情景所需的认知努力。总的来说，有大量研究表明，瞳孔直径会随着认知努力而增加。

虽然关于认知努力对瞳孔扩张影响的研究有许多，但这些研究并没有涉及 AD。据我们所知，甚至没有关于瞳孔扩张是否可以反映一般认知加工的已发表研究。因此，我们提供了第一项病例研究，其中我们评估了瞳孔扩张是否可以反映 AD 患者的认知努力。更具体地说，我们测量了一项需要认知努力的任务中的瞳孔直径（即从 100 开始以 7 递减倒数），同时也测量了不需要认知努力的对照组的瞳孔直径（该对照组是从 1 开始数数）。与对照组相比，我们预期在需要认知努力的任务中，瞳孔直径会更大。通过本项研究，我们旨在揭示瞳孔扩张是否具有反映 AD 患者认知加工的潜力。

第二节　方法

一、病例研究

L 先生今年 67 岁，接受过 10 年的正规教育，是右利手，母语是法语。L 先生与妻子一起居住在自己的家中。根据美美国国立神经、语言交流障碍和卒中研究 - 阿尔茨海默病及相关疾病协会（National Institute of Neurological and Communicative Disorders and Stroke and the Alzheimer's Disease and Related Disorders Association，NINCDS-ADRDA）的诊断标准[21]，L 先生于 2019 年被诊断为遗忘型轻度 AD。在研究期间，我们使用简明精神状态检查量表（MMSE）[22] 来评估 L 先生的认知表现，他在满分为 30 分的量表中得 24 分。

二、方法与步骤

L 先生接受了一个需要认知努力的任务和一个不需要认知努力的任务。在这两个任务中，他都戴着眼球追踪眼镜，面对着一堵白墙。这项实验是在南特医院神经科的一个安静的房间里进行的。为了确保瞳孔扩大的差异不是由视网膜照度的差异引起的，在两种情况下都关闭了百叶窗，并且房间的亮度（60 W 荧光灯）相同。在实验之前，L 先生被告知该实验一般与眼球追踪研究和认知有关。为了不影响 L 先生的表现，研究者没有给他关于瞳孔扩大及其与认知处理关系的更多细节。

在需要认知努力的情况下，我们应用简易精神状态检查量表，请 L 先生在

1 分钟内大声从 100 开始以 7 递减倒数（例如，93、86、79……）。在不需要认知努力的情况下，我们请 L 先生在 1 分钟内从 1 开始大声计数。采用瞳孔捕获软件记录这两种情况下的瞳孔直径。L 先生佩戴眼球追踪眼镜（瞳孔实验室），该眼镜包括一个远程瞳孔追踪系统，使用红外线照明，采样率为 200 Hz，注视位置精度为 < 0.1°。在每个任务之前，通过请 L 先生盯着一个黑色的十字架（一个 5 cm × 5 cm 的十字架，印在一张固定在墙壁中心的 A4 白纸上）作为校准参考；校准结束后，十字架会被撤走。在这两种情况下，L 先生坐在一堵白墙前，他与白墙之间的距离为 30~50 cm。我们请 L 先生不要看墙，但可以自由探索墙的各个部分。墙壁没有显示任何视觉刺激（例如，图纸、窗户）。对于因变量，我们计算了两种情况下瞳孔扩大的平均值（单位为毫米）。

三、结果

在需要认知努力的任务和不需要认知努力的任务中，L 先生的平均瞳孔直径分别为 3.3 mm 和 2.7 mm。换句话说，如图 4-1 所示，在需要认知努力的任务中的瞳孔比在不需要认知努力任务中的更大。

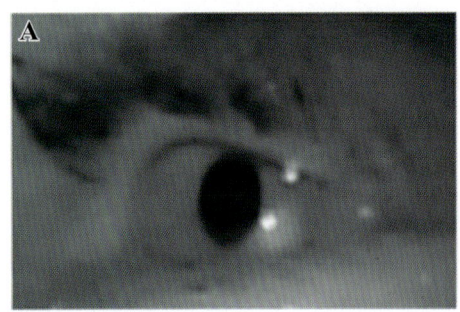 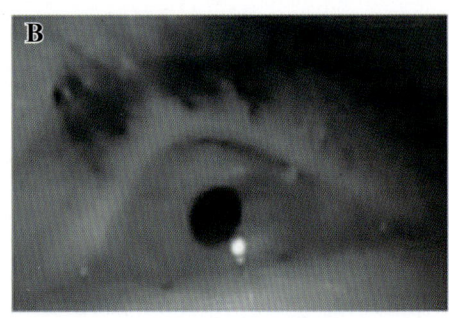

图 4-1　L 先生在需要认知努力（A）和不需要认知努力（B）任务中的瞳孔直径

第三节　讨论

我们提供了首例关于认知处理对 AD 患者瞳孔直径影响的研究。研究演示了如何在需要认知努力任务中观察到比在不需要认知努力任务中更大的瞳孔直径。这个方法展示了瞳孔直径如何反映 AD 患者的认知处理。

正如从 L 先生那观察到的那样，在需要认知努力任务中比在不需要认知努力任务中瞳孔更大，这可以归因于需要认知努力任务的认知负荷更大。这一假设可以得到大量表明瞳孔直径如何随着认知努力而增加[7-11,23-26]的研究的支持。这项研究支持了瞳孔直径可以提示认知负荷大小的假设。这种认知负荷假设符合我们的实验过程，因为与对照组相比，从 100 开始以 7 递减的反向计算需要更多的认知处理（即，激活工作记忆中的执行系统，以相反的顺序操纵和再现序列）。后一项任务需要更少的认知负荷，因为它只是涉及将一个点值归于数字"1"，以此类推。综上所述，观察到 L 先生在需要认知努力任务中瞳孔直径比不需认知努力任务中更大，可以归因于需要认知努力任务的认知负荷。

除了认知负荷的解释外，在 L 先生那观察到的瞳孔直径也可以归因于交感神经（即肾上腺素能）和副交感神经（即胆碱能）自主神经系统的活动。瞳孔扩大包括 Edinger-Westphal 核的抑制调节以及节前交感神经元的激活[3]。因此，正如在 L 先生那观察到的，在需要认知努力任务中比不需要认知努力任务中瞳孔直径更大，可归因于 Edinger-Westphal 核较高的抑制活性以及节前交感神经元的较高激活，导致在需要认知努力任务中括约肌活动的减少和开大肌活动减少。因此，两种实验条件下，瞳孔直径的变化可以反映肾上腺素能和胆碱能活动。这个问题很重要，因为 AD 与肾上腺素能活动缺陷[27,28]和胆碱能活动缺陷有关[29-32]。瞳孔测定法可作为 AD 患者肾上腺素能和胆碱能活性的生物标志物。重要的是，一项研究发现，AD 患者的瞳孔直径与脑脊液 Aβ 和 tau 水平之间存在显著相关性[33]。因此，瞳孔测量法可以反映 AD 的神经病理学，正如我们的案例研究中观察到的认知处理。我们认为，很少有研究评估瞳孔测量法和视网膜活动作为 AD 潜在生物标志物的价值，因此我们的研究为瞳孔测量法作为 AD 认知处理的潜在生物标志物的价值提供了证据。

诚然，案例研究的设计限制了我们发现的普遍性。虽然对产生创新研究很有用，但案例研究的实验设计没有严谨性的方法学水平去支持这些发现。因此，我们应该谨慎地看待这些发现的结论。我们相信，我们的案例研究为瞳孔测量法作为 AD 患者认知处理的一种实用且无创的生物标志物的设计和使用铺平了道路。这种生物标志物可能对寻求实现重大突破性技术和科学进展的精准医学做出重大贡献，尤其在神经科学领域，可以提供个性化的诊断[34]。

总之，瞳孔的直径提供了关于认知和神经处理的大量信息。正如我们的研究所提出的那样，瞳孔的直径可以作为 AD 患者的认知处理的一个有价值的生物标志物。鉴于 AD 缺乏有效的治疗方法，我们的研究案例为瞳孔测量法作为一种实用的、无创的认知处理生物标志物开启了创新研究，以便更好地诊断 AD。

参考文献

1. Kret, M. E., & Sjak-Shie, E. E. (2019). Preprocessing pupil size data: Guidelines and code. Behavior Research Methods, 51(3), 1336-1342. Available from https://doi.org/10.3758/s13428-018-1075-y.
2. Wyatt, H. J. (1995). The form of the human pupil. Vision Research, 35(14), 2021-2036.
3. Kawasaki, A. (1999). Physiology, assessment, and disorders of the pupil. Current Opinion in Ophthalmology, 10(6), 394-400.
4. Sirois, S., & Brisson, J. (2014). Pupillometry. Wiley Interdisciplinary Review of Cognitive Science, 5(6), 679-692. Available from https://doi.org/10.1002/wcs.1323.
5. Granholm, E., Morris, S., Galasko, D., Shults, C., Rogers, E., & Vukov, B. (2003). Tropicamide effects on pupil size and pupillary light reflexes in Alzheimer's and Parkinson's disease. International Journal of Psychophysiology: Official Journal of the International Organization of Psychophysiology, 47(2), 95-115. Available from https://doi.org/10.1016/s0167-8760(02)00122-8.
6. Murphy, C. (2019). Olfactory and other sensory impairments in Alzheimer disease. Nature Reviews Neurology, 15(1), 11-24. Available from https://doi.org/10.1038/s41582-018-0097-5.
7. Alnaes, D., Sneve, M. H., Espeseth, T., Endestad, T., van de Pavert, S. H., & Laeng, B. (2014). Pupil size signals mental effort deployed during multiple object tracking and predicts brain activity in the dorsal attention network and the locus coeruleus. Journal of Vision, 14(4), 1-6. Available from https://doi.org/10.1167/14.4.1.
8. Cabestrero, R., Crespo, A., & Quirós, P. (2009). Pupillary dilation as an index of task demands. Perceptual and Motor Skills, 109(3), 664-678. Available from https://doi.org/10.2466/pms.109.3.664-678.

9. Granholm, E., Asarnow, R. F., Sarkin, A. J., & Dykes, K. L. (1996). Pupillary responses index cognitive resource limitations. Psychophysiology, 33(4), 457-461.
10. Peavler, W. S. (1974). Pupil size, information overload, and performance differences. Psychophysiology, 11(5), 559-566.
11. Wahn, B., Ferris, D. P., Hairston, W. D., & Konig, P. (2016). Pupil sizes scale with attentional load and task experience in a multiple object tracking task. PLoS One, 11(12), e0168087. Available from https://doi.org/10.1371/journal.pone.0168087.
12. Just, M. A., & Carpenter, P. A. (1993). The intensity dimension of thought: Pupillometric indices of sentence processing. Canadian Journal of Experimental Psychology/Revue Canadienne de Psychologie Experimentale, 47(2), 310-339.
13. Porter, G., Troscianko, T., & Gilchrist, I. D. (2007). Effort during visual search and counting: Insights from pupillometry. Quarterly Journal of Experimental Psychology (Hove), 60(2), 211-229. Available from https://doi.org/10.1080/17470210600673818.
14. Brown, G. G., Kindermann, S. S., Siegle, G. J., Granholm, E., Wong, E. C., & Buxton, R. B. (1999). Brain activation and pupil response during covert performance of the Stroop Color Word task. Journal of the International Neuropsychological Society: JINS, 5(4), 308-319.
15. Brown, S. B., van Steenbergen, H., Kedar, T., & Nieuwenhuis, S. (2014). Effects of arousal on cognitive control: Empirical tests of the conflict-modulated Hebbianlearning hypothesis. Frontiers in Human Neuroscience, 8, 23. Available from https://doi.org/10.3389/fnhum.2014.00023.
16. Hasshim, N., & Parris, B. A. (2015). Assessing stimulus-stimulus (semantic) conflict in the Stroop task using saccadic two-to-one color response mapping and preresponse pupillary measures. Attention Perception Psychophysics, 77(8), 2601-2610. Available from https://doi.org/10.3758/s13414-015-0971-9.
17. Laeng, B., Orbo, M., Holmlund, T., & Miozzo, M. (2011). Pupillary Stroop effects. Cognitive Processing, 12(1), 13-21. Available from https://doi.org/10.1007/s10339-010-0370-z.
18. Steinhauer, S. R., Siegle, G. J., Condray, R., & Pless, M. (2004). Sympathetic and parasympathetic innervation of pupillary dilation during sustained processing. International Journal of Psychophysiology: Official Journal of the International Organization of Psychophysiology, 52(1), 77-86. Available from https://doi.org/10.1016/j.ijpsycho.2003.12.005.
19. El Haj, M., Janssen, S. M. J., Gallouj, K., & Lenoble, Q. (2019). Autobiographical memory iIncreases pupil dilation. Translational Neuroscience, 10, 280-287. Available from https://doi.org/10.1515/tnsci-2019-0044.

20. El Haj, M., & Moustafa, A. A. (2020). Pupil dilation as an indicator of future thinking. Neurological Sciences: Official Journal of the Italian Neurological Society and of the Italian Society of Clinical Neurophysiology. Available from https://doi.org/10.1007/s10072-020-04533-z.
21. McKhann, G., Knopman, D. S., Chertkow, H., Hyman, B. T., Jack, C. R., Jr., Kawas, C. H., & Phelps, C. H. (2011). The diagnosis of dementia due to Alzheimer's disease: Recommendations from the National Institute on Aging-Alzheimer's Association workgroups on diagnostic guidelines for Alzheimer's disease. Alzheimer's & Dementia: The Journal of the Alzheimer's Association, 7(3), 263-269. Available from https://doi.org/10.1016/j.jalz.2011.03.005.
22. Folstein, M. F., Folstein, S. E., & McHugh, P. R. (1975). Mini-mental state. A practical method for grading the cognitive state of patients for the clinician. Journal of Psychiatric Research, 12(3), 189-198.
23. Ahern, S., & Beatty, J. (1979). Pupillary responses during information processing vary with Scholastic Aptitude Test scores. Science (New York, N.Y.), 205(4412), 1289-1292.
24. Beatty, J. (1982). Task-evoked pupillary responses, processing load, and the structure of processing resources. Psychological Bulletin, 91(2), 276-292.
25. Karatekin, C., Couperus, J. W., & Marcus, D. J. (2004). Attention allocation in the dualtask paradigm as measured through behavioral and psychophysiological responses. Psychophysiology, 41(2), 175-185. Available from https://doi.org/10.1111/j.1469-8986.2004.00147.x.
26. Piquado, T., Isaacowitz, D., & Wingfield, A. (2010). Pupillometry as a measure of cognitive effort in younger and older adults. Psychophysiology, 47(3), 560-569. Available from https://doi.org/10.1111/j.1469-8986.2009.00947.x.
27. Kelly, S. C., He, B., Perez, S. E., Ginsberg, S. D., Mufson, E. J., & Counts, S. E. (2017). Locus coeruleus cellular and molecular pathology during the progression of Alzheimer's disease. Acta Neuropathologica Communications, 5(1), 8. Available from https://doi.org/10.1186/s40478-017-0411-2.
28. Prettyman, R., Bitsios, P., & Szabadi, E. (1997). Altered pupillary size and darkness and light reflexes in Alzheimer's disease. Journal of Neurology, Neurosurgery, and Psychiatry, 62(6), 665-668. Available from https://doi.org/10.1136/jnnp.62.6.665.
29. Ornek, N., Dag, E., & Ornek, K. (2015). Corneal sensitivity and tear function in neurodegenerative diseases. Current Eye Research, 40(4), 423-428. Available from https://doi.org/10.3109/02713683.2014.930154.
30. Scinto, L. F., Frosch, M., Wu, C. K., Daffner, K. R., Gedi, N., & Geula, C. (2001). Selective cell loss in Edinger-Westphal in asymptomatic elders and Alzheimer's patients.

Neurobiology of Aging, 22(5), 729-736. Available from https://doi.org/10.1016/s0197-4580(01)00235-4.

31. Shen, J., & Wu, J. (2015). Chapter Ten-Nicotinic cholinergic mechanisms in Alzheimer's disease. In M. De Biasi (Ed.), International Review of Neurobiology (Vol. 124, pp. 275-292). Academic Press.
32. Singh, A., & Verma, S. (2020). Use of ocular biomarkers as a potential tool for early diagnosis of Alzheimer's disease. Indian Journal of Ophthalmology, 68(4), 555-561. Available from https://doi.org/10.4103/ijo.IJO_999_19.
33. Frost, S., Kanagasingam, Y., Sohrabi, H. R., Taddei, K., Bateman, R., Morris, J., & Martins, R. N. (2013). Pupil response biomarkers distinguish amyloid precursor protein mutation carriers from non-carriers. Current Alzheimer Research, 10(8), 790-796. Available from https://doi.org/10.2174/15672050113109990154.
34. Hampel, H., Vergallo, A., Perry, G., Lista, S., & Alzheimer Precision Medicine, I. (2019). The Alzheimer Precision Medicine Initiative. Journal of Alzheimer's Disease: JAD, 68(1), 1-24. Available from https://doi.org/10.3233/JAD-181121.

第五章 维生素 D 缺乏与认知及神经的相关性：聚焦健康老龄化与阿尔茨海默病

Ahmed A. Moustafa，Wafa Jaroudi，Abdrabo Soliman 编
刘健菲，王铭子，刘梓轩，向智滔 译
陈仰昆 校

第一节 引言

维生素 D 缺乏指人体内和脑内的维生素 D 浓度低于所需的最低浓度，对身心均有影响，是一个全球公共健康问题。Holick 和 Chen[1] 研究估计全球有 10 亿人有维生素 D 缺乏。尽管对于维生素 D 缺乏的诊断标准仍未达成一致，但 Pettersen 等[2] 将维生素 D 的水平划分如下：< 50 nmol/L 为维生素 D 不足，在 50~75 nmol/L 之间为低度足量，在 75~100 nmol/L 之间为高度足量，≥ 100 nmol/L 是超足量[2]。

本文献综述纳入探讨血清 25- 羟基维生素 D[25（OH）D] 作用的流行病学、营养学和心理学的研究，包括研究血清 25（OH）D 与维生素 D 激素（Vitamin D hormone，VDH）的文献。此外，我们的综述还涵盖了一些探讨维生素 D 和认知功能相关性的研究。其中，有的研究提到认知功能整体水平可能受影响[3,4]，而其他研究则认为维生素 D 水平低下会影响特定的认知功能，包括语言流畅性[5,6]、情景记忆[7] 以及思维混乱与整体记忆问题[3-11]。Annweiler 等[3] 在 462 名 65 岁及以上的法国老年人的样本中，探讨了维生素 D 水平与整体认知功能之间的关系。通过几次认知测试（如时钟绘制测试）将参与者划分为认知功能正常组和受损组，结果显示，整体认知能力较差组的维生素 D 水平较低。然而，这些结果并不影响特定认知领域[3]。韩国最近的一项研究发现，在老年人样本

·第五章 维生素D缺乏与认知及神经的相关性：聚焦健康老龄化与阿尔茨海默病·

中维生素 D 水平与认知功能并没有明显相关性[12]。

有研究探讨了维生素 D 水平与大脑功能[13-17]、记忆[18-20]及语言流利性[2,20]之间的相关性。大部分研究发现，维生素 D 缺乏确实在认知和神经过程中发挥了作用[21]，特别是基于海马的认知过程[22]。维生素 D 水平的降低可能改变海马的功能，从而导致阿尔茨海默病（AD）[23-26]。

研究发现，多年来缺乏维生素 D 的患者，认知能力下降速度更快，尤其是在语言情景记忆领域。与缺乏维生素 D 的人相比，维生素 D 足量（超过 50 nmol/L）的老年人诊断为痴呆的风险更低，并且表现出更好的认知功能[7]。一项对象为啮齿动物的回顾研究发现，维生素 D 缺乏可能影响海马的结构和功能，从而导致认知功能受损。这不仅在早期出现，也可以在老年期出现，如潜伏抑制[27]。

一些研究重点探索维生素 D 水平在正常衰老中所起的作用[4,7,19]，以及探索在中老年人群中的作用[11,16]。例如，在一项纵向研究中，Bartali 等[4]探究了 1185 名 60~70 岁老年女性血浆维生素 D 水平与认知功能的关系。在这项研究中，1989—1990 年间测量参与者的血浆维生素 D 水平，通过 1999 年的电话访谈进行后续认知评估。虽然参与者血浆维生素 D 水平的测定早于认知评估约 9 年，但研究结果显示，维生素 D 水平较高者有更高的认知功能水平，这表明维生素 D 水平对认知能力的影响可以持续很长一段时间。因此，维生素 D 水平不仅在短期内对认知水平有促进作用[20]，在长期内也可能产生促进作用，其可以减慢同年龄相关的认知功能衰退[4]。

还有其他研究也探索了维生素 D 水平与某些大脑疾病之间的关系，其中包括痴呆与 AD[3,7,28-31]。Kandiah 等[29]强调了维生素 D 在轻度认知障碍（MCI）和 AD 中的作用，其使用简易精神状态检查量表（MMSE）和阿尔茨海默病评定量表-认知部分（Alzheimer's disease assessment scale-cognitive score，ADAS-Cog）等评估方法比较了认知功能正常和认知功能障碍（MCI 和 AD）参与者的认知能力，发现维生素 D 水平和认知能力之间有直接的联系。总之，认知功能正常者的维生素 D 水平高于认知障碍者的水平。Kandiah 等[29]通过在认知障碍组中进行比较，发现维生素 D 水平较低的个体的 MMSE 和 ADAS-Cog 评分也较差。Aguilar

Navarro 等[32] 与 Jeon 等[33] 的研究也有类似发现。这些研究表明，维生素 D 水平确实对认知功能有影响，并会导致认知障碍和 AD 等疾病的发展。

维生素 D 水平与认知过程之间的紧密联系，甚至发生在神经系统疾病（如阿尔茨海默病）发展之前，已经有研究证实了补充维生素 D 对大脑和认知的影响。例如，Pettersen[20] 研究了补充高剂量维生素 D_3 对维生素 D 不足（＜75 nmol/L）的年轻人的认知功能的影响。研究结果发现，高剂量的维生素 D 补充可以改善非语言（视觉）记忆。然而，语言记忆和其他认知领域并不受维生素 D 水平的影响。研究表明，维生素 D 水平可能是即时视觉空间记忆的独立预测指标，而即时视觉空间记忆也与执行力有关[20,34]。

此外，由于维生素 D 缺乏可能同神经系统疾病之间有联系，一些研究观察了补充维生素 D 的治疗效果。例如，Pettersen[20] 进行了一项为期 18 个月的研究，探索给 82 名健康参与者补充高剂量的维生素 D，是否可以改善认知功能，这些参与者的维生素 D 基线水平没有显著差异。在这项研究中，一些参与者补充了高剂量的维生素 D，其他参与者则给予低剂量的维生素 D。通过语言流畅度和数位跨度等评估参与者的认知功能。结果显示，接受高剂量维生素 D 的参与者的血清 25（OH）D 水平显著高于接受低剂量组。高剂量的维生素 D 补充剂改善了非语言（视觉）记忆，这在功效上有别于低剂量的维生素 D。因此，与低剂量维生素 D 相比，即使是在短时间内（如 18 个月），服用高剂量维生素 D 后记忆也能得到改善。

Annweiler 等[35] 研究了补充维生素 D_3 对记忆功能障碍的老年人认知功能（特别是执行能力）的长期影响。该研究的参与者是一家记忆诊所的门诊患者，他们口服了剂量约为 34 ng/mL 的维生素 D_3。使用 MMSE、认知评估量表（Cognitive Assessment Battery，CAB）以及额叶功能评定量表（Frontal Assessment Battery，FAB）等方法来评估整体认知水平。采用多元回归分析给予维生素 D_3 前后水平与认知水平的关系。在 16 个月的随访中，参与者的维生素 D_3 水平显著增加。与没有补充任何水平维生素 D_3 的对照组相比，补充维生素 D_3 可提高 MMSE、CAB 和 FAB 评分。此外，肝脏中产生的 VDH- 钙化二醇 [25（OH）D] 的增加

与补充维生素 D_3 的参与者的 FAB 评分相关。

在探索补充维生素 D 的剂量与改善认知之间的关系时,有研究发现,补充维生素 D 对改善认知的作用与个体之间的基因差异有关,这或许可以解释只有部分人可以因补充维生素 D 而获益的原因[36]。

Waterhouse 等[36]在 12 个月的时间里,使用血液样本测量 350 名老年人维生素 D 水平,通过 DNA 样本分析单核苷酸多态性(Single-nucleotide Polymorphisms,SNP)遗传变异,并通过问卷调查对他们的生活方式(如饮食、户外暴露)进行调查。两组患者补充的维生素 D_3 剂量不同,分别为 30 000 IU 和 60 000 IU。数据分析提示,维生素 D_3 的效应同体重指数、维生素 D 调节代谢相关的 SNP、阳光敏感性以及皮肤、眼睛和头发色素沉着相关。Waterhouse 等[36]发现,在 60 000 IU 组中,每天每摄入 100 IU 的维生素 D,则血液中维生素 D 浓度就会增加 1.8 nmol/L;在 30 000 IU 组中,每天每摄入 100 IU 维生素 D,则血液中维生素 D 浓度就会增加 2.2 nmol/L。这个发现进一步揭示,补充维生素 D_3 的反应性随着剂量的增加而降低。我们认为当维生素 D_3 在转化为 25(OH)D 时可能会趋于饱和,这可以解释维生素 D_3 增加与补充剂量之间的关系。研究发现,在遗传变异方面,维生素 D_3 转变为血清 25(OH)D 的羟基化反应中,*CYP2R1* 基因中的 rs10766197 和 rs10741657 等位基因比具有相同基因的其他等位基因更敏感。另外,在 *GC/DBP* 基因中发现的等位基因 rs2282679 与人们对维生素 D_3 的反应性较低有关。综上,该研究[36]解释了为什么有些人在补充不同剂量的维生素 D 时表现为反应更快及受益更多,而为什么有些人在基因上更容易缺乏维生素 D(关于类似的观点,请参见 Wang 等[37])。

本综述分为以下几个部分:①动物的认知功能与维生素 D 水平的关系;②正常衰老与 AD 患者的维生素 D 水平。在整个综述中,我们将讨论补充维生素 D(如添加富含维生素 D 的饮食)的影响,这对大脑和认知均有积极的影响。

第二节 关于认知功能与维生素 D 水平的动物实验

已经使用大鼠[17,18,38]和小鼠[9,15,38]进行了多种关于维生素 D 的研究。Becker 等[18]的包括产前阶段低维生素 D 水平的成年大鼠在内的研究结果显示,潜在抑制明显受损被认为是海马功能的生物标志物[39-41]。这表明,与产前阶段具有健康维生素 D 水平的成年大鼠相比,出生前具有低维生素 D 水平的成年大鼠可能具有较慢的学习能力[18]。这样的发现强调,维生素 D 水平不仅影响个体晚年的认知[4],还会影响出生前的认知[18]。

有研究表明,维生素 D 是大脑发育和成人大脑功能的重要组成部分。Minasyan 等[15]在 3~5 个月龄的维生素 D 受体(Vitamin D Receptor,VDR)突变雄性成年小鼠中探索了这一想法。他们使用 Y 迷宫测试评估了工作记忆功能,在该测试中,小鼠依靠其空间记忆在 30 分钟间隔的试验中完成迷宫。2 周后,在小鼠禁食 24 小时后要求它们完成另一个 Y 迷宫任务,其中使用食物强化 2 小时。通过比较及统计分析完成两个迷宫任务的表现,VDR 小鼠具有不变的空间和工作记忆。在情绪行为和运动缺陷方面,可以观察到情绪/焦虑状态,但未观察到抑郁。因此可以提出,尽管 VDR 会影响情绪状态(如焦虑),但它不会改变记忆的某些方面[15]。Minasyan 等[15]的研究结果与先前研究结果不同[6,18],其强调维生素 D 与认知功能之间的关联,导致关于维生素 D 和认知的研究之间的一致性存在差异。

动物研究表明,VDH 对认知功能很重要。Hua 等[13]对 46 只雄性大鼠(Sprague Dawley 品种)进行了一项动物研究,以研究何种水平的 VDH 和黄体酮剂量对治疗脑损伤最有效:低(1 μg/kg,VDH)、中(2.5 μg/kg,VDH)和高(5 μg/kg,VDH)。研究人员首先破坏了大鼠的内侧额叶皮质(Medial Frontal Cortex,MFC)。在手术损伤 MFC 10 天后,使其完成水迷宫任务,测量在迷宫外花费的时间作为大鼠的行为反应性、短期记忆和长期记忆的表示。在行为和学习评估之后,对大鼠的大脑结构进行分析,以检查神经元和脑组织的退化。结果发现,单独黄体酮不影响认知或空间记忆的保存,但联合使用 VDH

第五章　维生素D缺乏与认知及神经的相关性：聚焦健康老龄化与阿尔茨海默病

和黄体酮治疗会影响。具体而言，低剂量和中剂量的VDH和黄体酮在保持认知方面最有效，低剂量在改善学习方面有效。在行为上，通过观察大鼠接近水迷宫壁的倾向降低，注意到黄体酮和低VDH改善了大鼠的焦虑表现。在长期记忆方面，发现低VDH和黄体酮剂量最有效。因此，可以表明VDH能够在一定剂量下有效改善/保持具有脑损伤的动物的认知。这些发现可能适用于有认知障碍史的人，维生素D可能会逆转或至少改善他们的记忆衰退。此外，以正确的剂量（大鼠中的低剂量至中等剂量）联合黄体酮和维生素/激素D可能更有益。另一项研究有相似的发现，将维生素D与白藜芦醇联合可以在AD的小鼠模型中防止痴呆和AD的发展[42]。据我们所知，还没有在人类参与者中进行过类似的研究。最近，一项研究发现，维生素D水平升高可以增强AD大鼠模型中的海马功能并改善其记忆表现[43]。

其他研究调查了美金刚（一种常见的抗AD药物）与维生素D联合使用对认知的影响。在一项研究中，用美金刚治疗的患者显示出与用美金刚和维生素D补充剂治疗的患者相似的认知表现。也就是说，单独使用美金刚可以改善AD患者的认知，而维生素D补充剂并不能进一步显著改善认知[31]。因此，可以理解为，维生素D在认知疾病如AD的发展之前可能是重要的。而在发展为AD之后，仅用维生素D补充剂来改善认知可能为时已晚。相反，常见的抗AD药物干预可能更有益于改善认知。因此，提倡早期给予维生素D补充剂对避免认知问题、AD及相关AD药物干预具有重要意义。这表明，与白藜芦醇和黄体酮不同，美金刚与维生素D补充剂联合使用时可能会增强认知能力。其他研究还发现，维生素D补充剂在AD患者中会产生β-淀粉样蛋白[44]。

在评估维生素D状态和认知功能的研究中，Turner等[17]研究了发育性维生素D缺乏对使用五项选择系列反应时间任务（5-choice serial reaction time task，5-CSRT）和五项选择连续性能测试测量的注意力的影响。Turner等[17]通过测量母亲在妊娠期间缺乏维生素D的大鼠和对照组大鼠的视觉空间注意力，研究低维生素D水平对持续注意力和警惕性的影响。结果表明，妊娠期间维生素D水平低与注意力受损有关。根据妊娠期间低维生素D影响后代生活的想法，

Becker 等[18]研究了产前维生素 D 缺乏对潜在抑制(其是海马功能的量度)的影响。Becker 等[18]发现,产前维生素 D 缺乏与大鼠学习和记忆的细微和离散变化有关。因此,在妊娠期间,缺乏维生素 D 会影响未出生婴儿在学习和记忆方面的认知,这突出了维生素 D 在出生前的重要性,而不仅仅是随着年龄的增长而变化。

最近,一些研究调查了维生素 D 补充剂如何确切地对 AD 的发展具有神经保护作用。有一项研究分析了维生素 D_3 补充剂预处理对大鼠几种神经和行为指标的影响[45]。结果显示,维生素 D_3 改善了空间记忆(与海马功能有关)及乙酰胆碱的功能,并防止海马和皮质神经元坏死。这表明维生素 D_3 可以避免人们发展至 AD。

第三节 健康老龄化、痴呆及阿尔茨海默病

已有多项研究探索维生素 D 与痴呆、AD、健康老龄化之间的关联性[4,7,9,16,29-31,46-51],但 Duchaine 等[52]的研究则另有见解。在本节中,我们将先后讨论健康老龄化和 AD 的相关研究。

Breitling 等[5]探索在 65 岁及以上人群中,维生素 D_3 和不同认知功能之间的关系,对维生素 D 和认知功能的基线水平以及这两项指标在 5 年随访期的变化进行测量。研究使用认知电话采访(Cognition Telephone Interview,COGTEL)来评估认知功能并使用化学发光法测量维生素 D 水平。通过比较被试者的维生素 D 水平和认知功能,可得出维生素 D 水平较低的女性的认知功能更差,尤其是在语言流畅性和归纳推理方面。男性被试者中也存在类似的关系。因此,维生素 D 水平决定了整体认知表现的好坏[5]。

Przybelski 和 Binkley[6]探讨了血清中 25(OH)D 和维生素 B_{12} 的浓度对 80 岁以上老年人认知功能的影响。研究人员采用 MMSE 评估被试者的认知功能,并在完成评估的 6 小时内采样测量 25(OH)D 以及维生素 B_{12} 的浓度。经回归分析后发现,MMSE 评分与 25(OH)D 浓度呈正相关,而与维生素 B_{12} 浓度无关。提示维生素 D 浓度会影响认知,Shih 等[53]研究有同样发现。

第五章 维生素D缺乏与认知及神经的相关性：聚焦健康老龄化与阿尔茨海默病

最近，Pettersen[2]评估了142名健康成年人中维生素D对执行功能的影响。执行功能通过语言流畅性、倒背数字任务、剑桥自动化成套神经心理测试（Cambridge Neuropsychological Test Automated Battery，CANTAB）的空间再认记忆和剑桥一触式长袜测试评估。研究结果表明，维生素D水平是语言流畅性的一个重要独立预测因素。进一步的统计检验进行了样条分析，该分析显示，维生素D与执行功能呈正相关关系，并且25（OH）D在浓度100 nmol/L及以上接近线性相关[2]。因此，可以认为100 nmol/L的维生素D浓度可能是执行功能（如语言流畅性）的最佳水平[2]。

另一项基于人群的流行病学研究调查了45~60岁群体血浆25（OH）D浓度与认知的关系[54]。此研究应用多种神经心理学测试探讨认知表现与教育水平之间的关系，包括用语音和语义流畅性任务（如轨迹测试、数字正背和倒背任务）来评估言语记忆和短期/工作记忆。结果显示，在低文化程度人群中，25（OH）D水平与"短期/工作记忆"认知功能之间存在关联，特别表现在倒背数字任务里。同时，在受教育程度较高的被试者中，血浆维生素D水平只与语言流利性有关。因此，相较于受教育程度，血浆维生素D含量与个体认知功能的关系更密切。在年龄层面，即使年轻人的认知功能普遍比老年人更好，但血浆中维生素D含量充足的人比含量低的人在认知功能方面表现更好。

与前文研究相似[5,49]，Larsen[19]研究了维生素D摄入量与认知功能之间的关系。这项研究聚焦于1916名老年人（70~74岁）的饮食习惯与其认知功能之间的关系。在基线水平上，64%被试者摄入的维生素D低于每日所需量（即≥10 μg/d）。服用鱼肝油后，Larsen[19]发现被试者维生素D的摄入量增加了，约达到了每日所需量的76%。由以上研究结果可知，约38%的被试者食用鱼类（或鱼类相关产品）有助于维生素D的吸收。鱼类（或鱼类相关产品）不仅能提高被试者的维生素D水平，还能影响认知功能。也就是说，增加维生素D水平提高了被试者的言语流畅性（使用语义流畅性任务）和情景记忆（使用肯德里克目标学习测试）的评分。因此，我们认为食用鳕鱼等含脂肪量少的鱼类有助于提高维生素D水平，从而改善被试者的认知功能。

食用鱼类减缓认知能力下降的机制包括减轻炎症反应和氧化应激反应[55]，而正是这两者影响大脑正常运作，对其造成严重损害。鱼类可以提高认知能力，尤其是在言语、即时和延迟记忆方面[55]。此外，鱼类相关产品通常含有omega-3脂肪酸、二十碳五烯酸和二十二碳六烯酸，可减轻中枢神经系统的炎症反应和氧化应激反应[55]。因此，鱼类相关产品能维持和改善认知[56]。不管是鱼类相关产品还是鱼类本身都对认知有益。Nurk等[57]的研究也支持了这一观点，他们发现未经加工的高脂和低脂鱼类均可提高认知能力。

Prabhakar等[49]在140名60岁及以上的老年人群体样本中研究了维生素D的影响。作者假设，充足的维生素D可以预防血管性痴呆（VaD）的发生。结果显示，维生素D水平低（＜12 ng/ml）的个体患VaD的风险增加。该研究还发现，维生素D缺乏合并高血压患VaD的风险比以上单独任一因素患VaD的风险均高[49]。此外，最近一项研究发现，在不同亚型的痴呆患者中，包括AD、路易体痴呆、VaD和额颞叶痴呆，维生素D水平之间没有显著差异[58]。

许多研究揭示了维生素D与认知之间的关系[16,54]。在1652名年龄为45~65岁的不同肤色/种族被试者中，研究人员对25（OH）D浓度与认知之间的关联进行了数年研究[16]。研究选择不同肤色/种族作为研究对象是因为肤色深的人通常比肤色浅的人维生素D含量更低。测量被试者血清中25（OH）D的水平，以及钙、磷和甲状旁腺激素含量，并用延迟单词回忆测试（评估语言表达学习和近期记忆）、数字符号替换测试（测试执行功能和处理速度）和单词流畅度测试（测试执行功能和语言）来评估认知功能。结果显示，低水平25（OH）D与认知水平没关联。这一阴性结果可能与被试者的年龄有关，因为60岁及以上的人群中低水平25（OH）D更为常见。

Vieira等[11]评估了2型糖尿病、糖尿病前期和无糖尿病患者的维生素D水平与认知功能的关系。研究一共纳入37 973个被试者，平均年龄为（47±17）岁，目的是研究糖尿病如何影响躯体活动、记忆力以及维生素A、维生素E和维生素D水平。该研究还指出，40岁之前诊断为早期糖尿病的患者有记忆力问题，而且通常与维生素D水平低相关，但与维生素A和维生素E无关。这表明早期

第五章 维生素D缺乏与认知及神经的相关性：聚焦健康老龄化与阿尔茨海默病

糖尿病和低水平维生素 D 会导致认知问题，如思维混乱、记忆障碍以及身体活动耐受力下降（例如，不能长时间站立）[11]。根据 Vieira 等[11] 研究结果显示，与晚年发展为糖尿病且维生素 D 水平良好的人相比，中年早期发展为糖尿病且维生素 D 水平较低的人在晚年可能将面临更大的认知问题。认知问题结局可能与认知功能下降、痴呆和 AD 有关，因为糖尿病的病情进展和维生素 D 缺乏相关，进而导致认知问题[11]。维生素 D 缺乏也与痴呆和 AD 病情进展有关[59,60]，但维生素 D 缺乏与 AD 的病情进展的关系存在相悖的结论[61]。

Annweiler 等[3] 研究了 462 名 65 岁及以上老年人血清 25（OH）D 与情景记忆和容量规划的关系。参与这项研究的被试者根据三词表回忆测试和时钟绘图测试的整体认知评估被分为两组（认知受损组和正常组）。通过比较两组的表现得分，结果显示，整体认知的下降与较低浓度的 25（OH）D 有关，并不限于情景记忆、容量规划或空间安排功能的损害。

在一项基于人群的观察性研究中，Breitling 等[5] 对 1639 名年龄在 65 岁及以上的老年人进行了为期 5 年的认知功能评估（采用电话回访）。这项措施与 MMSE 非常相似，且其也可用于筛查 AD 等痴呆症。此外，如果需要额外的认知功能信息，被试者还需要完成标准化的问卷调查。Breitling 等[5] 发现，维生素 D 低水平与认知功能下降有关。然而，Walker[62] 对 2000—2010 年间发表的 5 篇文章进行了回顾，对老年人认知功能障碍与维生素 D 之间的关系得出了不同结论。与之相似，Luckhaus 等[63] 也没有发现维生素 D 和认知之间存在关系。在 47 名被试者（19 名轻度认知障碍患者，20 名 AD 患者，8 名认知正常者）的研究中，对他们的维生素 D 水平进行测量，并使用 MMSE 和临床痴呆评定量表等方法评估其认知能力。数据显示 3 组被试者的认知功能得分和维生素 D 水平在统计学上没有显著差异。

Bartali 等[4] 采用了一种更普遍的方法，调查了 1185 名年龄为 60~70 岁的女性的维生素 D 水平与认知功能之间的关系。这项纵向研究持续了 9 年，测量了被试者在 1989—1990 年的血浆 25（OH）D 水平，随后通过电话采访评估他们在 1999 年的认知功能，并在 1999 年至 21 世纪初完成其他认知评估（例如，电话版 MMSE，东波士顿记忆测试）。通过放射免疫分析法对维生素 D 进行评估。该研究发现，与血浆 25（OH）D 水平正常者相比，水平较低者的认知功能更差，而且在 9 年后的随访中也得到同样的结果。在研究的第 6 年有一项重要发现，被试者的维生素 D 水平与认知功能下降没有显著关联。然而，Assmann 等 [54] 认为，这一发现可能是由于人口的年龄差异造成的，年龄可能对结果有轻微的影响。因此，Bartali 等 [4] 这项长达 9 年的纵向随访研究中的结果可能有差异。

Feart 等 [7] 在 916 名 65 岁及以上的非痴呆人群中进行了一项与 Bartali 等 [4] 相似的研究，历时 12 年。研究采用 MMSE 和本顿视觉记忆测验（Benton Visual Retention test，BVRT）评估受试者的认知功能。另外，研究人员多年来通过收集被试者的血液样本并测量血浆中 25（OH）D 的浓度，来评估维生素 D 的水平。研究结果显示，在 12 年的随访研究中，缺乏维生素 D 者认知功能下降的速度更快，且患 AD 的风险也更高。另一角度来说，维生素 D 水平充足的人认知功能更好，这表明随着年龄和研究时间的推移，这类人群认知功能下降（如果有的话）的进展更慢，且患 AD 的可能性更低。因此，我们可以得出结论，特别对于老年人来说，适当摄入和维持维生素 D 在减缓认知衰退和痴呆的进展方面起着至关重要的作用 [7]，并能预防 AD 的发展。

Littlejohns 等 [60] 通过一项长达约 5.6 年的纵向研究，探讨了维生素 D 与老年人痴呆和 AD 之间的关系。采集血清 25（OH）D 测定维生素 D；采用多种方法筛查和评估痴呆和 AD 认知水平，包括磁共振成像、问卷调查和回顾既往认知表现等。Littlejohns 等 [60] 发现，患有痴呆症和 AD 的被试者缺乏或严重缺乏维生素 D。缺乏维生素 D 的被试者患痴呆症的可能性增加 51%，而严重缺乏维生素 D 者的可能性增加高达 121%。在 AD 发展的过程中也有类似的发现。作者认为，维生素 D 水平 < 50 nmol/L 是患痴呆和 AD 的一个危险因素。多项研究表明，维生素 D 缺乏与认知问题相关 [4,7]，并且 Littlejohns 等 [60] 也表明，维生素 D 缺乏可能导致认知损害，增加患痴呆症的风险（但 Nourhashemi 等 [64] 有不同的结论）。在另一项对 1700 多名非痴呆老年人的纵向研究（约 6 年）中，Zhao 等 [51] 发现，高水平维生素 D 与患痴呆症可能性降低有关。

第四节 结论

维生素 D 水平在公众健康尤其是在衰老和 AD 方面至关重要,这一点已经在上述研究中得到了解释。几项动物和人体研究报告显示,充足的维生素 D 水平对各种健康促成都很重要,尤其是在改善和保持认知功能与减少与痴呆和 AD 发展相关的风险因素上[6,7]。正如 San Martin 等[65]强调的,为健康老年人和有 MCI 的个体补充维生素 D 可能对 AD 的进展有保护性作用,这一观点值得重视。同时,维生素 D 不仅对晚年有影响,而且对出生前和生命的早期阶段的学习和记忆也有影响[18]。重要的是,维生素 D 缺乏确实见于老年甚至在 AD 出现之前的阶段[7]。根据广泛的文献检索和回顾,在 AD 发生之前使用维生素 D 是更为重要的,因为补充维生素 D 对认知功能的作用在 AD 发生后较弱(如果不是最小的话)。

第五节 展望

为了进一步探讨维生素 D 与健康和健康老龄化以及痴呆和 AD 认知之间的关系,回顾与维生素 D 缺乏相关的性别比例的探索很重要。回顾维生素 D 缺乏症、痴呆和阿尔茨海默病的性别比例,可以更好地了解哪种性别更容易缺乏维生素 D,使他们更容易患脑部疾病(痴呆与阿尔茨海默病)。

了解维生素 D 与年轻人认知功能的关系和影响也很重要,有助于明确后期导致认知疾病发展的因素,并促进认知的改善和维生素 D 水平的提高。这种探索势在必行,因为年轻人群(青少年与婴儿)的维生素 D 状况评估存在明显差距,会对认知产生不利的影响。重要的是,与动物研究一样,对老年人和阿尔茨海默病患者的研究,应着重调查维生素 D 与白藜芦醇[42]或黄体酮[13]对大脑和认知的综合影响。

伦理审批及知情同意： 本综述无需审查申请。

出版的同意： 所有作者均同意本研究的出版。

数据和材料的获取： 由于本文为综述，我们的研究不包括任何数据和材料。

利益冲突： 我们无任何利益冲突。

基金资助： 本研究无任何基金资助。

作者贡献： AS 撰写初稿。然后，AAM 和 WJ 对本综述的稿件进行了数次修改。本文所有的思路均由 AAM、WJ 和 AS 设计。

参考文献

1. Holick, M. F., & Chen, T. C. (2008). Vitamin D deficiency: A worldwide problem with health consequences. The American Journal of Clinical Nutrition, 87(4), 1080S-1086S.

2. Pettersen, J. A. (2016). Vitamin D and executive functioning: Are higher levels better? Journal of Clinical and Experimental Neuropsychology, 38(4), 467-477. Available from https://doi.org/10.1080/13803395.2015.1125452.

3. Annweiler, C., Fantino, B., Le Gall, D., & Beauchet, O. (2011). Which cognitive function is influenced by vitamin D among older high-functioning community-dwellers? Alzheimer's & Dementia, 7(4), S590-S591.

4. Bartali, B., Devore, E., Grodstein, F., & Kang, J. H. (2014). Plasma vitamin D levels and cognitive function in aging women: The Nurses' Health Study. The Journal of Nutrition, Health & Aging, 18(4), 400-406.

5. Breitling, L. P., Perna, L., Muller, H., Raum, E., Kliegel, M., & Brenner, H. (2012). Vitamin D and cognitive functioning in the elderly population in Germany. Experimental Gerontology, 47(1), 122-127. Available from https://doi.org/10.1016/j.exger.2011.11.004.

6. Przybelski, R. J., & Binkley, N. C. (2007). Is vitamin D important for preserving cognition? A positive correlation of serum 25-hydroxyvitamin D concentration with cognitive function. Archives of Biochemistry and Biophysics, 460(2), 202-205. Available from https://doi.org/10.1016/j.abb.2006.12.018.

7. Feart, C., Helmer, C., Merle, B., Herrmann, F. R., Annweiler, C., Dartigues, J. F., & Samieri, C. (2017). Associations of lower vitamin D concentrations with cognitive decline and long-term risk of dementia and Alzheimer's disease in older adults. Alzheimer's & Dementia, 13(11), 1207-1216. Available from https://doi.org/10.1016/

j.jalz.2017.03.003.

8. Brouwer-Brolsma, E. M., de Groot, L. C. P. G. M., & van de Rest, O. (2015). Chapter 63-Vitamin D and the association with cognitive performance, cognitive decline, and dementia. In Diet and Nutrition in Dementia and Cognitive Decline, pp. 679-700.

9. Brouwer-Brolsma, E. M., Schuurman, T., de Groot, L. C., Feskens, E. J., Lute, C., Naninck, E. F., & Steegenga, W. T. (2014). No role for vitamin D or a moderate fat diet in aging induced cognitive decline and emotional reactivity in C57BL/6 mice. Behavioural Brain Research, 267, 133-143. Available from https://doi.org/10.1016/j.bbr.2014.03.038.

10. Van der Schaft, J., Koek, H. L., Dijkstra, E., Verhaar, H. J., Van der Schouw, Y. T., & Emmelot-Vonk, M. H. (2013). The association between vitamin D and cognition: A systematic review. Ageing Research Reviews, 12(4), 1013-1023. Available from https://doi.org/10.1016/j.arr.2013.05.004.

11. Vieira, E. R., Mendy, A., Prado, C. M., Gasana, J., & Albatineh, A. N. (2015). Falls, physical limitations, confusion and memory problems in people with type II diabetes, undiagnosed diabetes and prediabetes, and the influence of vitamins A, D and E. Journal of Diabetes and Its Complications, 29(8), 1159-1164. Available from https://doi.org/10.1016/j.jdiacomp.2015.08.005.

12. Lee, D. H., Chon, J., Kim, Y., Seo, Y. K., Park, E. J., Won, C. W., & Soh, Y. (2020). Association between vitamin D deficiency and cognitive function in the elderly Korean population: A Korean frailty and aging cohort study. Medicine (Baltimore), 99 (8), e19293. Available from https://doi.org/10.1097/MD.0000000000019293.

13. Hua, F., Reiss, J. I., Tang, H., Wang, J., Fowler, X., Sayeed, I., & Stein, D. G. (2012). Progesterone and low-dose vitamin D hormone treatment enhances sparing of memory following traumatic brain injury. Hormones and Behavior, 61(4), 642-651. Available from https://doi.org/10.1016/j.yhbeh.2012.02.017.

14. McCann, J. C., & Ames, B. N. (2008). Is there convincing biological or behavioral evidence linking vitamin D deficiency to brain dysfunction? The FASEB Journal, 22(4),982-1001.

15. Minasyan, A., Keisala, T., Lou, Y. R., Kalueff, A. V., & Tuohimaa, P. (2007). Neophobia, sensory and cognitive functions, and hedonic responses in vitamin D receptor mutant mice. The Journal of Steroid Biochemistry and Molecular Biology, 104(3-5), 274-280. Available from https://doi.org/10.1016/j.jsbmb.2007.03.032.

16. Schneider, A. L., Lutsey, P. L., Alonso, A., Gottesman, R. F., Sharrett, A. R., Carson, K. A., & Michos, E. D. (2014). Vitamin D and cognitive function and dementia risk in a biracial cohort: The ARIC Brain MRI Study. European Journal of Neurology, 21(9),

1211-1218. Available from https://doi.org/10.1111/ene.12460, e1269-1270.
17. Turner, K. M., Young, J. W., McGrath, J. J., Eyles, D. W., & Burne, T. H. (2013). Cognitive performance and response inhibition in developmentally vitamin D (DVD)-deficient rats. Behavioural Brain Research, 242, 47-53. Available from https://doi.org/10.1016/j.bbr.2012.12.029.
18. Becker, A., Eyles, D. W., McGrath, J. J., & Grecksch, G. (2005). Transient prenatal vitamin D deficiency is associated with subtle alterations in learning and memory functions in adult rats. Behavioural Brain Research, 161(2), 306-312. Available from https://doi.org/10.1016/j.bbr.2005.02.015.
19. Larsen, L. (2010). Intake of vitamin D in relation to cognition in the elderly. Master's thesis, University of Oslo.
20. Pettersen, J. A. (2017). Does high dose vitamin D supplementation enhance cognition?: A randomized trial in healthy adults. Experimental Gerontology, 90, 90-97. Available from https://doi.org/10.1016/j.exger.2017.01.019.
21. Sultan, S., Taimuri, U., Basnan, S. A., Ai-Orabi, W. K., Awadallah, A., Almowald, F., & Hazazi, A. (2020). Low vitamin D and its association with cognitive impairment and dementia. Journal of Aging Research, 2020, 6097820. Available from https://doi.org/10.1155/2020/6097820.
22. Croll, P. H., Boelens, M., Vernooij, M. W., van de Rest, O., Zillikens, M. C., Ikram, M. A., & Voortman, T. (2020). Associations of vitamin D deficiency with MRI markers of brain health in a community sample. Clinical Nutrition (Edinburgh, Scotland), 40 (1), 72-78. Available from https://doi.org/10.1016/j.clnu.2020.04.027.
23. Apostolova, L. G., Dutton, R. A., Dinov, I. D., Hayashi, K. M., Toga, A. W., Cummings, J. L., & Thompson, P. M. (2006). Conversion of mild cognitive impairment to Alzheimer disease predicted by hippocampal atrophy maps. Archives of Neurology, 63(5), 693-699.
24. Dhikav, V., & Anand, K. (2011). Potential predictors of hippocampal atrophy in Alzheimer's disease. Drugs & Aging, 28(1), 1-11. Available from https://doi.org/10.2165/11586390-000000000-00000, 1 [pii].
25. Hyman, B. T., Van Hoesen, G. W., Damasio, A. R., & Barnes, C. L. (1984). Alzheimer'sdisease: Cell-specific pathology isolates the hippocampal formation. Science (New York, N.Y.), 225(4667), 1168-1170.
26. Jaroudi, W., Garami, J., Garrido, S., Hornberger, M., Keri, S., & Moustafa, A. A. (2017). Factors underlying cognitive decline in old age and Alzheimer's disease: The role of the hippocampus. Reviews in the Neurosciences, 28(7), 705-714. Available from https://doi.org/10.1515/revneuro-2016-0086.

27. Lardner, A. L. (2015). Vitamin D and hippocampal development-the story so far. Frontiers in Molecular Neuroscience, 8, 58. Available from https://doi.org/10.3389/fnmol.2015.00058.

28. Annweiler, C., Montero-Odasso, M., Llewellyn, D. J., Richard-Devantoy, S., Duque, G., & Beauchet, O. (2013). Meta-analysis of memory and executive dysfunctions in relation to vitamin D. Journal of Alzheimer's Disease, 37(1), 147-171.

29. Kandiah, N., Jion, Y., & Ng, A. (2011). Severity of cognitive impairment is correlated to levels of vitamin D. Alzheimer's & Dementia, 7(4), S612-S613.

30. Llewellyn, D. J., Lang, I. A., Langa, K. M., & Melzer, D. (2010). Vitamin D and cognitive impairment in NHANES III. Alzheimer's & Dementia, 6(4), S81.

31. Wong, D., Bellyou, M., Beauchet, O., Montero-Odasso, M., Annweiler, C., & Bartha, R. (2017). Combined memantine and vitamin d treatment provides the same cognitive benefit as memantine alone in a chronically vitamin D deficient double-transgenic mouse model of Alzheimer's disease. Alzheimer's & Dementia, 13(7), P269-P270.

32. Aguilar-Navarro, S. G., Mimenza-Alvarado, A. J., Jimenez-Castillo, G. A., BrachoVela, L. A., Yeverino-Castro, S. G., & Avila-Funes, J. A. (2019). Association of vitamin D with mild cognitive impairment and Alzheimer's dementia in older Mexican adults. Revista de Investigacion Clinica; Organo del Hospital de Enfermedades de la Nutricion, 71(6), 381-386. Available from https://doi.org/10.24875/RIC.19003079.

33. Jeon, Y. J., Jung, S. J., & Kim, H. C. (2020). Does serum vitamin D level affect the association between cardiovascular health and cognition? Results of the Cardiovascular and Metabolic Diseases Etiology Research Center (CMERC) study. European Journal of Neurology: The Official Journal of the European Federation of Neurological Societies, 28(1), 48-55. Available from https://doi.org/10.1111/ene.14496.

34. Zugic Soares, J., Pettersen, R., Saltyte Benth, J., Knapskog, A. B., Selbaek, G., & Bogdanovic, N. (2019). Higher vitamin D levels are associated with better attentional functions: Data from the NorCog Register. The Journal of Nutrition, Health & Aging, 23(8), 725-731. Available from https://doi.org/10.1007/s12603-019-1220-z.

35. Annweiler, C., Rolland, Y., Schott, A. M., Blain, H., Vellas, B., Herrmann, F. R., et al. (2012). Higher vitamin D dietary intake is associated with lower risk of Alzheimer's disease: a 7-year follow-up. The Journals of Gerontology. Series A, Biological Sciences and Medical Sciences, 67, 1205-1211. https://doi.org/10.1093/gerona/gls107.

36. Waterhouse, M., Tran, B., Armstrong, B. K., Baxter, C., Ebeling, P. R., English, D. R., & Neale, R. E. (2014). Environmental, personal, and genetic determinants of response to vitamin D supplementation in older adults. The Journal of Clinical Endocrinology and Metabolism, 99(7), E1332 E1340. Available from https://doi.org/10.1210/jc.2013-4101.

37. Wang, L., Qiao, Y., Zhang, H., Zhang, Y., Hua, J., Jin, S., & Liu, G. (2020). Circulating vitamin D levels and Alzheimer's disease: A Mendelian randomization study in the IGAP and UK biobank. Journal of Alzheimer's Disease: JAD, 73(2), 609-618. Available from https://doi.org/10.3233/JAD-190713.

38. Erbas, O., Solmaz, V., Aksoy, D., Yavasoglu, A., Sagcan, M., & Taskiran, D. (2014). Cholecalciferol (vitamin D 3) improves cognitive dysfunction and reduces inflammation in a rat fatty liver model of metabolic syndrome. Life Sciences, 103(2), 68-72. Available from https://doi.org/10.1016/j.lfs.2014.03.035.

39. Grecksch, G., Bernstein, H. G., Becker, A., Hollt, V., & Bogerts, B. (1999). Disruption of latent inhibition in rats with postnatal hippocampal lesions. Neuropsychopharmacology: Official Publication of the American College of Neuropsychopharmacology, 20(6), 525-532.

40. Moustafa, A. A., Myers, C. E., & Gluck, M. A. (2009). A neurocomputational model of classical conditioning phenomena: A putative role for the hippocampal region in associative learning. Brain Research, 1276, 180-195.

41. Schmajuk., Larrauri., & Labar. (2007). Reinstatement of conditioned fear and the hippocampus: An attentional-associative model. Behavioural Brain Research, 177(2), 242-253.

42. Cheng, J., Rui, Y., Qin, L., Xu, J., Han, S., Yuan, L., & Wan, Z. (2017). Vitamin D combined with resveratrol prevents cognitive decline in SAMP8 mice. Current Alzheimer Research, 14(8), 820-833. Available from https://doi.org/10.2174/1567205014666170207093455.

43. Mehri, N., Haddadi, R., Ganji, M., Shahidi, S., Soleimani Asl, S., Taheri Azandariani, M., & Ranjbar, A. (2020). Effects of vitamin D in an animal model of Alzheimer's disease: Behavioral assessment with biochemical investigation of hippocampus and serum. Metabolic Brain Disease, 35(2), 263-274. Available from https://doi.org/10.1007/s11011-019-00529-7.

44. Jia, J., Hu, J., Huo, X., Miao, R., Zhang, Y., & Ma, F. (2019). Effects of vitamin D supplementation on cognitive function and blood Abeta-related biomarkers in older adults with Alzheimer's disease: A randomised, double-blind, placebo-controlled trial. Journal of Neurology, Neurosurgery, and Psychiatry, 90(12), 1347-1352. Available from https://doi.org/10.1136/jnnp-2018-320199.

45. Yamini, P., Ray, R. S., & Chopra, K. (2018). Vitamin D3 attenuates cognitive deficits and neuroinflammatory responses in ICV-STZ induced sporadic Alzheimer's disease. Inflammopharmacology, 26(1), 39-55. Available from https://doi.org/10.1007/s10787-017-0372-x.

46. Ertilav, E., Barcin, N. E., & Ozdem, S. (2020). Comparison of serum free and bioavailable 25-hydroxyvitamin D levels in Alzheimer's disease and healthy control patients. Laboratory Medicine. https://doi.org/10.1093/labmed/lmaa066.

47. Eymundsdottir, H., Chang, M., Geirsdottir, O. G., Gudmundsson, L. S., Jonsson, P. V., Gudnason, V., & Ramel, A. (2020). Lifestyle and 25-hydroxy-vitamin D among community-dwelling old adults with dementia, mild cognitive impairment, or normal cognitive function. Aging Clinical and Experimental Research, 32(12), 2649-2656. Available from https://doi.org/10.1007/s40520-020-01531-1.

48. Kalra, A., Teixeira, A. L., & Diniz, B. S. (2020). Association of vitamin D levels with incident all-cause dementia in longitudinal observational studies: A systematic review and meta-analysis. The Journal of Prevention of Alzheimer's Disease, 7(1), 14-20. Available from https://doi.org/10.14283/jpad.2019.44.

49. Prabhakar, P., Chandra, S. R., Supriya, M., Issac, T. G., Prasad, C., & Christopher, R. (2015). Vitamin D status and vascular dementia due to cerebral small vessel disease in the elderly Asian Indian population. Journal of the Neurological Sciences, 359(1-2), 108-111. Available from https://doi.org/10.1016/j.jns.2015.10.050.

50. SanMartín, C., Ponce, D., Salech, F., & Behrens, M. (2015). Correction of vitamin D status improves lymphocyte susceptibility to oxidative cell death in mild cognitive impairment patients. Journal of the Neurological Sciences, 357, e137-e138.

51. Zhao, C., Tsapanou, A., Manly, J., Schupf, N., Brickman, A. M., & Gu, Y. (2020). Vitamin D intake is associated with dementia risk in the Washington Heights-Inwood Columbia Aging Project (WHICAP). Alzheimer's & Dementia. Available from https://doi.org/10.1002/alz.12096.

52. Duchaine, C. S., Talbot, D., Nafti, M., Giguere, Y., Dodin, S., Tourigny, A., & Laurin, D.(2020). Vitamin D status, cognitive decline and incident dementia: The Canadian study of health and aging. Canadian Journal of Public Health. Revue Canadienne de Sante Publique, 111(3), 312-321. Available from https://doi.org/10.17269/s41997-019-00290-5.

53. Shih, E. J., Lee, W. J., Hsu, J. L., Wang, S. J., & Fuh, J. L. (2020). Effect of vitamin D on cognitive function and white matter hyper intensity in patients with mild Alzheimer''s disease. Geriatrics & Gerontology International, 20(1), 52-58. Available from https://doi.org/10.1111/ggi.13821.

54. Assmann, K. E., Touvier, M., Andreeva, V. A., Deschasaux, M., Constans, T., Hercberg, S., & Kesse-Guyot, E. (2015). Midlife plasma vitamin D concentrations and performance in different cognitive domains assessed 13 years later. The British Journal of Nutrition, 113(10), 1628-1637. Available from https://doi.org/10.1017/

S0007114515001051.
55. Qin, B., Plassman, B. L., Edwards, L. J., Popkin, B. M., Adair, L. S., & Mendez, M. A. (2014). Fish intake is associated with slower cognitive decline in Chinese older adults. The Journal of Nutrition, 144(10), 1579-1585. Available from https://doi.org/10.3945/jn.114.193854.
56. O'Connor, E. M., Power, S. E., Fitzgerald, G. F., & O'Toole, P. W. (2012). Fish-oil consumption is inversely correlated with depression and cognition decline in healthy irish elderly adults. Proceedings of the Nutrition Society, 71(1).
57. Nurk, E., Drevon, C. A., Refsum, H., Solvoll, K., Vollset, S. E., Nygard, O., & Smith, A.D. (2007). Cognitive performance among the elderly and dietary fish intake: The Hordaland Health Study. The American Journal of Clinical Nutrition, 86(5), 1470-1478. Available from https://doi.org/10.1093/ajcn/86.5.1470.
58. Soysal, P., Dokuzlar, O., Erken, N., Dost Gunay, F. S., & Isik, A. T. (2020). The relationship between dementia subtypes and nutritional parameters in older adults. Journal of the American Medical Directors Association, 21(10), 1430-1435. Available from https://doi.org/10.1016/j.jamda.2020.06.051.
59. Chai, B., Gao, F., Wu, R., Dong, T., Gu, C., Lin, Q., & Zhang, Y. (2019). Vitamin D deficiency as a risk factor for dementia and Alzheimer's disease: An updated metaanalysis. BMC Neurology, 19(1), 284. Available from https://doi.org/10.1186/s12883- 019-1500-6.
60. Littlejohns, T. J., Henley, W. E., Lang, I. A., Annweiler, C., Beauchet, O., Chaves, P. H., & Llewellyn, D. J. (2014). Vitamin D and the risk of dementia and Alzheimer disease. Neurology, 83(10), 920-928. Available from https://doi.org/10.1212/WNL.0000000000000755.
61. Yang, K., Chen, J., Li, X., & Zhou, Y. (2019). Vitamin D concentration and risk ofAlzheimer disease: A meta-analysis of prospective cohort studies. Medicine (Baltimore), 98(35), e16804. Available from https://doi.org/10.1097/MD.0000000000016804.
62. Walker, E. (2010). The relationship between vitamin D deficiency and cognitive decline in the geriatric population. Paper 194, MSc thesis, Pacific University.
63. Luckhaus, C., Mahabadi, B., Grass-Kapanke, B. et al. (2009). Blood biomarkers of osteoporosis in mild cognitive impairment and Alzheimer's disease. Journal of Neural Transmission, 116(7), 905-911.
64. Nourhashemi, F., Hooper, C., Cantet, C., Feart, C., Gennero, I., Payoux, P., ... Multidomain Alzheimer Preventive Trial/Data Sharing Alzheimer (DSA) study group. (2018). Cross-sectional associations of plasma vitamin D with cerebral beta-amyloid in

older adults at risk of dementia. Alzheimer's Research & Therapy, 10(1), 43. Available from https://doi.org/10.1186/s13195-018-0371-1.
65. SanMartin, C. D., Henriquez, M., Chacon, C., Ponce, D. P., Salech, F., Rogers, N. K., & Behrens, M. I. (2018). Vitamin D increases Abeta140 plasma levels and protects lymphocytes from oxidative death in mild cognitive impairment patients. Current Alzheimer Research, 15(6), 561-569. Available from https://doi.org/10.2174/1567205015666171227154636.

第六章 阿尔茨海默病对丘脑的影响

Rasu Karki，Ahmed A. Moustafa 编
刘勇林，卢志豪 译
肖卫民 校

第一节 引言

丘脑是位于前脑内的大灰质核团，主要由两部分组成，即背侧丘脑和腹侧丘脑[1]。背侧丘脑包括一组核团，这些核团将初级感觉信息传递到大脑皮质[1]。在发育的早期阶段，丘脑被划分为两个祖区，即尾侧区域和头侧区域。尾侧区域负责不同丘脑核中谷氨酸能神经元的发育[2]。头侧区域负责丘脑网状核的形成。

丘脑的主要核群分为中继核群、联合核群、中线/板内核群及网状核[2-4]，它们充当传入感觉信息的特异中继站[5-7]。中继核群在中枢神经系统中充当运动和感觉信息的中继站，包括外侧膝状体和内侧膝状体[2]。外侧膝状体接收来自视网膜神经节的感觉输入，并其将投射到初级视觉皮层，而内侧膝状体则接收来自内耳的输入并将信号通过神经轴索投射到初级听觉复合体[5]。

联合核群主要与边缘系统建立联系，负责调节感觉信息。此外，联合核群在高级认知功能中也很重要[2]。板内核群由背侧组和腹侧组构成。背侧组包括带旁核和丘脑室旁核，而丘脑腹侧的中线核群包括联结核和菱形核[2,8]。这些核团构成皮质-丘脑-皮质通路，并参与到记忆和注意力的加工处理过程[9]。最后，网状核在丘脑核群周围形成一层外壳，并负责调节丘脑和皮质之间的信息处理[2,10]。

丘脑的边缘核或称边缘丘脑，包括内侧背核、外侧背核、前核及中线核群[11,12]。这些核群与几个皮质和皮质下区域有密切联系，同时它们对于昼夜节律的调节和睡眠调节也很重要[11]。丘脑对于注意力集中至关重要，并有助于信息处理、记忆、情绪、动机和联结认知过程[5,13-16]。丘脑还参与意识和睡眠的调节[17]。此外，丘

脑的前核、内侧背核、板内核和中线核对记忆功能十分重要[13,18]。

阿尔茨海默病（AD）是一种神经系统退行性疾病，伴有记忆力下降及语言、执行功能损害。它是最常见的一种痴呆，全世界有超过5000万人受其影响[19,20]。AD以大脑皮质和海马内锥体神经元的持续丢失为特征[21]，其病因是大脑中细胞内神经质纤维缠结的形成和细胞外β-淀粉蛋白（Aβ）斑块的堆积[13,22,23]。上述病理改变会导致神经退行性变，从而导致神经元的丢失、神经元功能受损以及突触和神经元的损失[22,24]。此外，结构成像研究表明，神经元纤维缠结和淀粉样斑块的形成会导致海马、杏仁核、内侧颞叶、楔前叶和全脑灰质萎缩[13]。

多个有关AD患者淀粉样蛋白的影像研究显示，淀粉样蛋白沉积发生在丘脑[25]。其中几项研究还发现，在AD中胆碱能系统也受到影响[26,27]。重要的是，一些研究表明胆碱能系统在丘脑的活动中起着关键的作用[28-30]。然而，一些研究表明，向丘脑投射的胆碱能系统与AD无关[31,32]。

第二节　阿尔茨海默病对丘脑的影响

在本节中，我们讨论AD如何影响丘脑，包括体积减小和几个丘脑区域的神经损伤。

一、体积减小

AD由丘脑边缘核中神经原纤维缠结和淀粉样斑块增加以及突触丧失引起[13,33]。根据Zarei等[33]研究，丘脑前背侧、中央内侧及枕部核群是丘脑退化的主要部位。丘脑体积的减小是认知功能下降的早期迹象，同时伴随着灰质和白质的体积减小[34]。

AD患者存在明显的丘脑体积减小[13]。研究发现，在校正年龄、性别、脑室体积和新皮质灰质体积后，丘脑体积的减小与老年患者认知功能损害有关[13]。Zidan等[34]研究显示，丘脑体积减小是AD患者淀粉样蛋白积聚和轴突变性的结果。研究发现，AD患者丘脑的前部和背部体积明显较健康人小。然而，丘脑体积减小不仅仅归因于前部核团的减小，这提示丘脑其他部分也发生了萎缩[13]。这些神经元纤维缠结和淀粉样斑块见于丘脑所有边缘核团，其中以背内侧核团的缠结最严重。

此外，Xuereb 等[35]发现，除后外侧核群和中央外侧核群外，所有丘脑核群在 AD 中均出现某种程度的体积减小，尽管这些减小在个体上并不具有统计学显著性。他们发现只有网状核和背核表现明显的体积减小。此外，Low 等[36]发现，AD 患者左后腹外侧丘脑和腹内侧丘脑比其他脑区显示出更严重的萎缩。左腹外侧丘脑在言语流畅度方面发挥作用，该脑区的损伤可能解释 AD 患者所面临的问题，如言语受损、言语输出减少以及其他言语问题[36]。网状核体积的减小可能反映了整个丘脑的萎缩，因为网状核由形成围绕丘脑核团核心的外层的神经细胞构成，如果丘脑核团核心出现一些萎缩，那么周围的网状核将向内收缩，这样就反映了丘脑的萎缩。

二、神经细胞丢失

丘脑前部核团分为前腹侧、前内侧和前背侧核。前背侧核是前部核团中神经元纤维变性和神经元丢失主要部位，神经元丢失率达 80%[33,35,37]。Xuereb 等[35]研究认为，前部核团的前腹侧和前内侧核以及背外侧核并不出现神经元丢失。此外，中央中核和丘脑枕核也出现神经元丢失[33]。前背侧核严重神经细胞丢失的解剖学/化学基础以及由细胞丢失造成的行为方面的后果已得到了完全证实。此外，Xuereb 等[35]的研究表明，中央内侧核也会发生神经元丢失，但与前背侧核不同，这与显著的神经原纤维缠结形成无关。与 Xuereb 等[35]的研究结果相反，Aggleton 等[37]认为 AD 患者的丘脑前外侧核也会出现神经元丢失。此外，根据 Xuereb 等[35]研究，丘脑中央中核是神经退行性变的主要部位。残存的神经细胞退化成不规则的、暗的、萎缩的结构，这些结构位于中央中核的神经细胞内。这与星形胶质细胞数量增加有关，表明凋亡前存在神经损伤。然而，Xuereb 等[35]发现，这种神经变性在老年对照组和 AD 组中同样严重，提示其不能仅归因于 AD。中央中核缺乏神经纤维缠结的研究发现证实了这一点。然而，研究发现，背内侧核和腹后内侧核周围的神经细胞不受 AD 影响[35]。

此外还发现，丘脑的形态也随 AD 的进展而变化。由于前背侧核围绕前腹侧核弯曲，且它只占丘脑体积的很小一部分，因此提示内侧髓质层也发生了变性[33]。

所观察到的丘脑体积的变化不能仅用神经细胞丢失来解释，因为前侧核群仅占整个丘脑体积的一小部分[33]。Iglesias 等[17]提出假说，丘脑体积变化可能为细胞神经突起的丢失或神经胶质细胞数量改变所导致。

第三节　丘脑与脑部其他部分之间的联系

在这一节中，我们将讨论与丘脑连接的区域受损与 AD 发病机制之间的关系，这些区域包括海马、Papez 环路、扣带回后部皮质、丘脑皮质网络及前额叶-纹状体环路。

一、海马

情景记忆的缺失是 AD 发病早期的表现之一，海马被认为是调节情景记忆的重要部位[37]。

海马通过穹窿直接与前丘脑相连，通过颞穹窿束与丘脑枕相连。海马还通过乳头体间接与前丘脑相连。海马-前丘脑通路对情景记忆至关重要[33]。海马输入的信息通过穹窿达到丘脑。然而，在 AD 患者中，穹窿出现神经元丢失及神经纤维缠结形成，乃至萎缩，从而导致其与海马信息连接的中断，引起情景记忆障碍[37]。海马信息输入来源于海马下托。在 AD 患者中，海马下托会出现神经元丢失和神经纤维变性。这会导致左侧海马与前丘脑核团之间的联系中断，从而引起情景记忆损害[38,39]。沿着这些思路，Jenkins 等[40]发现，海马病变降低了前丘脑核群的基因活性。

二、Papez 环路

Papez 与边缘丘脑相连，该网络对记忆和情绪过程具有重要意义。边缘丘脑包括前丘脑核群、背外侧核和背内侧核[37,41]。边缘丘脑是空间定向和情景记忆的中枢。AD 患者由于边缘丘脑和 Papez 环路的损伤，会出现情景记忆和空间定向损害。Aggleton 等[37]发现，情景记忆的缺失反映神经退行性病变程度较重，其中包括 Papez 环路和边缘丘脑。前丘脑核群在这一系统中具有至关重要的作用。

AD 患者脑部萎缩的主要部位之一是扣带回后部区域[42,43]。Nestor 等[44]发现在 AD 中情景记忆损害与间脑和后扣带回网络功能障碍有关。根据 Aggleton 和 Brown[38]研究，Papez 环路包括海马、穹窿、乳头体、前丘脑核和后扣带回，它对情景记忆具有重要意义。AD 患者的穹窿发生萎缩，丘脑与海马的功能连接减弱，从而导致情景记忆损害。Hornberger 等[42]指出，在 AD 患者中，除前扣带回外，Papez 环路所有区域均出现变性。

此外，Papez 环路中的前丘脑还会通过穹窿向海马发出纤维。这3个区域（海马、前丘脑和穹窿）在 AD 中都会发生萎缩。由于海马和后扣带回都与前丘脑核相连，是 Papez 环路的一部分，且均因 AD 而发生萎缩，因此这可以看作是 Papez 环路的受损。

三、压后皮质

压后皮质（retrosplenial cortex）包括后扣带回区域，在 AD 早期，该区域容易出现萎缩和体积变化[37]。当一个人执行需要自我产生思维的任务时，如对未来的思考、情景记忆和空间导航，后扣带回区域就会变得活跃[41]。丘脑的前核及背内侧核与后扣带回区域有很紧密的连接。在 AD 中，左侧丘脑前部的病变会损害默认模式网络的后扣带回[41]。

丘脑前核和压后皮质对情景记忆至关重要，并由密集的连接相连[38]。它们在空间学习、情景记忆和注意力方面也相互依赖[37]。Robertson 和 Kaitz[45]发现，丘脑前背核与枕后边缘区有联系，前腹侧核与扣带回有联系[33]。丘脑前部的病变会导致压后皮质的慢性功能障碍[46]。这种功能障碍导致了基因转录的中断，从而降低了海马中的即时早期基因表达。它还会导致代谢活性降低和某些形式的神经元可塑性丧失[37]。

AD 患者很难改变空间方向，这与压后皮质/后扣带回萎缩有关[37]。这印证了空间定向改变的决定需要海马、后扣带皮质、丘脑前部协同工作，而这一相互作用的核心是压后皮质。

四、丘脑 - 皮质网络

丘脑 - 皮质网络由丘脑核群与大脑皮质相互连接组成[47]。这种连接由丘脑网状核调节[10]。网状神经元是围绕丘脑前部和外侧部的一层抑制性神经元，对丘脑神经元的振荡非常重要[10]。这些神经元抑制功能的破坏会影响它们的振荡[47]。丘脑皮质振荡在调节认知过程和身体活动中起着关键作用。Abuhassan 等[47]发现，AD 患者中这些神经元的振荡活动异常。他们还认为 AD 的认知障碍是由于丘脑 - 皮质网络连接受损引起的，该网络主要连接丘脑内侧及皮质区域、颞叶、额叶和枕叶[47]。

感官信息在传递到皮质之前必须通过丘脑，因此丘脑 - 皮质网络对注意力过程以及睡眠和清醒状态之间的转换也很重要[10]。在 AD 患者中，当网状核体积减小时，它们的活动性严重下降，这损害了丘脑和皮质之间的通信。网状核也有大量代谢异常的神经突触，代表损伤的末端轴突。因此，AD 引起的丘脑 - 皮质网络的破坏会导致注意为缺陷。另外，丘脑 - 皮质网络的失调还会产生尖波放电，导致 AD 患者有明显的非惊厥性癫痫发作[10]。此外，Abuhassan 等[47]发现，部分丘脑 - 皮质失神经后，丘脑活动性严重下降。这让人猜测丘脑体积的减小可能是丘脑 - 皮质失神经支配的结果。除此以外，部分丘脑 - 皮质失神经支配也导致丘脑振荡活动的减少。

第四节　前额叶 - 纹状体环和内侧前额皮质

前额叶 - 纹状体网络是一个前馈环路，从前额叶皮质到纹状体（基底节区的输入结构），然后投射到丘脑，再返回到前额叶区域[48]。这个网络对于目标导向的行为和执行功能至关重要。这个网络的受损会引起认知和情绪处理障碍，导致淡漠和同理心的下降[49,50]。Bertoux等[51]发现，AD患者前额叶背外侧后部有明显的退行性改变，但前额叶-纹状体萎缩相对较小。AD引起的丘脑退行性变影响了前额叶-纹状体网络的连接，这可能导致AD患者的认知障碍和淡漠。此外，纹状体在认知和行为中具有关键作用，在促进自愿运动中也很重要[51]。纹状体包括双侧尾状核和壳核。AD患者纹状体出现萎缩[51,52]。Jeong等[48]的研究发现，与无淡漠的AD患者相比，淡漠的AD患者眶额皮质、丘脑、壳核、伏隔核和岛叶的脑灌注降低。研究还发现，区域脑血流量的减少与严重的淡漠有直接关系。

眶额皮质与边缘/旁边缘结构有紧密的联系，可以接收来自大脑区域的信号，包括初级感觉器官、下丘脑和边缘系统[53,54]。眶额皮质是前额叶-纹状体网络的组成部分[48]，它涉及日常决策，并在奖励过程中起重要作用[55-59]。此外，它还结合感官、情感和动机信息来评价行动和奖励[60]。眶额皮质受损导致日常决策能力受损，并抑制反应[50]，这些都是淡漠的特征。有研究显示，眶额皮质的低灌注、低代谢和萎缩与AD患者的淡漠有关[50]。

内侧前额叶皮质（Medial Prefrontal Cortex，mPFC）整合了来自不同皮质和皮质下区域的信息。它对认知过程、情绪调节、动机和工作记忆等不同功能至关重要[23]。mPFC沿背侧和腹侧轴分为四个亚区：内侧中央前区、前扣带皮质、前边缘皮质和下边缘皮质[61]。mPFC主要由锥体神经元组成。PL和IL中的锥体神经元接收来自丘脑中线、杏仁核基底外侧、海马腹侧和对侧mPFC等区域的输入[23]。丘脑投射到背侧和腹侧PFC的第一层。

已有研究表明，AD的症状与mPFC的病理/功能改变有关。默认模式网络与mPFC、后扣带皮质、丘脑前核和背内侧核有结构上的连接[23,41]。早期AD患者默认模式网络与丘脑核和mPFC的功能连通性及其活性均下降[23]。AD导致mPFC细胞外Aβ斑块积聚。斑块的存在导致大鼠不良的行为表现，并导致工作记忆缺陷[23]。AD导致的背内侧丘脑和mPFC之间的联系减少，也会导致工作记忆的损害。此外，AD 患者的工作、记忆和认知缺陷也是由 mPFC 锥体神经元和海马树突棘密度的降低造成的。记忆巩固后树突棘密度增加，但随着树突棘密度的下降导致工作记忆的下降[23]。

第五节 讨论

AD 是一种常见的神经退行性病变，导致大脑中形成神经纤维缠结和淀粉样斑块[13]。丘脑是 AD 中最早受淀粉样蛋白沉积影响的脑区之一[25]。综述分析结果显示，AD 不仅影响丘脑本身（例如，体积减小和细胞丢失），也影响丘脑与其他大脑区域的连接，包括海马、Papez 环路、压后皮质和其他皮质区域。在 AD 中，丘脑的核群受到影响严重，其发生体积减小和退化。Zidan 等[34]认为，AD 患者的丘脑体积减小可归因于淀粉样蛋白沉积和轴突变性。Xuereb 等[35]认为，AD 患者丘脑除后外侧核群和中央外侧核群外，其余核体积均减少，其中网状核、背核和丘脑腹侧核体积显著减小[36]。研究还发现，前核组的前背核以及中央内侧核和枕核的神经细胞损失最为严重。中央内侧核缺乏明显的神经纤维缠结形成，而这在前核组中很明显[33,35,37]。

然而，神经细胞丢失的潜在影响因素及其后果仍是未知的，需要进行大量的研究以更好地了解[33,35]。存在于丘脑中央内侧核群的神经细胞退化变暗和结构萎缩与星形胶质细胞数量增加有关，这表明死者生前存在神经损伤。然而，这一发现并不能仅仅归咎于 AD 的进展，因为健康的老年人在同一丘脑区域也有同样严重的神经细胞丢失[35]。Aggleton 等[37]研究认为，丘脑前腹侧核群也有神经细胞丢失，这与 Xuereb 等[35]的丘脑前腹侧核群和前内侧核群没有神经细胞丢失结论相反。Zarei 等[33]也发现，在 AD 早期丘脑髓板内核群有变性发生。而丘脑髓板内核群参与记忆过程和注意力，形成皮质 - 丘脑 - 皮质通路[9]。此外，丘脑与大脑的其他区域（如海马、压后皮质）相连接，而该连接在 AD 中受到影响。海马通过穹窿与丘脑前部直接相连，通过颞枕区与丘脑枕区直接相连。这种连接对情景记忆的再现很重要，也涉及 Papez 环路[33,37]。然而，在 AD 中，穹窿细胞丢失、神经纤维缠结形成和萎缩都很明显，这导致海马输入中断，造成情景记忆的中断[37]。

包含后扣带回区域的压后皮质对情景记忆至关重要[37,38]。在阿尔茨海默病的早期，后扣带回区域会出现萎缩和体积变化[37]，而后扣带回区域与前丘脑核群具有密集的连接[38]。AD会引起前丘脑损伤，从而导致后扣带回皮质的慢性功能障碍，进一步破坏情景记忆。此外，确定空间方位的变化需要海马、扣带回皮质和前丘脑协同工作。由于AD中这些区域的连接受损，故患者难以适应空间定位的改变[37]。

边缘丘脑对空间定位至关重要，并且情景记忆与Papez环路相连。Papez环路包含了海马和后扣带回区域，在维持情景记忆中也起着重要作用[37,41]。Aggleton等[38]和Hornberger等[42]研究认为，丘脑中的海马连接减少导致情景记忆中断。这显示AD对Papez环路及其连接存在间接影响。研究还发现，AD患者除前扣带回区域外，Papez环路的所有区域都发生变性[42]。最后，丘脑-皮质网络连接丘脑核群和皮质，该网络由丘脑网状核调节[10,47]。AD患者网状核体积减小。这种网状核体积的变化造成丘脑和皮质之间的通信中断[10]。这引起丘脑皮质网络和皮质之间的连接受损，从而导致认知障碍。这些网状核群对维持丘脑振荡至关重要，而他们在AD患者中存在异常[10]。丘脑振荡在调节认知和功能活动中发挥着关键作用[47]。此外，丘脑-皮质网络对注意力的产生也很重要。因此，丘脑-皮质网络的受损会导致AD患者的注意力缺陷[10]。

此外,淡漠已被认为是AD的症状之一。前额叶-纹状体网络是一个前馈回路，投射到丘脑，参与执行功能。AD引起的丘脑变性破坏了与前额叶-纹状体网络的连接，导致认知障碍和淡漠[49,50]。眶额皮质是前额纹状体网络的重要组成部分，在日常决策中起着重要作用[48,60]。因此，眶额皮质受损会导致反应抑制和决策困难[50]。

mPFC可以将来自不同输入区域的信息进行整合，并将更新后的信息传递到输出区域。它在许多大脑功能中发挥重要作用，包括认知过程、情绪调节和工作记忆[23]。默认模式网络与mPFC、后扣带皮质、丘脑前核群和背内侧核群有很紧密的结构连接。上述结构连接性的下降和因 AD 导致的 mPFC 中淀粉样斑块的形成会造成行为表现和工作记忆的恶化[23]。对工作记忆的影响也与 AD 导致 mPFC 锥体神经元树突棘密度的下降有关[23]。因此，AD 通过引起神经细胞丢失、体积减小而极大地破坏丘脑，并影响其相关网络。然而，还需要开展更多的研究，以更好地了解 AD 对丘脑的影响。

第六节 未来的工作

AD 对丘脑的影响大多被忽视，尚未得到广泛研究。目前仍认为丘脑功能障碍是颞叶内侧受损的继发性反应，并且丘脑功能障碍导致的认知丧失的结果被低估[37]。边缘丘脑至海马结构投射的重要性也被忽视，需要进一步的研究。目前，已经对丘脑核进行了磁共振成像，以更好地了解丘脑的体积、神经元丢失和退化。未来对 AD 患者模型中皮质-丘脑功能的细胞、分子和环路方面的研究有助于更深入地阐述其机制[10]。此外，还需要进行更多的研究来了解 Papez 环路的淀粉样蛋白病理学。为了获得更广泛的知识和更好地了解丘脑在 AD 中的作用，还需要进行大量的研究。需要对所有年龄段，包括青年、中年和老年人的丘脑进行定量研究，并与诊断为 AD 的患者进行对比[35]。

第七节 结论

综上所述，丘脑作为传入的感觉信息的中转站，在 AD 的影响下，会形成神经元纤维缠结和淀粉样斑块，并伴有突触丢失。AD 还导致丘脑体积减小（主要在网状核和背核），这与认知功能损害有关。AD 还可导致神经细胞的丢失，而这种退行性变主要发生在前背侧丘脑核。

此外，丘脑与大脑的其他部分（如海马、压后皮质和大脑皮质）有紧密联系，并在 Papez 环路、默认模式网络、海马、丘脑皮质网络和前额叶-纹状体网络中发挥重要作用。当丘脑和其他参与不同过程的大脑部位因 AD 而出现萎缩，所有这些微妙的过程都会被破坏。

关于 AD 引起的丘脑萎缩的研究还没有得到足够的重视，如果我们要充分深入地探索和了解丘脑对 AD 的作用，还需要进行更多的研究。

参考文献

1. Murray Sherman S. 2006. Thalamus, Scholarpedia, viewed April 6, 2020, http://www.scholarpedia.org/article/Thalamus.
2. Blumenfeld, H., & Gummadavelli, A. 2018, Thalamus, Encyclopædia Britannica.
3. Li, Y., Lopez-Huerta, V. G., Adiconis, X., Levandowski, K., Choi, S., Simmons, S. K., et al. (2020). Distinct subnetworks of the thalamic reticular nucleus. Nature, 583, 819-824.
4. Moustafa, A. A., Mcmullan, R. D., Rostron, B., Hewedi, D. H., & Haladjian, H. H. (2017). The thalamus as a relay station and gatekeeper: Relevance to brain disorders. Reviews in the Neurosciences, 28(2), 203-218.
5. Gazzaniga, M., Ivry, R., & Mangun, G. (1998). Cognitive neuroscience (4th ed., pp. 45-46). New York: W.W. Norton and Company.
6. Pelzer, E. A., Pauls, K. A. M., Braun, N., Tittgemeyer, M., & Timmermann, L. (2020). Probabilistic tractography in the ventrolateral thalamic nucleus: Cerebellar and pallidal connections. Brain Structure and Function, 225, 1685-1689.
7. Sheridan, N., & Tadi, P. (2020). Neuroanatomy, thalamic nuclei. Treasure Island, FL: StatPearls.
8. Cassel, J., Pereira De Vasconcelos, A., Loureiro, M., Cholvin, T., Dalrymple-Alford, J., & Vertes, R. (2013). The reuniens and rhomboid nuclei: Neuroanatomy, electrophysiological characteristics and behavioral implications. Progress in Neurobiology, 111, 34-52.
9. De Medeiros Silva, A., De Santana, M., De Góis Morais, P., De Sousa, T., Januário Engelberth, R., De Souza Lucena, E., et al. (2014). Serotonergic fibers distribution in the midline and intralaminar thalamic nuclei in the rock cavy (Kerodon rupestris). Brain Research, 1586, 99-108.
10. Jagirdar, R., & Chin, J. (2019). Corticothalamic network dysfunction and Alzheimer's disease. Brain Research, 1702, 38-45.
11. Taber, K., Wen, C., Khan, A., & Hurley, R. (2015). The limbic thalamus. Journal of Neuropsychiatry, 16(2), 127-132.
12. Vertes, R., Linley, S., & Hoover, W. (2015). Limbic circuitry of the midline thalamus.

Neuroscience & Biobehavioral Reviews, 54, 89-107.

13. De Jong, L. W., Van Der Hiele, K., Veer, I. M., Houwing, J. J., Westendorp, R. G., Bollen, E. L., et al. (2008). Strongly reduced volumes of putamen and thalamus in Alzheimer's disease: An MRI study. Brain: A Journal of Neurology, 131(12), 3277-3285.

14. Fama, R., & Edith, V. S. (2015). Thalamic structures and associated cognitive functions: Relations with age and aging. Neuroscience and Biobehavioral Reviews, 54, 29-37.

15. Koyama, M. S., Molfese, P. J., Milham, M. P., Mencl, W. E., & Pugh, K. R. (2020). Thalamus is a common locus of reading, arithmetic, and IQ: Analysis of local intrinsic functional properties. Brain and Language, 209, 104835.

16. Li, X., Xia, J., Ma, C., Chen, K., Xu, K., Zhang, J., et al. (2020). Accelerating structural degeneration in temporal regions and their effects on cognition in aging of MCI patients. Cerebral Cortex, 30, 326-338.

17. Iglesias, J., Insausti, R., Usabiaga, G., Bocchetta, M., Leemput, K., Greve, D., et al. (2018). A probabilistic atlas of the human thalamic nuclei combining ex vivo MRI and histology. Neuroimage, 183, 314-326.

18. Štillová, K., Jurák, P., Chládek, J., Chrastina, J., Halámek, J., Bočková, M., et al. (2015). The role of anterior nuclei of the thalamus: A subcortical gate in memory processing: An intracerebral recording study. PLoS One, 10(11), e0140778.

19. Cutsuridis, V., & A.A. Moustafa 2014. Computational modes of Alzheimer's disease, Scholarpedia, viewed April 8, 2020.

20. Hodson, R. (2018). Alzheimer's disease. Nature, 559(7715).

21. Minter, M., Taylor, J., & Crack, P. (2015). The contribution of neuroinflammation to amyloid toxicity in Alzheimer''s disease. Journal of Neurochemistry, 136(3), 457-474.

22. Aisen, P., Cummings, J., Jack, C., Morris, J., Sperling, R., Frölich, L., et al. (2017). On the path to 2025: Understanding the Alzheimer's disease continuum. Alzheimer's Research & Therapy, 9(1).

23. Xu, P., Chen, A., Li, Y., Xing, X., & Lu, H. (2019). Medial prefrontal cortex in neurological diseases. Physiological Genomics, 51(9), 432-442.

24. Lane, C., Hardy, J., & Scott, J. (2018). Alzheimer's disease. European Journal of Neurology, 25, 59-70.

25. Ryan, N., Keihaninejad, S., Shakespeare, T., Lehmann, M., Crutch, S., Malone, I., et al. (2013). Magnetic resonance imaging evidence for presymptomatic change in thalamus and caudate in familial Alzheimer's disease. Brain, 136(5), 1399-1414.

26. Hampel, H., Mesulam, M. M., Cuello, A. C., Farlow, M. R., Giacobini, E., Grossberg, G. T., et al. (2018). The cholinergic system in the pathophysiology and treatment of

Alzheimer's disease. Brain, 141, 1917-1933.

27. Kanel, P., Muller, M., Van Der Zee, S., Sanchez-Catasus, C. A., Koeppe, R. A., Frey, K. A., & Bohnen, N. I. (2020). Topography of cholinergic changes in dementia with Lewy bodies and key neural network hubs. The Journal of Neuropsychiatry and Clinical Neurosciences, 32(4), 370-375, appineuropsych19070165.

28. Huerta-Ocampo, I., Hacioglu-Bay, H., Dautan, D., & Mena-Segovia, J. (2020). Distribution of midbrain cholinergic axons in the thalamus. eNeuro, 7.

29. Noftz, W. A., Beebe, N. L., Mellott, J. G., & Schofield, B. R. (2020). Cholinergic projections from the pedunculopontine tegmental nucleus contact excitatory and inhibitory neurons in the inferior colliculus. Frontiers in Neural Circuits, 14, 43.

30. Pita-Almenar, J. D., Yu, D., Lu, H. C., & Beierlein, M. (2014). Mechanisms underlying desynchronization of cholinergic-evoked thalamic network activity. The Journal of Neuroscience, 34, 14463-14474.

31. Kotagal, V., Muller, M. L., Kaufer, D. I., Koeppe, R. A., & Bohnen, N. I. (2012). Thalamic cholinergic innervation is spared in Alzheimer disease compared to parkinsonian disorders. Neuroscience Letters, 514(2), 169-172. Available from https://doi.org/10.1016/j.neulet.2012.02.083.

32. Mega, M. S. (2000). The cholinergic deficit in Alzheimer's disease: Impact on cognition, behaviour and function. The International Journal of Neuropsychopharmacology/Official Scientific Journal of the Collegium Internationale Neuropsychopharmacologicum (CINP), 3(7), 3-12. Available from https://doi.org/10.1017/S1461145700001942.

33. Zarei, M., Patenaude, B., Damoiseaux, J., Morgese, C., Smith, S., Matthews, P., et al. (2010). Combining shape and connectivity analysis: An MRI study of thalamic degeneration in Alzheimer's disease. Neuroimage, 49(1), 1-8.

34. Zidan, M., Boban, J., Bjelan, M., Todorović, A., Stankov Vujanić, T., Semnic, M., et al. (2019). Thalamic volume loss as an early sign of amnestic mild cognitive impairment. Journal of Clinical Neuroscience, 68, 168-173.

35. Xuereb, J. H., Perry, R. H., Candy, J. M., Perry, E. K., Marshall, E., & Bonham, J. R. (1991). Nerve cell loss in the thalamus in Alzheimer's and Parkinson's disease. Brain, 114(Pt 3), 1363-1379.

36. Low, A., Mak, E., Malpetti, M., Chouliaras, L., Nicastro, N., Su, L., et al. (2019). Asymmetrical atrophy of thalamic subnuclei in Alzheimer's disease and amyloid-positive mild cognitive impairment is associated with key clinical features. Alzheimer's & Dementia: Diagnosis, Assessment & Disease Monitoring, 11(1), 690-699.

37. Aggleton, J., Pralus, A., Nelson, A., & Hornberger, M. (2016). Thalamic pathology and memory loss in early Alzheimer's disease: Moving the focus from the medial temporal

lobe to Papez circuit. Brain, 139(7), 1877-1890.

38. Aggleton, J., & Brown, M. (1999). Episodic memory, amnesia, and the hippocampal anterior thalamic axis. Behavioral and Brain Sciences, 22(3), 425-444.
39. Feng, F., Zhou, B., Wang, L., Yao, H., Guo, Y., An, N., et al. (2019). The correlation of functional connectivity and structural connectivity between hippocampus and thalamus in Alzheimer's disease and amnestic mild cognitive impairment. Zhonghua Nei Ke Za Zhi (Chinese Journal of Internal Medicine), 58(9), 662-667.
40. Jenkins, T., Amin, E., Brown, M., & Aggleton, J. (2006). Changes in immediate early gene expression in the rat brain after unilateral lesions of the hippocampus. Neuroscience, 137(3), 747-759.
41. Jones, D., Mateen, F., Lucchinetti, C., Jack, C., & Welker, K. (2011). Default mode network disruption secondary to a lesion in the anterior thalamus. Archives of Neurology, 68(2).
42. Hornberger, M., Wong, S., Tan, R., Irish, M., Piguet, O., Kril, J., et al. (2012). In vivo and post-mortem memory circuit integrity in frontotemporal dementia and Alzheimer's disease. Brain, 135(10), 3015-3025.
43. Zhou, B., Liu, Y., Zhang, Z., An, N., Yao, H., Wang, P., et al. (2013). Impaired functional connectivity of the thalamus in Alzheimer's disease and mild cognitive impairment: A resting-state fMRI study. Current Alzheimer Research, 10(7), 754-766.
44. Nestor, P., Fryer, T., & Hodges, J. (2006). Declarative memory impairments in Alzheimer's disease and semantic dementia. Neuroimage, 30(3), 1010-1020.
45. Robertson, R., & Kaitz, S. (1981). Thalamic connections with limbic cortex. I. Thalamocortical projections. The Journal of Comparative Neurology, 195(3), 501-525.
46. Torso, M., Serra, L., Giulietti, G., Spanò, B., Tuzzi, E., Koch, G., et al. (2015). Strategic lesions in the anterior thalamic radiation and apathy in early Alzheimer's disease. PLoS One, 10(5), e0124998.
47. Abuhassan, K., Coyle, D., & Maguire, L. (2014). Compensating for thalamocortical synaptic loss in Alzheimer"s disease. Frontiers in Computational Neuroscience, 8, 65.
48. Jeong, H., Kang, I., Im, J., Park, J., Na, S., Heo, Y., et al. (2018). Brain perfusion correlates of apathy in Alzheimer's disease. Dementia and Neurocognitive Disorders, 17(2), 50.
49. Levy, R., & Dubois, B. (2005). Apathy and the functional anatomy of the prefrontal cortex basal ganglia circuits. Cerebral Cortex, 16(7), 916-928.
50. Theleritis, C., Politis, A., Siarkos, K., & Lyketsos, C. (2013). A review of neuroimaging findings of apathy in Alzheimer's disease. International Psychogeriatrics, 26(2), 195-207.
51. Bertoux, M., O'callaghan, C., Flanagan, E., Hodges, J., & Hornberger, M. (2015). Fronto-striatal atrophy in behavioral variant frontotemporal dementia and Alzheimer's

disease. Frontiers in Neurology, 6, 147.

52. Yi, D., Bertoux, M., Mioshi, E., Hodges, J., & Hornberger, M. (2013). Fronto-striatal atrophy correlates of neuropsychiatric dysfunction in frontotemporal dementia (FTD) and Alzheimer's disease (AD). Dementia and Neuropsychologia, 7(1), 75-82.

53. Kobayashi, S. (2009). Reward neurophysiology and primate cerebral cortex. Encyclopedia of Neuroscience (pp. 325-333). Academic Press.

54. Naish, K., & Balodis, I. (2019). Reward processing in food addiction and overeating. In P. Cottone, C. Moore, V. Sabino, & G. Koob (Eds.), Compulsive eating behavior and food addiction (pp. 217-249). Elsevier.

55. Balasubramani, P. P., Chakravarthy, S., Balaraman, R., & Moustafa, A. A. (2014). An extended reinforcement learning model of basal ganglia to understand the contribution of serotonin and dopamine in risk-based decision making, reward prediction, and punishment learning. Frontiers in Computational Neuroscience, 8, 47.

56. Balasubramani, P. P., Chakravarthy, S., Balaraman, R., & Moustafa, A. A. (2015). A network model of basal ganglia for understanding the roles of dopamine and serotonin in reward-punishment-risk based decision making. Frontiers in Computational Neuroscience, 9, 76.

57. Mandali, A., Rengaswamy, M., Chakravarthy, S., & Moustafa, A. A. (2015). A spikingbasal ganglia model of synchrony, exploration and decision making. Frontiers in Neuroscience, 9, 191.

58. Moustafa, A. A., & Gluck, M. A. (2011a). Computational cognitive models of prefrontal striatal-hippocampal interactions in Parkinson's disease and schizophrenia. Neural Networks, 24(6), 575-591.

59. Moustafa, A. A., & Gluck, M. A. (2011b). A neurocomputational model of dopamine and prefrontal-striatal interactions during multi-cue category learning by Parkinson's patients. Journal of Cognitive Neuroscience, 23(1), 51-67.

60. Wallis, J. (2007). Orbitofrontal cortex and its contribution to decision-making. Annual Review of Neuroscience, 30(1), 31-56.

61. Heidbreder, C., & Groenewegen, H. (2003). The medial prefrontal cortex in the rat: Evidence for a dorso-ventral distinction based upon functional and anatomical characteristics. Neuroscience & Biobehavioral Reviews, 27(6), 555-579.

第七章 利用大数据方法去理解阿尔茨海默病

Samuel L. Warren,Ahmed A. Moustafa,Hany Alashwal 编
屈剑锋,胡伟东,刘晓汶 译
陈仰昆 校

第一节 引言

阿尔茨海默病(AD)是最常见的痴呆症,其影响着全世界 5000 万人[1]。全球范围内被确诊的痴呆症预计在未来 30 年将增加至 1.32 亿例[2],最终导致阿尔茨海默病全球性流行。由于阿尔茨海默病目前无法治愈,并且最终导致死亡,故痴呆症病例的迅速增加成为目前一个值得关注的问题[3]。因此,阿尔茨海默病被认为是全球第五大死亡原因[3,4]。不得不说,阿尔茨海默病是现代最大的医学难题之一。因此,迫切需要对其进行相关研究,以预防阿尔茨海默病成为全球流行性的疾病。

本章主要探讨大数据如何分析和克服复杂性问题以及如何将大数据应用于阿尔茨海默病的研究。目标是提供对阿尔茨海默病的一般认识,并概述痴呆症研究中常用的大数据分析方法。同时探讨大数据收集和陈述数据库技术相对于标准心理学研究的优势。在本章的最后,我们提议将阿尔茨海默病神经影像学计划(the Alzheimer's Disease Neuroimaging Initiative,ADNI)数据库作为阿尔茨海默病研究中大数据分析的具体例子。因此,本章旨在强调突出大数据分析的独特优势,并讨论研究人员应如何利用大数据来预防阿尔茨海默病。

本章包括 4 个部分:广泛讨论阿尔茨海默病、大数据方法、预测建模和 ADNI。具体来说,每个部分讨论以下主题:①"什么是阿尔茨海默病"的部分简要介绍了阿尔茨海默病,并探讨了该病的病因、治疗方法、诊断和相关研究;

②"大数据方法"的部分突出了大数据方法的优势,概述了数据库在阿尔茨海默病研究中的作用;③"大数据分析"的部分讨论了预测模型(统计模型和计算模型)在阿尔茨海默病研究中的重要性;④"示例:阿尔茨海默病神经影像学计划"的部分探讨了 ADNI 数据库的方法和影响。总而言之,我们的目标是提供一个关于如何将大数据应用于阿尔茨海默病研究的整体认识。

第二节　什么是阿尔茨海默病

阿尔茨海默病是指由于大脑逐渐死亡而导致的精神和身体功能丧失的一类疾病[5]。阿尔茨海默病患者通常会出现记忆丧失、沟通困难、思维混乱和行动不便等症状[6]。记忆丧失是阿尔茨海默病患者的大脑与记忆功能相关的区域开始衰退的典型特征[7,8]。而且,其他许多认知和身体功能(如语言和运动技能)也受到影响。随着阿尔茨海默病病程的进展,疾病的症状变得更加严重。例如,晚期阿尔茨海默病患者通常无法完成行走或说话等任务。此外,随着阿尔茨海默病的进展,发生并发症(如肺炎)的机会也会增加[9,10]。因此,阿尔茨海默病患者将会经历功能逐渐丧失,直至死亡。

一、阿尔茨海默病的病因是什么?

阿尔茨海默病的病因目前尚不清楚。然而,目前的理论,如淀粉样蛋白级联假说,为阿尔茨海默病的发展提供了很好的见解。淀粉样蛋白级联假说认为,阿尔茨海默病的发展与老年斑和神经元纤维缠结等有毒物质的聚集和形成有关[11]。据推测,高浓度的阿尔茨海默病 β-淀粉蛋白(Aβ)导致老年斑的形成[12]。老年斑具有持续的毒性,当其累积时会导致神经元(脑细胞)坏死[13],同时也会改变 tau 蛋白,导致神经原纤维缠结的形成[14]。然后神经元纤维缠结会损害神经元的结构完整性,导致细胞坏死和进一步的毒性[15]。因此,Aβ 和 tau 都延续了神经毒性的循环,并损害神经元直至坏死。

淀粉样蛋白级联假说还指出,神经元损失开始于海马,然后逐渐扩展到更宽的内侧颞叶和大脑皮质区域[16]。在本章中呈现出来的这种级联变性现象，是目前对阿尔茨海默病进展理解的基础[17]。因此，淀粉样蛋白级联假说是目前大多数阿尔茨海默病研究的理论基础。然而，淀粉样蛋白级联假说并不是阿尔茨海默病的全面理论。例如，研究表明，健康的成年人可以有高水平的 Aβ 而不会患上阿尔茨海默病[18]。此外，造成 Aβ 和 tau 聚集的原因也是未知的。因此，阿尔茨海默病发展的其他理论也会被应用于医学研究（如胆碱能假说）[19,20]。然而，其他理论超出了本章的讨论范围。

二、阿尔茨海默病有治疗方法吗？

虽然阿尔茨海默病没有治愈的方法，但有可用的治疗方法。药物和老年护理通常用于缓解阿尔茨海默病的症状[21]。老年护理的重点是帮助因阿尔茨海默病而难以完成日常任务的患者[22]。例如，护理人员通常会帮助阿尔茨海默病患者进食、清理和服药。根据阿尔茨海默病的严重程度，患者们需要不同程度的护理。通过老年护理援助，阿尔茨海默病患者可以在舒适的环境中生存更长的时间（如退休村），并保持一定的自主权[23]。因此，老年护理有助于延长和改善阿尔茨海默病患者的生命及生活质量。

药物也被用于治疗阿尔茨海默病的症状。例如，胆碱酯酶抑制剂是一种常用于治疗阿尔茨海默病认知症状（如记忆丧失）的药物[24]。胆碱酯酶抑制剂通过调节神经化学物质乙酰胆碱起作用，乙酰胆碱是一种有助于认知功能的物质，其在阿尔茨海默病中会减少[25]。胆碱酯酶抑制剂通过调节乙酰胆碱，有助于维持认知功能，减缓阿尔茨海默病的症状进展[26]。然而，胆碱酯酶抑制剂的效果取决于不同个体、疾病阶段和诊断时间[27]。在治疗阿尔茨海默病时，很少有可以替代胆碱酯酶抑制剂的药物[28]。因此，阿尔茨海默病的药物治疗亟需更进一步的发展。然而，目前对阿尔茨海默病的诊断却限制了药物治疗。

目前阿尔茨海默病是通过临床评估来诊断的。医生使用多种心理和生理测试（例如，记忆、语言、注意力、平衡、反应和运动技能）来评估阿尔茨海默病的症状[29]。但是，阿尔茨海默病的诊断只能在患者死亡后通过尸检得到完全证实。此外，由于阿尔茨海默病涉及与其他形式的痴呆症重叠的临床症状（如血管性痴呆），导致了其诊断非常受限[30,31]。因此，目前的阿尔茨海默病诊断常在疾病的后期，此时脑损伤已经不可逆转，大多数药物在很大程度上已无效[32]。目前的治疗方法，如胆碱酯酶抑制剂，可以极大地治疗阿尔茨海默病的症状（如记忆和运动功能丧失），但不能逆转或预防疾病[24,33]。因此，目前的研究应积极探索在早期阶段诊断阿尔茨海默病的方法，以改善治疗策略。

三、研究人员如何研究阿尔茨海默病？

目前的心理学研究使用预测方法来了解阿尔茨海默病的进展。反过来，这些阿尔茨海默病的预测因素为诊断策略和潜在的治疗提供信息。研究人员通常通过研究那些逐渐过渡到阿尔茨海默病的疾病来预测其进展。具体来说，阿尔茨海默病协会和国家老龄化研究所认为，阿尔茨海默病是一种连续性疾病，有3个不同的阶段，分别是临床前阿尔茨海默病、轻度认知障碍（MCI）和阿尔茨海默病痴呆[34]。临床前阿尔茨海默病是阿尔茨海默病发展的初始阶段，是一种无症状状态，可以持续数十年，然后过渡到轻度认知障碍或阿尔茨海默病[5]。由于临床前阿尔茨海默病的性质隐匿，故在阿尔茨海默病的研究中，轻度认知障碍更容易预测、识别和研究。

轻度认知障碍是指至少有一种认知功能的非痴呆性受损，如语言或记忆[35]。这些损伤在轻度认知障碍中并不会使人衰弱。衰弱性损伤通常提示另一些疾病，如痴呆或帕金森病。此外，轻度认知障碍并不是阿尔茨海默病发展的唯一原因。然而，轻度认知障碍确实与阿尔茨海默病有许多共同特征，并转化为阿尔茨海默病的概率较高[36]。具体来说，患有轻度认知障碍的个体有10%~15%的概率转变为阿尔茨海默病，而一般人群只有2%~4%的概率会发展为阿尔茨海默病[37]。因此，通过研究轻度认知障碍，研究人员可以保证有更大、更可靠的阿尔茨海默病转化人群用于研究。

四、阿尔茨海默病标准研究的问题

然而，研究患有阿尔茨海默病和轻度认知障碍的参与者可能非常复杂。因此，阿尔茨海默病和轻度认知障碍的研究非常复杂，通常受到 3 个主要因素的限制。首先，组织和招募弱势群体（如痴呆症患者）进行研究非常困难。例如，神经系统方面的参与者（如阿尔茨海默病的参与者），随着疾病症状的恶化，可能会退出研究[38]。其次，阿尔茨海默病的检测方法往往需要很高的经济和管理成本，这限制了它们的使用。例如，磁共振成像（Magnetic Resonance Imaging，MRI）技术可以高精度地测量神经元损失，但该设备使用起来非常昂贵，而且很难获得[39]。因此，由于无法获得创新技术，阿尔茨海默病的研究进展可能会推迟。

最后，纵向（长期）研究阿尔茨海默病进展和轻度认知障碍转化需要巨大的资源，超出了一些实验室的范围。大多数（如果不是全部的话）实验室都负担不起投入数年的时间来纵向收集阿尔茨海默病的数据。因此，像阿尔茨海默病进展这样的纵向课题可能缺乏足够的研究。然而，阿尔茨海默病研究的这些资源、时间和招募障碍问题往往可以通过大数据来克服。

第三节　大数据方法

阿尔茨海默病是一种内在复杂的疾病，发生在整个生命周期。例如，一些研究假设阿尔茨海默病的预兆（如神经原纤维缠结），可以在疾病发病前几十年观察到[40]。因此，纵向收集阿尔茨海默病数据需要大量的资源和专门的方法。在阿尔茨海默病研究中，大数据通常使用数据库来记录和维护复杂的纵向数据集。反过来，这些数据库使研究人员能够分析阿尔茨海默病在整个生命周期中的发展。在本节中，我们将讨论数据库在阿尔茨海默病研究中的背景和优势。

一、什么是数据库？

数据库是研究人员可以在其中上传、合并、共享和访问阿尔茨海默病数据的信息中心[41]。数据库通常由寻求促进数据协作收集的大学和组织运行。这些数据库是持续的，因此随着时间的推移建立了大型纵向数据集。通常研究人员可以自由地使用和贡献数据库。因此，数据库本质上是大型协作数据集，为研究人员提供丰富的纵向数据。数据库还为研究人员提供了大量访问阿尔茨海默病的样本和通常单个实验室无法获得的大量变量的机会。因此，数据库中包含的复杂数据使研究人员能够纵向评估和了解阿尔茨海默病。

例如，ADNI 是阿尔茨海默病研究中使用的最大数据库。作为一个组织，ADNI 试图通过疾病生物标志物（阿尔茨海默病的生物指标）来了解、检测和观察阿尔茨海默病的进展[42]。具体而言，ADNI 收集对照（没有神经系统疾病的人群）、轻度认知障碍和阿尔茨海默病参与者的神经影像学、生物标志物、心理和人口统计学指标[43]。对研究人员来说最重要的是，ADNI 遵循信息共享政策，这使得任何获得机构伦理批准的研究都可以使用 ADNI 数据。通过 ADNI，研究人员可以在克服上述组织管理、时间和经济限制的同时研究阿尔茨海默病。因此，像 ADNI 这样的数据库在促进和加速阿尔茨海默病的研究方面发挥着重要作用。

二、数据库的优势

数据库具有独一无二的优势，通常可以克服标准阿尔茨海默病研究的资源、人员招募和时间的限制。具体而言，协作和信息共享的优势使研究人员能够克服资源限制、招募障碍，从而进行纵向研究。

标准的心理学研究常常受到阿尔茨海默病研究的高昂经济和管理成本的限制。然而，大数据研究往往通过数据库就可以克服这些资源限制。数据库具有通过协作在短时间内收集大量数据的独特能力[44]。协作数据收集涉及多个研究小组在创建一个总体数据库方面的合作。通过合作，结果数据库包含的数据比任何一项研究都要多[45]。因此，研究人员可以克服资源限制进而访问更多的数据。通过数据库，研究人员还能够利用难以负担或获取的技术和资源来研究阿尔茨海默病[46]。例如，研究人员可能存在设备不良或无法进行腰椎穿刺（用于收集 Aβ 和 tau）等侵入性手术的情况。其可以通过数据库访问类似的数据，从而继续他们的工作。因此，通过协作研究和数据库，在文献中推广了昂贵而耗时的研究。

数据库还可以克服招募障碍（例如，招募弱势群体，其通常限制了阿尔茨海默病的研究）。具体来说，数据库可以通过信息共享来克服招募障碍[47]。利用大数据方法了解阿尔茨海默病，以及阿尔茨海默病数据的分布。利用数据库与更广泛的科学界免费共享数据以加速对阿尔茨海默病的研究是很常见的。通过信息共享，研究人员可以访问预先存在的大型数据库，避免发生参与者招募障碍[48]。作为回报，数据库可以确保对阿尔茨海默病进行彻底和有组织的调查。虽然信息共享并不能消除对数据收集的需要，但确实减少了单个研究对人员招募参与者的需要。在某种程度上，由于协作收集和数据库对数据的有效重用，单个研究人员可以收集更少的数据。因此，信息共享使研究人员能够将资源集中在阿尔茨海默病的治疗、诊断和理解上，而非数据收集上[49]。

标准心理学研究的另一个问题是无法对阿尔茨海默病进行纵向观察。以目前的数据收集方法，研究阿尔茨海默病的进展可能真的需要整个生命周期的时间，因为阿尔茨海默病的纵向研究获得稳定的资金也非常困难。在大数据研究中，数据库可以通过协作高效地收集阿尔茨海默病纵向数据[47,50]。很显然，当倡议和组织承担协作负担时，个体研究人员不需要花费数年时间来用于数据收集[49]。反过来，研究人员可以通过数据库纵向研究阿尔茨海默病，而不必担心数据收集困难问题[51]。因此，数据库通过其数据的可及性、数量和质量来积极促进复杂的纵向研究。

三、使用数据库的常见困难

显然，数据库在帮助推进阿尔茨海默病研究方面具有独特的优势。然而，数据库本身也非常复杂，需要持续组织管理。在阿尔茨海默病的研究中，数据库包含大量的信息，这些信息很容易存在管理不善的问题。例如，当数据由不同的研究组收集时，测量值和变量可能不兼容或产生冲突。数据收集中的组织故障直接威胁到数据库的协作概念，并可能限制大数据分析。例如，在进行大数据分析时，数据缺失限制了统计能力和可用的方法[52]。因此，数据库统一数据收集策略以确保高效的研究十分重要。

标准化是使所有科学措施符合同一规则和程序的过程。度量标准的标准化使得数据收集和数据库构建的一致性得以实现[44]。因此，拥有多个贡献者的数据库应该定义一套研究人员在收集数据时必须遵循的措施和规则。通过遵循相同的规则，研究可以确保所有的测量都以类似的方式收集，并结合起来形成一个有凝聚力的数据集[53]。标准化的措施和变量也确保了统计能力，并降低了分析过程中出现偏倚的可能性。此外，通过标准化概述的数据收集规则和方法也可以使未来的研究人员复制和确认研究结果。因此，实施标准化的研究人员可以确保大数据收集的效率，减少大数据分析过程中的复杂性，并确保未来复制的透明度。

第四节　大数据分析

大数据分析是对大数据集的调查和解释[54]。在阿尔茨海默病研究中，大数据通常分析从数据库中获得的复杂的纵向数据集。例如，预测模型通常用于研究从 ADNI 数据库获得的复杂纵向数据集[55]。预测模型的使用并不是大数据分析所独有的，而是在整个研究中广泛使用的。然而，大数据确实使用了独特的统计和计算技术，专门用于分析大量数据[49]。本节讨论了如何使用统计和计算模型来研究阿尔茨海默病，以及如何在临床实践中使用大数据分析来帮助诊断和治疗阿尔茨海默病。

一、统计模型

在大数据分析中，统计模型是使用数学模式来预测未来的结果[56]。在阿尔茨海默病研究中，统计模型通常用于确定疾病发展中变量的重要性。例如，研究人员经常会随着时间的推移来观察疾病生物标志物（如 Aβ 累积）以预测阿尔茨海默病的进展[57]。组成统计模型的预测变量通常是由理论或前期的研究结果来决定的。在进行分析时，统计模型的准确性和有效性是通过将模型与数据集中的观察结果进行检验来确定的[58]。例如，如果研究人员试图预测阿尔茨海默病的进展，统计模型将与数据集中观察到的疾病进展进行比较。因此，研究人员可以了解一个变量在多大程度上可以预测阿尔茨海默病及其与该疾病的总体联系。

有多种统计技术用于创建预测模型。然而，阿尔茨海默病研究中的大多数统计模型使用回归分析（见 Doody 等[59]）。在最简单的形式中，回归分析使用2个历史变量来预测它们未来的相互作用[60]。对于不同类型的数据，有许多类型的回归。例如，存在线性和非线性数据、单一和多个测量以及分类和数值变量的回归[61,62]。回归分析在心理学研究中使用广泛。然而，当使用大型数据集时，大多数回归分析是不可行的。因此，大数据分析通常使用多元回归分析，专门分析多变量和模拟复杂现象，如阿尔茨海默病[63-65]。而多元回归分析背后的数学原理超出了本章讨论的范围。

统计建模方法是目前阿尔茨海默病研究中最常用的大数据分析方法；但是与其他大数据方法相比（如计算模型和机器学习），这些统计技术过于简单[66]。例如，统计方法往往难以处理大量数据，因为它们受到计算能力或数学假设的限制[54]。即使是可以处理大数据的统计技术，如多元回归分析，也受到其计算能力和潜在假设的限制。例如，多元回归分析对抑制效应是开放的，有时会影响变量[67]。抑制变量是一种较差的预测指标，仅包含在混合模型中，因为其他指标掩盖了较差的预测指标的影响[68]。抑制变量对模型是有害的，因为它们没有提供任何益处，并且可能混淆结果。这些抑制效应是可以克服的，但代价是限制变量和使分析复杂化[69]。因此，研究人员逐渐选择使用计算模型而非传统的统计方法来研究阿尔茨海默病。

二、计算模型

计算模型是通过数据分析来模拟和分析复杂的系统（如大脑、神经元）。在大数据研究中，研究人员通过构建计算模型来理解复杂系统的组成部分。通过理解这些组成部分，计算模型使研究人员能够回答有关复杂系统潜在机制的问题。在阿尔茨海默病研究中，计算模型可以制定比统计模型更复杂的分析，也可以创建阿尔茨海默病的模型[70]。统计模型和计算模型在数学上是相似的，其区别在于处理能力、科学方法和技术[71]。统计模型是对数据的数学分析和解释，而计算模型是对数据的技术分析和模拟。因此，计算模型可以执行与统计模型相同的任务，同时也擅长执行更复杂的分析和模拟[72]。例如，计算模型通常使用回归树来提供比标准统计分析更复杂和详细的数据解释[73,74]。模拟在安全测试研究假设和探索阿尔茨海默病的机制方面表现出色。例如，疾病生物标志物模型可用于测试阿尔茨海默病的新疗法[75]。因此，计算模型提供了阿尔茨海默病的复杂预测，并可以实现基础探索性研究。

例如，Petrella 等[76]开发了阿尔茨海默病生物标志物级联的计算模型。该模型由 Aβ、tau、认知衰退和神经退行性标志物组成，用于模拟不同人群（早期、常染色体显性和晚期阿尔茨海默病）的阿尔茨海默病进展。在数学软件 MATLAB 中采用因果建模方法和常微分方程建立计算模型。Petrella 等[76]发现，他们的级联模型准确地模拟了阿尔茨海默病的认知能力下降以及 tau 和 Aβ 的进展。他们还发现，生物标志物之间的相互作用准确地模拟了文献中进行的临床试验。他们的结论是，他们的模型是一个强有力的概念证明，并在未来的改进过程中，可用于评估阿尔茨海默病的因果性质。同时，Petrella 等[76]也强调，生物标志物级联模型只是探索性的，高度依赖于此前的理论假设。计算模型非常通用，可以从单细胞模拟到大规模的基于人群的诊断模型[75]。计算模型在阿尔茨海默病研究中也取得了不同程度的成功。具体来说，在制定生化、单细胞和系统级模型（单个大脑区域）方面已经取得很大成功；但目前的计算模型往往难以模拟出阿尔茨海默病的发生、进展等复杂现象[70,75]。这些复杂的计算模型受到我们目前对阿尔茨海默病和大脑理解的限制。尽管如此，计算模型仍是了解阿尔茨海默病的理想方法，对痴呆症的研究是无价的。随着进一步的研究和理论的发展，计算模型将继续推进我们对阿尔茨海默病的理解。

三、预测模型的临床应用

以上讨论的大多数预测模型都集中在高度复杂的研究课题上，如阿尔茨海默病的病因和进展；同时，研究人员也在开发疾病预测模型，可以直接帮助阿尔茨海默病的临床诊断和治疗。本节主要探讨研究人员如何使用电子健康记录和患者自我监测技术来创建可供临床使用的预测模型。

电子健康记录是政府（或机构）运行的数据库，其中包含公民的医疗数据[77]。电子健康记录通常是半自动化的系统，允许从医疗机构自动检索健康记录，也允许医生和患者手动输入信息。近年来，电子健康记录越来越受欢迎，因为这些数据库是收集医疗信息和简化医疗保健实践的有效方法。重要的是，研究人员可以访问未识别版本的电子健康记录进行研究[78]。在阿尔茨海默病研究中，电子健康记录被用于创建预测模型，以识别普通人群中阿尔茨海默病风险个体[79]。具体来说，预测分析和机器学习正被用于分析电子健康记录，并识别与阿尔茨海默病进展相关的健康模式（例如心血管健康、压力、头部创伤、年龄和家族史）[80]。因此，这种预测模型可以用来识别有阿尔茨海默病进展风险的个体，并为早期诊断和治疗计划提供信息。

预测分析还可用于监测有阿尔茨海默病风险的患者，并制定适当的治疗计划。具体来说，智能手机应用程序等技术使研究人员能够轻松有效地收集患者数据并监测有阿尔茨海默病风险的参与者[81]。这些应用使用游戏、测验和谜题来定期收集参与者的数据进行分析[82]。通过预测分析，这些应用程序能够向医生提供参与者的健康概况。反过来，医生在决定诊断或治疗阿尔茨海默病患者时，也有更多的可用信息[83,84]。例如，诊断应用程序CogniSense被临床医生用于监测阿尔茨海默病患者并指导治疗[85]。CogniSense是一款iPad应用程序，包含一系列评估阿尔茨海默病症状的问题和任务（如记忆丧失），完整的认知评估大约需要10分钟，测试结果会立即提供给医生。因此，患者监测技术为医生提供了更多的信息，可以帮助加快阿尔茨海默病的诊断和治疗。

另外需要注意的是，在预测模型应用于临床实践之前，必须克服重大的伦理界限。也就是说，电子健康记录和数据监测技术必须克服数据安全和患者同意方面的问题，才能在临床上可行[84]。数据泄露和安全的历史问题严重限制了电子健康记录的采用。例如，澳大利亚政府的"我的健康记录"一直受到安全问题的困扰,这导致公民大规模退出该计划[86]。如果机构想要使用电子健康记录,必须使个人感受到他们的数据是安全的。此外,预测模型在知情同意与信息可及性方面也存在问题[87,88]。如果一个算法标记出一个人患有阿尔茨海默病,谁来告诉这个人呢?患者想知道吗?研究人员能让患者去看病吗?因此,在临床实践中,建立基于个人数据的诊断和治疗项目的伦理问题可能会显得突兀和混乱。显然,当前伦理方面的困境将决定未来大数据在临床实践中的应用情况。

第五节　举例：阿尔茨海默病神经影像计划

本章简要地讨论了 ADNI 作为阿尔茨海默病研究中大数据收集的一个例子。第二节阐述了数据库,如 ADNI 是如何克服干扰阿尔茨海默病标准研究的运行、时间和经济等方面的限制(如基于实验室的小型研究)。第三节讨论了数据库如何使用预测模型。与标准分析方法(如 t 检验和简单线性回归)相比,预测模型更适合阿尔茨海默病的研究。本节将深入了解 ADNI 如何收集和分析大数据。我们还旨在提供一个贯穿本章讨论的关于大数据概念的简要示例。因此,本节概述了 ADNI 的背景、数据收集方法、常见分析实践以及对阿尔茨海默病研究的影响。

ADNI 成立于 2004 年,是一个由政府和私人组织共同资助的项目,致力于探索阿尔茨海默病的生物标志物和疾病预测策略。如上文所述,ADNI 向研究人员免费提供所有数据。ADNI 在其历史上研究了 4 个队列,参与者都是从先前的研究中继承的,并且在每个新计划的开始添加了新参与者。ADNI 研究通常持续 5 年,以便对参与者进行纵向评估。截至到目前,ADNI 队列依次为 ADNI-1、ADNI-GO、ADNI-2 和 ADNI-3 队列[42]。在启动新的 ADNI 队列后,将添加新的生物标志物和研究方法,以使该计划与当前阿尔茨海默病文献保持同步[43]。然而,计划的迭代有时很难审查 ADNI 的措施。

从 2016 年开始,ADNI-3 队列是最近正在进行的队列,并且 ADNI-2 队列是最近完成的研究[89]。ADNI-2 队列从 2011—2016 年持续了 5 年,参与者的数据每隔 1 年或 2 年记录 1 次，具体取决于所讨论的措施。ADNI-2 队列包括来自先前计划的 700 名参与者和 150 名认知健康对照组，100 名早期轻度认知障碍，150 名晚期轻度认知障碍，150 名阿尔茨海默病参与者，以及 107 名具有显著记忆问题（Significant Memory Concern，SMC）的新标准参与者[43]。有显著记忆问题的参与者在健康老龄化和 MCI 个体之间的阿尔茨海默病谱上出现疾病转化风险较高的控制组。

一、数据类型

阿尔茨海默病的研究通常分为神经影像学、生物标志物和心理学研究 3 个领域。ADNI 数据库收集来自这些领域的数据，以预测阿尔茨海默病的进展并识别该疾病的标志物。ADNI 根据与之相关的文献选择标志物和方法。然而，ADNI 数据库的普及和可访问性也显著影响了文献中某些指标的流行程度。

传统的生物标志物研究评估与阿尔茨海默病相关的大脑生化变化。例如，阿尔茨海默病生物标志物研究通常研究 APOE4、tau、Aβ42 和早老素 -1 等基因、蛋白质和肽[12,90]。ADNI 数据库收集了大量用于阿尔茨海默病研究的生物标志物。因此，ADNI 收集血液、脑脊液（CSF）和尿液样本，以研究血浆、酶、蛋白质、氨基酸和基因作为阿尔茨海默病的生物标志物。传统生物标志物在预测模型中的使用存在争议，因为它们是早期阿尔茨海默病的弱预测因子。然而，生物标志物是当前阿尔茨海默病发展理论的基础，如淀粉样蛋白级联假说[91]。因此，生物标志物为阿尔茨海默病的进展提供了很好的见解，并在疾病发展的混合预测模型中发挥着重要作用。

神经影像学研究通常使用电磁信号来无创性测量阿尔茨海默病的神经变性和代谢变化（例如，MRI 测量海马萎缩）。神经影像学研究在某种程度上是生物标志物研究的一种形式，但由于该领域的规模和独特的方法，因此通常与传统的生物标志物分开。MRI 和正电子发射断层扫描（Positron Emission Tomography，PET）是神经影像学研究中最常用的方法。在 ADNI 数据库中，MRI 测量广泛应用于评估脑萎缩、脑体积和神经元连接性状，而 PET 测量则用来评估脑代谢和 Aβ 病理[92-94]。神经影像技术的使用是所有 ADNI 研究的基础，因为该技术用于预测阿尔茨海默病时非常准确。因此，ADNI 有助于巩固脑容量和萎缩的 MRI 测量作为阿尔茨海默病发展和进展的最佳预测指标。

心理学研究主要侧重于测量认知和功能能力（如运动技能和记忆）。因此，书面测试通常用于诊断阿尔茨海默病和监测高危患者（如轻度认知障碍患者）。ADNI 目前使用 11 项认知测试和 10 项功能和行为测试来监测所有阿尔茨海默病、轻度认知障碍和对照组参与者。根据具体测试的性质和使用，认知测试可以进一步分为 3 类[30]。在阿尔茨海默病研究中，认知测试大致可分为以下几种：用于筛查阿尔茨海默病的简短问卷（如简短的智力测试），用于区分血管性痴呆和阿尔茨海默病等类似疾病的高度特异性测试（如时钟绘制测试），以及通常用于阿尔茨海默病诊断的一般多域测试（如简易精神状态检查）[30,95,96]。认知测试应用是阿尔茨海默病的诊断、治疗和研究的基础。因此，ADNI 研究通常在预测研究和临床评估中使用心理测量方法。

二、混合预测模型

ADNI 数据库拥有大量的数据，涵盖了阿尔茨海默病研究的各个学科。因此，大多数 ADNI 研究经常在混合预测模型（如情景记忆和海马萎缩模型）中同时评估多个变量[97]。混合预测模型很受欢迎，因为它们是一种可以同时研究多种生物标志物的有效方法（如多元回归分析）。同时研究多种生物标志物很重要，因为阿尔茨海默病被视为一种多病因疾病。大多数 ADNI 研究结合了 MRI 测量（如脑容量或萎缩）、记忆评分和 Aβ 以及 tau 等生物标志物[92]。例如，研究人员发现内侧颞叶萎缩（海马和内嗅区体积/萎缩）与记忆衰退生物标志物之间存在密切关系[55,98]。然而，目前还没有一个突出的混合模型可以更好地预测阿尔茨海默病。实际上，有少数生物标志物可以根据疾病的阶段精确地预测阿尔茨海默病的发展。

比如说，Huang 等[99]的研究使用 ADNI 数据库和混合预测模型来检测阿尔茨海默病的发展。该研究[99]评估了 290 名轻度认知障碍参与者的脑脊液、神经影像学和认知标志物来预测阿尔茨海默病转化的能力。研究结果[99]发现，混合预测模型优于所有独立预测模型。与其他模型相比，由遗传、Aβ、大脑皮质和功能活动问卷测量组成的混合模型是疾病转化的最佳预测因子。基于他们的结果，Huang 等[99]将他们的混合预测模型发展成一个量表，临床医生可以用它来评估阿尔茨海默病的发展。据此，Huang 等[99]强调了混合预测模型的优势，以及阿尔茨海默病生物标志物在疾病诊断中的重要性。

ADNI 数据和预测模型使研究人员在阿尔茨海默病研究方面取得了重大突破。在对使用 ADNI 数据发表的所有期刊文章的回顾中，Weiner 等[100]概述了基于 ADNI 的研究的突破。该研究[100]详细介绍了 ADNI 数据在用于以诊断为目的的关于神经影像技术（如 MRI 和 PET）的发展，早期阿尔茨海默病生物标志物（CSF 生物标志物）的发现以及阿尔茨海默病发展的潜在预测因素（血液生物标志物）的研究中发挥了重要的作用[100,101]。通过在健康科学领域开创大数据技术，该计划本身也对研究产生了重大影响。例如，ADNI 激发了世界各地许多其他阿尔茨海默病计划的发展，如澳大利亚衰老成像、生物标志物和生活方式旗舰研究（Australian Imaging, Biomarker and Lifestyle Flagship Study of Ageing）。显然，ADNI 数据库已经帮助推动、激励和加速了阿尔茨海默病的研究。

第六节　结论

大数据正在积极改变阿尔茨海默病的研究范围。通过数据库和预测建模，大数据已经克服了标准阿尔茨海默病研究的许多限制。像 ADNI 这样的数据库在推进痴呆症研究和实现复杂的大数据分析方面发挥了重要作用[100]。随着时间的推移，预测模型也改变了研究人员研究阿尔茨海默病的方式。计算和统计方法都导致了阿尔茨海默病复杂混合预测模型的形成。随着技术不断发展，这些混合预测模型将帮助临床医生更好地诊断、治疗和了解阿尔茨海默病。然而，大数据阿尔茨海默病研究仍有重大的障碍需要克服。研究人员必须克服限制大数据研究的伦理和组织界限。因此，研究人员必须不断创新，并将大数据技术应用于阿尔茨海默病的研究。我们希望可以利用大数据改善阿尔茨海默病患者的生活，并最终治愈这种疾病。

参考文献

1. World Health Organization. (2017). Global action plan on the public health response to dementia 2017-2025. https://www.who.int/mental_health/neurology/dementia/action_plan_2017_2025/en/.
2. Alzheimer's Disease International. (2019). Dementia statistics. Alzheimer's Disease International. https://www.alz.co.uk/research/statistics.
3. Alzheimer's Association. (2018). 2018 Alzheimer's disease facts and figures. Alzheimer's & Dementia, 14(3), 367-429.
4. World Health Organization. (2018). Global Health Estimates 2016: Deaths by cause, age, sex, by country and by region, 2000-2016. https://www.who.int/gho/mortality_burden_disease/causes_death/top_10/en/.
5. Dubois, B., Feldman, H. H., Jacova, C., Cummings, J. L., DeKosky, S. T., Barberger Gateau, P., ... Scheltens, P. (2010). Revising the definition of Alzheimer's disease: A new lexicon. The Lancet Neurology, 9(11), 1118-1127. Available from https://doi.org/10.1016/S1474-4422(10)70223-4.
6. American Psychiatric Association. (2013). Diagnostic and Statistical Manual of Mental Disorders (5th Ed.). American Psychiatric Publishing.
7. Bastin, C., & Salmon, E. (2014). Early neuropsychological detection of Alzheimer's disease. European Journal of Clinical Nutrition, 68(11), 1192-1199. Available from https://doi.org/10.1038/ejcn.2014.176.
8. Perry, R. J., Watson, P., & Hodges, J. R. (2000). The nature and staging of attention dysfunction in early (minimal and mild) Alzheimer's disease: Relationship to episodic and semantic memory impairment. Neuropsychologia, 38(3), 252-271. Available from https://doi.org/10.1016/S0028-3932(99)00079-2.
9. Doraiswamy, P. M., Leon, J., Cummings, J. L., Marin, D., & Neumann, P. J. (2002). Prevalence and impact of medical comorbidity in Alzheimer's disease. The Journals of Gerontology: Series A, Biological Sciences and Medical Sciences, 57(3), M173-M177. Available from https://doi.org/10.1093/gerona/57.3.M173.
10. Wada, H., Nakajoh, K., Satoh-Nakagawa, T., Suzuki, T., Ohrui, T., Arai, H., & Sasaki, H. (2001). Risk factors of aspiration pneumonia in Alzheimer's disease patients. Gerontology, 47(5), 271-276. Available from https://doi.org/10.1159/000052811.

11. Bloom, G. S. (2014). Amyloid-β and tau: The trigger and bullet in Alzheimer disease pathogenesis. JAMA Neurology, 71(4), 505-508. Available from https://doi.org/10.1001/jamaneurol.2013.5847.
12. Sharma, N., & Singh, A. N. (2016). Exploring biomarkers for Alzheimer's disease. Journal of Clinical and Diagnostic Research: JCDR, 10(7), KE01 KE06. Available from https://doi.org/10.7860/JCDR/2016/18828.8166.
13. Yankner, B. A., Duffy, L. K., & Kirschner, D. Λ. (1990). Neurotrophic and neurotoxic effects of amyloid beta protein: Reversal by tachykinin neuropeptides. Science (New York, N.Y.), 250(4978), 279-282. Available from https://doi.org/10.1126/ science.2218531.
14. Iqbal, K., Liu, F., Gong, C.-X., & Grundke-Iqbal, I. (2010). Tau in Alzheimer disease and related tauopathies. Current Alzheimer Research, 7(8), 656-664.
15. Jack, C. R., Knopman, D. S., Jagust, W. J., Shaw, L. M., Aisen, P. S., Weiner, M. W., ... Trojanowski, J. Q. (2010). Hypothetical model of dynamic biomarkers of the Alzheimer's pathological cascade. Lancet Neurology, 9(1), 119. Available from https://doi.org/10.1016/S1474-4422(09)70299-6.
16. El Haj, M., Antoine, P., Amouyel, P., Lambert, J.-C., Pasquier, F., & Kapogiannis, D. (2016). Apolipoprotein E (APOE) ε4 and episodic memory decline in Alzheimer's disease: A review. Ageing Research Reviews, 27, 15-22. Available from https://doi.org/10.1016/j.arr.2016.02.002.
17. Murphy, M. P., & LeVine, H. (2010). Alzheimer's disease and the β-amyloid peptide. Journal of Alzheimer's Disease: JAD, 19(1), 311. Available from https://doi.org/10.3233/JAD-2010-1221.
18. Rodrigue, K. M., Kennedy, K. M., Devous, M. D., Rieck, J. R., Hebrank, A. C., DiazArrastia, R., ... Park, D. C. (2012). β-Amyloid burden in healthy aging. Neurology,78(6), 387-395. Available from https://doi.org/10.1212/WNL.0b013e318245d295.
19. Bartus, R. T., Dean, R. L., Beer, B., & Lippa, A. S. (1982). The cholinergic hypothesis of geriatric memory dysfunction. Science (New York, N.Y.), 217(4558), 408-414. Available from https://doi.org/10.1126/science.7046051.
20. Craig, L. A., Hong, N. S., & McDonald, R. J. (2011). Revisiting the cholinergic hypothesis in the development of Alzheimer's disease. Neuroscience & Biobehavioral Reviews, 35(6), 1397-1409. Available from https://doi.org/10.1016/ j.neubiorev.2011.03.001.
21. Feldman, H., Gauthier, S., Hecker, J., Vellas, B., Emir, B., Mastey, V., ... Group, T. D. M. S. I. (2003). Efficacy of donepezil on maintenance of activities of daily living in patients with moderate to severe Alzheimer's disease and the effect on caregiver burden. Journal of the American Geriatrics Society, 51(6), 737-744. Available from https://doi.org/10.1046/j.1365-2389.2003.51260.x.

22. Bradway, C., Trotta, R., Bixby, M. B., McPartland, E., Wollman, M. C., Kapustka, H., ... Naylor, M. D. (2012). A qualitative analysis of an advanced practice nurse-directed transitional care model intervention. The Gerontologist, 52(3), 394 -407. Available from https://doi.org/10.1093/geront/gnr078.

23. Edvardsson, D., Fetherstonhaugh, D., & Nay, R. (2010). Promoting a continuation of self and normality: Person-centred care as described by people with dementia, their family members and aged care staff. Journal of Clinical Nursing, 19(17-18), 2611-2618. Available from https://doi.org/10.1111/j.1365-2702.2009.03143.x.

24. Tan, C.-C., Yu, J.-T., Wang, H.-F., Tan, M.-S., Meng, X.-F., Wang, C., ... Tan, L. (2014). Efficacy and safety of donepezil, galantamine, rivastigmine, and memantine for the treatment of Alzheimer's disease: A systematic review and meta-analysis. Journal of Alzheimer's Disease, 41(2), 615-631. Available from https://doi.org/10.3233/JAD-132690.

25. Cummings, J., Lai, T., Hemrungrojn, S., Mohandas, E., Yun Kim, S., Nair, G., & Dash, A.(2016). Role of donepezil in the management of neuropsychiatric symptoms in Alzheimer's disease and dementia with Lewy bodies. CNS Neuroscience & Therapeutics, 22(3), 159-166. Available from https://doi.org/10.1111/cns.12484.

26. Ma, Y., Ji, J., Li, G., Yang, S., & Pan, S. (2018). Effects of donepezil on cognitive functions and the expression level of β-amyloid in peripheral blood of patients with Alzheimer's disease. Experimental and Therapeutic Medicine, 15(2), 1875-1878.

27. Small, G., & Bullock, R. (2011). Defining optimal treatment with cholinesterase inhibitors in Alzheimer's disease. Alzheimer's & Dementia, 7(2), 177-184. Available from https://doi.org/10.1016/j.jalz.2010.03.016.

28. Yiannopoulou, K. G., & Papageorgiou, S. G. (2013). Current and future treatments for Alzheimer's disease. Therapeutic Advances in Neurological Disorders, 6(1), 19-33. Available from https://doi.org/10.1177/1756285612461679.

29. McKhann, G. M., Knopman, D. S., Chertkow, H., Hyman, B. T., Jack, C. R., Jr., Kawas,C H., ... Phelps, C. H. (2011). The diagnosis of dementia due to Alzheimer's disease: Recommendations from the National Institute on Aging-Alzheimer's Association workgroups on diagnostic guidelines for Alzheimer's disease. Alzheimer's & Dementia, 7(3), 263-269. Available from https://doi.org/10.1016/j.jalz.2011.03.005.

30. Brown, J. (2015). The use and misuse of short cognitive tests in the diagnosis of dementia. Journal of Neurology, Neurosurgery & Psychiatry, 86(6), 680-685. Available from https://doi.org/10.1136/jnnp-2014-309086.

31. Larner, A. J. (2019). Evaluating cognitive screening instruments with the "likelihood to be diagnosed or misdiagnosed" measure. International Journal of Clinical Practice, 73(2), e13265. Available from https://doi.org/10.1111/ijcp.13265.

32. Kalat, J. W. (2018). Biological psychology (13th ed). Cengage.
33. Edvardsson, D., Winblad, B., & Sandman, P. (2008). Person-centred care of people with severe Alzheimer's disease: Current status and ways forward. The Lancet Neurology, 7(4), 362-367. Available from https://doi.org/10.1016/S1474-4422(08)70063-2.
34. Jack, C. R., Albert, M., Knopman, D. S., McKhann, G. M., Sperling, R. A., Carillo, M., ... Phelps, C. H. (2011). Introduction to revised criteria for the diagnosis of Alzheimer's disease: National Institute on Aging and the Alzheimer Association Workgroups. Alzheimer's & Dementia, 7(3), 257-262. Available from https://doi.org/10.1016/j.jalz.2011.03.004.
35. Csukly, G., Sirály, E., Fodor, Z., Horváth, A., Salacz, P., Hidasi, Z., ... Szabó, Á. (2016). The differentiation of amnestic type MCI from the non-amnestic types by structural MRI. Frontiers in Aging Neuroscience, 8. Available from https://doi.org/10.3389/fnagi.2016.00052.
36. Albert, M. S., DeKosky, S. T., Dickson, D., Dubois, B., Feldman, H. H., Fox, N. C., ... Phelps, C. H. (2011). The diagnosis of mild cognitive impairment due to Alzheimer's disease: Recommendations from the National Institute on Aging-Alzheimer's Association workgroups on diagnostic guidelines for Alzheimer's disease. Alzheimer's & Dementia, 7(3), 270-279. Available from https://doi.org/10.1016/j.jalz.2011.03.008.
37. Roberts, R., Geda, Y., Knopman, D., Cha, R., Pankratz, V., Boeve, B., ... Rocca, W. (2008). The Mayo Clinic Study of Aging: Design and sampling, participation, baseline measures and sample characteristics. Neuroepidemiology, 30(1), 58-69. Available from https://doi.org/10.1159/000115751.
38. Watson, J. L., Ryan, L., Silverberg, N., Cahan, V., & Bernard, M. A. (2014). Obstacles and opportunities in Alzheimer's clinical trial recruitment. Health Affairs (Project Hope), 33(4), 574-579. Available from https://doi.org/10.1377/hlthaff.2013.1314.
39. Stites, S. D., Milne, R., & Karlawish, J. (2018). Advances in Alzheimer's imaging are changing the experience of Alzheimer's disease. Alzheimer's & Dementia: Diagnosis, Assessment & Disease Monitoring, 10, 285-300. Available from https://doi.org/10.1016/j.dadm.2018.02.006.
40. Braak, H., & Del Tredici, K. (2011). The pathological process underlying Alzheimer's disease in individuals under thirty. Acta Neuropathologica, 121(2), 171-181. Available from https://doi.org/10.1007/s00401-010-0789-4.
41. Mueller, S. G., Weiner, M. W., Thal, L. J., Petersen, R. C., Jack, C., Jagust, W., ... Beckett, L. (2005). The Alzheimer's Disease Neuroimaging Initiative. Neuroimaging Clinics of North America, 15(4), 869. Available from https://doi.org/10.1016/j.nic.2005.09.008, xii.

42. Alzheimer's Disease Neuroimaging Initiative. (2017a). ADNI about. Alzheimer's Disease Neuroimaging Initiative. http://adni.loni.usc.edu/about/.
43. Alzheimer's Disease Neuroimaging Initiative. (2017b). ADNI data types. Alzheimer's Disease Neuroimaging Initiative. http://adni.loni.usc.edu/data-samples/data-types/.
44. Papale, D., Agarwal, D. A., Baldocchi, D., Cook, R. B., Fisher, J. B., & van Ingen, C. (2012). Database maintenance, data sharing policy, collaboration. In M. Aubinet, T. Vesala, & D. Papale (Eds.), Eddy covariance: a practical guide to measurement and data analysis (pp. 399-424). Netherlands: Springer. Available from https://doi.org/10.1007/978-94-007-2351-1_17.
45. Pearlson, G. (2009). Multisite collaborations and large databases in psychiatric neuroimaging: Advantages, problems, and challenges. Schizophrenia Bulletin, 35(1), 1-2. Available from https://doi.org/10.1093/schbul/sbn166.
46. Olfson, M., Wall, M. M., & Blanco, C. (2017). Incentivizing data sharing and collaboration in medical research-The S-index. JAMA Psychiatry, 74(1), 5-6. Available from https://doi.org/10.1001/jamapsychiatry.2016.2610.
47. Toga, A. W., Bhatt, P., & Ashish, N. (2016). Global data sharing in Alzheimer's disease research. Alzheimer Disease and Associated Disorders, 30(2), 160-168. Available from https://doi.org/10.1097/WAD.0000000000000121.
48. Martone, M. E., Garcia-Castro, A., & VandenBos, G. R. (2018). Data sharing in psychology. The American Psychologist, 73(2), 111-125. Available from https://doi.org/10.1037/amp0000242.
49. Geerts, H., Dacks, P. A., Devanarayan, V., Haas, M., Khachaturian, Z. S., Gordon, M. F., ... Stephenson, D. (2016). Big data to smart data in Alzheimer's disease: The brain health modeling initiative to foster actionable knowledge. Alzheimer's & Dementia, 12(9), 1014-1021. Available from https://doi.org/10.1016/j.jalz.2016.04.008.
50. Vikström, P., Edvinsson, S., & Brändström, A. (2002). Longitudinal databases-Sources for analyzing the life-course: Characteristics, difficulties and possibilities. History and Computing, 14(12), 109-128. Available from https://doi.org/10.3366/hac.2002.14.1-2.109.
51. Cook, D. A., Andriole, D. A., Durning, S. J., Roberts, N. K., & Triola, M. M. (2010). Longitudinal research databases in medical education: Facilitating the study of educational outcomes over time and across institutions. Academic Medicine, 85(8), 1340-1346. Available from https://doi.org/10.1097/ACM.0b013e3181e5c050.
52. Nakagawa, S., & Freckleton, R. P. (2008). Missing inaction: The dangers of ignoring missing data. Trends in Ecology & Evolution, 23(11), 592-596. Available from https://doi.org/10.1016/j.tree.2008.06.014.
53. Schmitt, C. P., & Burchinal, M. (2011). Data management practices for collaborative

research. Frontiers in Psychiatry, 2. Available from https://doi.org/10.3389/fpsyt.2011.00047.

54. Fan, J., Han, F., & Liu, H. (2014). Challenges of big data analysis. National Science Review, 1(2), 293-314. Available from https://doi.org/10.1093/nsr/nwt032.

55. Moradi, E., Hallikainen, I., Hänninen, T., Tohka, J., & Alzheimer's Disease Neuroimaging Initiative. (2017). Rey's Auditory Verbal Learning Test scores can be predicted from whole brain MRI in Alzheimer's disease. NeuroImage. Clinical, 13, 415-427. Available from https://doi.org/10.1016/j.nicl.2016.12.011.

56. Eaton, M. L. (2001). Invariance in statistics. In N. J. Smelser, & P. B. Baltes (Eds.), International encyclopedia of the social & behavioral sciences (pp. 7893-7897). Pergamon. Available from https://doi.org/10.1016/B0-08-043076-7/00529-5.

57. Forlenza, O. V., Diniz, B. S., Talib, L. L., Radanovic, M., Yassuda, M. S., Ojopi, E. B., & Gattaz, W. F. (2010). Clinical and biological predictors of Alzheimer's disease in patients with amnestic mild cognitive impairment. Revista Brasileira De Psiquiatria, 32(3), 216-222.

58. Mayer, D. G., & Butler, D. G. (1993). Statistical validation. Ecological Modelling, 68(1), 21-32. Available from https://doi.org/10.1016/0304-3800(93)90105-2.

59. Doody, R. S., Pavlik, V., Massman, P., Rountree, S., Darby, E., & Chan, W. (2010). Predicting progression of Alzheimer's disease. Alzheimer's Research & Therapy, 2(1), 2. Available from https://doi.org/10.1186/alzrt25.

60. Ethington, C. A., Thomas, S. L., & Pike, G. R. (2002). Back to the basics: Regression as it should be. In J. C. Smart, & W. G. Tierney (Eds.), Higher education: handbook of theory and research (pp. 263-293). Netherlands: Springer. Available from https://doi.org/10.1007/978-94-010-0245-5_6.

61. Schneider, A., Hommel, G., & Blettner, M. (2010). Linear regression analysis. Deutsches Ärzteblatt International, 107(44), 776-782. Available from https://doi.org/10.3238/arztebl.2010.0776.

62. Yoo, C., Ramirez, L., & Liuzzi, J. (2014). Big data analysis using modern statistical and machine learning methods in medicine. International Neurourology Journal, 18(2), 50-57. Available from https://doi.org/10.5213/inj.2014.18.2.50.

63. Leech, N. L., Gliner, J. A., Morgan, G. A., & Harmon, R. J. (2003). Use and interpretation of multiple regression. Journal of the American Academy of Child & Adolescent Psychiatry, 42(6), 738-740. Available from https://doi.org/10.1097/01.CHI.0000046845.56865.22.

64. Pandis, N. (2016). Multiple linear regression analysis. American Journal of Orthodontics and Dentofacial Orthopedics, 149(4), 581. Available from https://doi.org/10.1016/

j.ajodo.2016.01.012.
65. Passamonti, L., Tsvetanov, K. A., Jones, P. S., Bevan-Jones, W. R., Arnold, R., Borchert, R. J., ... Rowe, J. B. (2019). Neuroinflammation and functional connectivityin Alzheimer's disease: Interactive influences on cognitive performance. Journal of Neuroscience, 39(36), 7218-7226. Available from https://doi.org/10.1523/ JNEUROSCI.2574-18.2019.
66. Gandomi, A., & Haider, M. (2015). Beyond the hype: Big data concepts, methods, and analytics. International Journal of Information Management, 35(2), 137-144. Available from https://doi.org/10.1016/j.ijinfomgt.2014.10.007.
67. MacKinnon, D. P., Krull, J. L., & Lockwood, C. M. (2000). Equivalence of the mediation, confounding and suppression effect. Prevention Science, 1(4), 173-181. Available from https://doi.org/10.1023/A:1026595011371.
68. Beckstead, J. W. (2012). Isolating and examining sources of suppression and multicollinearity in multiple linear regression. Multivariate Behavioral Research, 47(2), 224-246. Available from https://doi.org/10.1080/00273171.2012.658331.
69. Kraha, A., Turner, H., Nimon, K., Zientek, L., & Henson, R. (2012). Tools to support interpreting multiple regression in the face of multicollinearity. Frontiers in Psychology, 3. Available from https://doi.org/10.3389/fpsyg.2012.00044.
70. Saraceno, C., Musardo, S., Marcello, E., Pelucchi, S., & Diluca, M. (2013). Modeling Alzheimer's disease: From past to future. Frontiers in Pharmacology, 4. Available from https://doi.org/10.3389/fphar.2013.00077.
71. Hunt, C. A., Ropella, G. E. P., Park, S., & Engelberg, J. (2008). Dichotomies between computational and mathematical models. Nature Biotechnology, 26(7), 737-738. Available from https://doi.org/10.1038/nbt0708-737.
72. Geerts, H., Hofmann-Apitius, M., Anastasio, T. J., & Brain Health Modeling Initiative. (2017). Knowledge-driven computational modeling in Alzheimer's disease research: Current state and future trends. Alzheimer's & Dementia, 13(11), 1292-1302. Available from https://doi.org/10.1016/j.jalz.2017.08.011.
73. Kumar, A., & Singh, T. R. (2017). A new decision tree to solve the puzzle of Alzheimer's disease pathogenesis through standard diagnosis scoring system. Interdisciplinary Sciences, Computational Life Sciences, 9(1), 107-115. Available from https://doi.org/10.1007/s12539-016-0144-0.
74. Loh, W.-Y. (2011). Classification and regression trees. WIREs Data Mining and Knowledge Discovery, 1(1), 14-23. Available from https://doi.org/10.1002/widm.8.
75. Hassan, M., Abbas, Q., Seo, S.-Y., Shahzadi, S., Ashwal, H. A., Zaki, N., ... Moustafa, A. (2018). Computational modeling and biomarker studies of pharmacological treatment of Alzheimer's disease. Molecular Medicine Reports, 18(1), 639-655. Available from

https://doi.org/10.3892/mmr.2018.9044.

76. Petrella, J. R., Hao, W., Rao, A., & Doraiswamy, P. M. (2019). Computational causal modeling of the dynamic biomarker cascade in Alzheimer's disease. Computational and Mathematical Methods in Medicine, 2019, 6216530, Hindawi. Available from https://doi.org/10.1155/2019/6216530.

77. Häyrinen, K., Saranto, K., & Nykänen, P. (2008). Definition, structure, content, use andimpacts of electronic health records: A review of the research literature. International Journal of Medical Informatics, 77(5), 291-304. Available from https://doi.org/10.1016/j.ijmedinf.2007.09.001.

78. Jensen, P. B., Jensen, L. J., & Brunak, S. (2012). Mining electronic health records: Towards better research applications and clinical care. Nature Reviews. Genetics, 13(6), 395-405. Available from https://doi.org/10.1038/nrg3208.

79. Amra, S., O'Horo, J. C., Singh, T. D., Wilson, G. A., Kashyap, R., Petersen, R., ... Gajic, O. (2017). Derivation and validation of the automated search algorithms to identify cognitive impairment and dementia in electronic health records. Journal of Critical Care, 37, 202-205. Available from https://doi.org/10.1016/j.jcrc.2016.09.026.

80. Perera, G., Pedersen, L., Ansel, D., Alexander, M., Arrighi, H. M., Avillach, P., ... Stewart, R. (2018). Dementia prevalence and incidence in a federation of European Electronic Health Record databases: The European Medical Informatics Framework resource. Alzheimer's & Dementia, 14(2), 130-139. Available from https://doi.org/10.1016/j.jalz.2017.06.2270.

81. Sabbagh MN, Boada M, Borson S, Chilukuri M, Dubois B, Ingram J, ... Hampel H. (2020). Early detection of mild cognitive impairment (MCI) in primary care. https://doi.org/10.14283/JPAD.2020.21.

82. Clionsky, M., & Clionsky, E. (2012). P4-277: The MOST-96120 iPad app improves PCP Alzheimer's disease screening. Alzheimer's & Dementia, 8(4 Suppl. Part 20), S755-S756. Available from https://doi.org/10.1016/j.jalz.2013.08.058.

83. Clionsky, M., & Clionsky, E. (2016). Dementia and the brain-breathing connection. Journal of Alzheimer's Disease & Parkinsonism, 06(06). Available from https://doi.org/10.4172/2161-0460.1000e135.

84. Ienca, M., Vayena, E., & Blasimme, A. (2018). Big data and dementia: Charting the route ahead for research, ethics, and policy. Frontiers in Medicine, 5. Available from https://doi.org/10.3389/fmed.2018.00013.

85. Quest Diagnostics. (2015). CogniSense™ iPad App for cognitive impairment screening. CogniSense. http://www.questcognisense.com/.

86. McCall, C. (2018). Opt-out digital health records cause debate in Australia. The Lancet,

392(10145), 372. Available from https://doi.org/10.1016/S0140-6736(18)31726-4.
87. Arribas-Ayllon, M. (2011). The ethics of disclosing genetic diagnosis for Alzheimer's disease: Do we need a new paradigm? British Medical Bulletin, 100(1), 7-21. Available from https://doi.org/10.1093/bmb/ldr023, http://orca.cf.ac.uk/view/cardiffauthors/A063035C.html.
88. Post, S. G., Whitehouse, P. J., Binstock, R. H., Bird, T. D., Eckert, S. K., Farrer, L. A., ... Zinn, A. B. (1997). The clinical introduction of genetic testing for Alzheimer disease: An ethical perspective. JAMA: The Journal of the American Medical Association, 277(10), 832-836. Available from https://doi.org/10.1001/jama.1997.03540340066035.
89. Alzheimer's Disease Neuroimaging Initiative. (2016). ADNI3 protocol. http://adni.loni.usc.edu/wp-content/themes/freshnews-dev-v2/documents/clinical/ADNI3_Protocol.pdf.
90. Natelson Love, M., Clark, D. G., Cochran, J. N., Den Beste, K. A., Geldmacher, D. S., Benzinger, T. L., ... Roberson, E. D. (2017). Clinical, imaging, pathological, and biochemical characterization of a novel presenilin 1 mutation (N135Y) causing Alzheimer's disease. Neurobiology of Aging, 49, 216.e7-216.e13. Available from https://doi.org/10.1016/j.neurobiolaging.2016.09.020.
91. Cui, Y., Liu, B., Luo, S., Zhen, X., Fan, M., Liu, T., ... Alzheimer's Disease Neuroimaging Initiative. (2011). Identification of conversion from mild cognitive impairment to Alzheimer's disease using multivariate predictors. PLoS One, 6(7), e21896. Available from https://doi.org/10.1371/journal.pone.0021896.
92. Davatzikos, C., Bhatt, P., Shaw, L. M., Batmanghelich, K. N., & Trojanowski, J. Q. (2011). Prediction of MCI to AD conversion, via MRI, CSF biomarkers, and pattern classification. Neurobiology of Aging, 32(12), 2322. Available from https://doi.org/10.1016/j.neurobiolaging.2010.05.023, e19-27.
93. Ewers, M., Brendel, M., Rizk-Jackson, A., Rominger, A., Bartenstein, P., Schuff, N., ... Alzheimer's Disease Neuroimaging Initiative (ADNI). (2014). Reduced FDG-PET brain metabolism and executive function predict clinical progression in elderly healthy subjects. NeuroImage. Clinical, 4, 45-52. Available from https://doi.org/10.1016/j.nicl.2013.10.018.
94. Landau, S. M., Mintun, M. A., Joshi, A. D., Koeppe, R. A., Petersen, R. C., Aisen, P. S., ... Jagust, W. J. (2012). Amyloid deposition, hypometabolism, and longitudinal cognitive decline. Annals of Neurology, 72(4), 578-586. Available from https://doi.org/10.1002/ana.23650.
95. Kato, Y., Narumoto, J., Matsuoka, T., Okamura, A., Koumi, H., Kishikawa, Y., ... Fukui, K. (2013). Diagnostic performance of a combination of Mini-Mental State Examinationand Clock Drawing Test in detecting Alzheimer's disease. Neuropsychiatric

Disease and Treatment, 9, 581-586. Available from https://doi.org/10.2147/NDT.S42209.

96. Swain, D. G., O'Brien, A. G., & Nightingale, P. G. (1999). Cognitive assessment in elderly patients admitted to hospital: The relationship between the Abbreviated Mental Test and the Mini-Mental State Examination. Clinical Rehabilitation, 13(6), 503-508. Available from https://doi.org/10.1191/026921599670895633.

97. Ramanan, V., Shen, L., Risacher, S., Kim, S., Boddu, M., West, J., ... Saykin, A. (2012). Hippocampal subfield atrophy in the Alzheimer's Disease Neuroimaging Initiative (ADNI) cohort: Relationships to diagnosis and memory impairment. Alzheimer's & Dementia, 8(4 Suppl.), P533 P534. Available from https://doi.org/10.1016/j.jalz.2012.05.1434.

98. Ihara, R., Iwata, A., Suzuki, K., Ikeuchi, T., Kuwano, R., & Iwatsubo, T. (2018). Clinical and cognitive characteristics of preclinical Alzheimer's disease in the Japanese Alzheimer's disease neuroimaging initiative cohort. Alzheimer's & Dementia: Translational Research & Clinical Interventions, 4, 645-651. Available from https://doi.org/10.1016/j.trci.2018.10.004.

99. Huang, K., Lin, Y., Yang, L., Wang, Y., Cai, S., Pang, L., ... Huang, L. (2020). A multipredictor model to predict the conversion of mild cognitive impairment to Alzheimer's disease by using a predictive nomogram. Neuropsychopharmacology: Official Publication of the American College of Neuropsychopharmacology, 45(2), 358-366. Available from https://doi.org/10.1038/s41386-019-0551-0.

100. Weiner, M. W., Veitch, D. P., Aisen, P. S., Beckett, L. A., Cairns, N. J., Cedarbaum, J., ... Alzheimer's Disease Neuroimaging Initiative. (2015). 2014 Update of the Alzheimer's Disease Neuroimaging Initiative: A review of papers published since its inception. Alzheimer's & Dementia, 11(6). Available from https://doi.org/10.1016/j.jalz.2014.11.001,e1-120.

101. Weiner, M. W., Veitch, D. P., Aisen, P. S., Beckett, L. A., Cairns, N. J., Green, R. C., ... Alzheimer's Disease Neuroimaging Initiative. (2013). The Alzheimer's Disease Neuroimaging Initiative: A review of papers published since its inception. Alzheimer's & Dementia, 9(5), e111-e194. Available from https://doi.org/10.1016/j.jalz.2013.05.1769.

第八章 阿尔茨海默病的深度学习方法概况

Samuel L. Warren, Ahmed A. Moustafa, Dustin van der Haar 编

成蔚阳, 梁灼源 译

屈剑锋 校

第一节 引言

阿尔茨海默病（AD）以严重的认知功能下降和神经退行性病变为特征, 是痴呆最常见的类型[1]。近数十年来, 尽管针对阿尔茨海默病的诊断和治疗已进行了广泛的研究, 但仍远远不够。例如, 目前容易将其他不同形式的痴呆诊断为阿尔茨海默病（如将血管性痴呆诊断为阿尔茨海默病）, 同时缺乏针对疾病早期或潜在可逆性阶段进行检测的方法[2,3]。现阶段尚没有治愈阿尔茨海默病的方法, 该病仍然是全球范围内死亡的主要原因之一[4]。因此, 在阿尔茨海默病早期及可治疗阶段找到明确疾病诊断的方法显得尤为迫切。

既往研究者利用统计模型（如线性回归）来预测阿尔茨海默病的早期阶段, 以实现在可治疗阶段对疾病的识别(详见Xu等[5])。然而, 这些模型往往过于简单, 并不能完全概括阿尔茨海默病复杂且多因素的本质。因此, 神经科学研究正逐步从统计学诊断方法过渡到计算机处理的诊断方法（如机器学习和深度学习）。计算机辅助诊断（Computer-assisted Diagnosis, CAD）的兴起得益于多种技术和科学的进步。例如, 计算机辅助诊断的发展与人工智能（Artificial Intelligence, AI）、计算机硬件（如计算机处理单元）、数据共享、开源软件、神经影像技术[如磁共振成像（MRI）]以及阿尔茨海默病生物标志物的发现息息相关[6-8]。通过这些先进技术的应用, 计算机辅助诊断方法已经能够克服以往统计学方法中存在的一些局限性（例如, 简化阿尔茨海默病的表现, 诊断准确性不高）。

在阿尔茨海默病的研究中，CAD通常分为机器学习和深度学习两大领域。无论机器学习，还是深度学习，两者都属于对数据进行计算处理和分类的人工智能技术。但两者的复杂性、方法论和独立性是不同的。机器学习方法相对传统且简单。这种传统计算机辅助诊断方法通过使用多个统计学测试来识别、提取和分类数据[9]。然而，该分法存在着一定的局限性。例如，需要耗费大量时间，需要进行监督，并且缺乏临床实践应用[10]。与之相反，深度学习方法是使用神经网络模仿人类学习的新技术[11]。其优于传统的计算机辅助诊断方法，因为深度学习更高效，可以在不需要监督的情况下运行，并且对阿尔茨海默病的识别有更高的准确度[12]。因此，基于深度学习的计算机辅助诊断系统正在给阿尔茨海默病研究带来革命性的变化。

本章描述了深度学习方法在阿尔茨海默病研究中的应用和操作。将对以下几个问题进行论述：①传统CAD方法及其对深度学习计算机辅助诊断系统的启示；②深度学习方法在阿尔茨海默病研究中的应用；③深度学习方法在阿尔茨海默病研究中的优势和局限性。希望读者可以对基于深度学习的计算机辅助诊断系统有一个深入的了解，从而促进对阿尔茨海默病诊断和治疗的进一步研究。

第二节　传统阿尔茨海默病CAD方法的趋势

一、引言

传统的CAD方法使用统计学和机器学习技术来检测阿尔茨海默病[9]。因其具备分析大数据集和准确检测阿尔茨海默病的性能而在研究中备受欢迎。因此，传统的CAD模型普遍应用于精简数据分析并为阿尔茨海默病诊断提供信息（例如，提供次选意见）[13]。然而，传统CAD方法存在一定的局限性（例如，缺乏自主性和可推广性），导致其临床应用受限[10,14]。

因此，在阿尔茨海默病的研究中，传统的CAD模型正在被深度学习方法所取代。深度学习模型之所以备受青睐，是因为它们准确性较高，并且可以克服传统CAD模型的许多限制[12]。例如，与大多数传统方法不同[15]，深度学习模型无须在监督下运行。尽管如此,传统的 CAD 模型仍然发挥着作用,其与深度学习方法也有许多相似之处。因此,在了解新兴的深度学习模型之前,我们有必要回顾、梳理传统的 CAD 方法。本节将讨论传统 CAD 研究的常用方法和步骤。

二、传统 CAD 方法在阿尔茨海默病研究中的应用

传统的 CAD 模型包括 3 个步骤:数据预处理、特征提取以及分类(图 8-1)[16]。数据预处理的目的是对数据集进行清理和归一化;特征提取是为了识别和分离出感兴趣的变量;分类则旨在训练、测试和评估诊断模型[17]。每个步骤采用不同的统计和计算方法处理 AD 数据。在这些方法中,研究人员通常会根据收集的数据类型选择特定的分析方法。例如,采用统计转换预处理脑影像(如磁共振成像)的方法不同于研究脑电信号(如脑电图)的方法[18]。

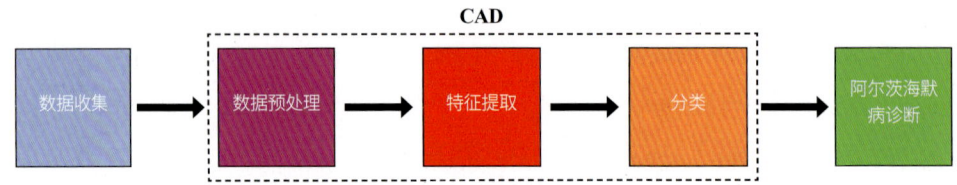

图 8-1 传统的计算机辅助诊断流程

由于技术和数据收集方法的普及,某些方法更容易受到研究者们青睐。例如,在传统的 CAD 研究中,神经影像学生物标志物常用于阿尔茨海默病的诊断(例如,MRI 脑体积测量)。这些成像方法因直观、无创、诊断准确率高等优点而备受青睐[10,17]。因此,在阿尔茨海默病研究中 CAD 方法大多侧重于神经影像学数据的处理和分析。少数研究使用其他阿尔茨海默病诊断方法(例如,记忆测试)进行诊断。然而,这些非成像方法是极其少的[19]。因此,本节概述了传统 CAD 研究的 3 个阶段,重点是神经影像学方法。

(一)数据预处理

数据预处理是传统计算机辅助诊断方法的第一步。在预处理阶段,研究者需对数据进行清理、归一化和转换,以便于进行特征提取[20]。数据预处理阶段

是 CAD 模型建立的基础，对 CAD 模型的分类精度起到至关重要的作用。因此，在预处理过程中必须恰当地对数据进行获取、清理和管理。在计算机辅助诊断研究中，数据预处理通常涉及简化和标准化神经影像的统计或计算变换。

统计参数图（Statistical Parametric Mapping，SPM）和基于体素的形态测量学（Voxel-based Morphometry，VBM）是使用最广泛的技术[21]。SPM 通过对各组图像进行统计分析和比较，以突出神经系统的差异[22]，其还通常涉及图像的比对、均化和单变量分析。与之类似，VBM 利用 SPM 技术比较图像，但通过脑组织体素的计算比较来突出神经系统差异（体素是大脑的计算像素或三维表征）[23]。SPM 和 VBM 技术都有相应的软件（如 SPM12 和 Free Surfer）可以精简和半自动化数据预处理。

（二）特征提取

特征提取是 CAD 方法学的第二步。在特征提取阶段，对感兴趣的变量进行识别、分离和处理[19]。该阶段旨在检测和细化变量以便于下一步分类，通常分为三个步骤，即特征选择、提取和降维（也称维数约化）[24]。首先，特征选择对感兴趣的区域或变量进行识别和分类。接下来，特征提取将感兴趣的区域或变量从图像或数据中分离出来。最后，特征降维通过对数据进行压缩，以减轻分类过程中的数据处理负荷（特征降维主要用于成像数据）。

一些常用的特征提取处理方法有离散波变换、傅里叶分析、偏最小二乘法和主成分分析（Principal Component Analysis，PCA）[21]。这些方法大多使用数学转化或相关分析来处理特征。例如，PCA 是一种统计检验方法，根据相似变量之间的相互关系以实现对变量的识别和分组[25,26]。选择正确的特征提取技术对 CAD 模型的清晰度和准确性起到至关重要的作用。因此，理想的特征提取处理方法往往通过先前的研究和测试合适的数据集来确定。通过对多种特征提取技术进行对比，以确定哪种方法得到的 CAD 模型最准确，这也是研究中常见的方法[21]。

（三）分类

分类是传统 CAD 方法论的第三步，也是最后阶段。在分类阶段，通过对不同 CAD 方法的迭代训练、测试和评估，建立诊断模型[27]。这些训练、测试和评估的步骤都是环环相扣的，并且不断完善，从而构建出高精度的 CAD 模型。分类的初始步骤是对数据集进行分区，分别用于训练和测试诊断模型。有多种机器学习方法可用于训练和测试分类模型，如支持向量机、随机森林、逻辑回归等[16,17,28]。每个分类模型使用相似的分类技术以区分不同的诊断组（如 AD 组与对照组）。例如，支持向量机通过将数据（如脑容量）绘制在一个平面上，并根据数据点之间的关系来确定诊断（以训练类别为参考）[16,20]。

交叉验证技术通常用于确定训练和分类数据的特定机器学习方法。交叉验证技术贯穿在整个分类过程中，并通过比较不同的训练/测试标准和诊断方法来评估模型[29]。这种分类技术的评估一般是通过划分数据集并比较不同方法学（如支持向量机和逻辑回归）的结果来完成。例如，10 倍交叉验证将数据集分为 10 个偶数组，每组交替作为训练或测试组。同时，研究中也对一系列不同的分类方法进行了测试和比较。结果将指出哪种训练/测试组合和分类方法具备最高的诊断精度[30]。

三、外部因素对模型应用的影响

值得注意的是，数据预处理、特征提取和分类这些步骤并不是影响 CAD 模型精度和应用的唯一因素。数据质量和临床意见（例如，临床医生使用模型的意愿）等外部因素也会影响 CAD 模型的应用。在数据收集方面，重要的是明白数据集的质量和清晰度将直接影响 CAD 模型是否成功。在不考虑数据预处理和特征提取技术的前提下，一个弱类型数据集会导致 CAD 模型欠佳。另外，样本量小会导致模型不具有代表性且分类效果差。

因此，数据的质量高（例如，极少的缺失数据）及是否能代表 AD 患者的特征显得尤为重要。获得这些具有代表性和高质量数据往往比较困难。而大多数研究人员可以通过使用协作数据库来克服这些障碍。在具备高质量数据的数据集前提下，大多数 CAD 研究会取得成功（详见 Bi 等[15]，Ding 等[31]）。大部分的 AD 数据是从以下数据库中获取的，如阿尔茨海默病神经影像倡议（Alzheimer's

Disease Neuroimaging Initiative）等数据库；澳大利亚衰老成像、生物标志物和生活方式旗舰研究；英国生物银行和全球阿尔茨海默病协会互动网络（The Global Alzheimer's Association Interactive Network）。

同样重要的是，要了解临床医生对 CAD 模型的准确性和应用的影响。传统的 CAD 模型只能在监督下运行，而且依赖临床医生进行验证和诊断。因此，CAD 方法的成功取决于临床医生信任、使用和解释模型的能力[32]。如果临床医生认为一个模型不准确或时效性差，他们就不会使用它。因此，必须对 CAD 模型进行优化，以便临床医生找到可靠、对用户友好且易于解释的模型[14]。研究者在模型制作过程中应考虑到临床医生这一因素。研究人员还应该确保 CAD 模型在临床样本中的可靠性，并提供足够的训练资源。通过管理 CAD 模型和临床医生之间的关系，研究人员可以提高 CAD 的准确性和应用。

四、结论

本节概述了传统 CAD 的常见步骤以及影响诊断模型的外部因素。我们还讨论了用于预处理、提取和分类诊断数据的常用方法。虽然其中一些方法可能不会直接应用到深度学习模型中，但重要的是掌握其首要主题。传统 CAD 在诊断模型的可推广性和可监督性方面存在一定的局限性，但其复杂性和迭代性值得学习。因此，新兴的 CAD 方法应该借鉴传统 CAD 的迭代性和系统性。深度学习模型还应考虑到影响 CAD 应用的外部因素。如果能克服这些障碍，CAD 将给 AD 诊断带来革命性的变化。

第三节 深度学习情境下的阿尔茨海默病

一、引言

深度学习使 CAD 系统发生了革命性的变化。更多的数据获取、更好的硬件和创新的神经网络使得深度学习方法在许多领域都处于领先地位。深度学习开创了一个行业级方法的时代。这些方法不仅准确，而且能够容纳 CAD 系统中通常会发现的诸多有问题的数据。本节内容将对基于 AD 的深度学习进行拆解，并阐述传统方法向深度学习方法过渡的背景、深度学习方法的通常应用及其与传统方法的区别。最后探讨在 CAD 系统中使用的最流行模型结构和通用模型结构。

二、转变

传统的 CAD 方法是侧重于利用领域知识并最大化提高辨别能力的特征工程。例如，可以在 MRI 上概括内侧颞叶萎缩的特征[33]并进行分类。这些方法的性能取决于特征是如何设计的，以及机器学习模型是否适合区分 AD 的阳性和阴性病例。然而，传统方法可能会出现问题，因其需要专门的知识和多个优化阶段，这可能很耗时[11]。

深度学习方法采用不同的方式去构建特征和分类。它使用表征学习，在训练时间内"动态"生成特征，从而消除了需要创建专门的特征预处理和特征处理的过程，并实现了最先进的性能[34]。它使用人工神经网络（Artificial Neural Network，ANN），该网络由连接的神经元组成，这些神经元通过单独权重方法将每个神经元中发现的输入与后续输出对应，并通过使用激活函数进行调制，如图 8-2 所示。普通的 ANN[多层感知器（Multilayer Perceptron，MLP）]由输入层、中间层和输出层组成。然而，深度学习网络有更多的隐藏层，也由各种其他参数、层类型和架构组成，这将在"通用模型体系结构"一节中讨论。在这之前，将先讨论深度学习方法在典型 CAD 阶段运行，以及它与传统机器学习方法的比较。

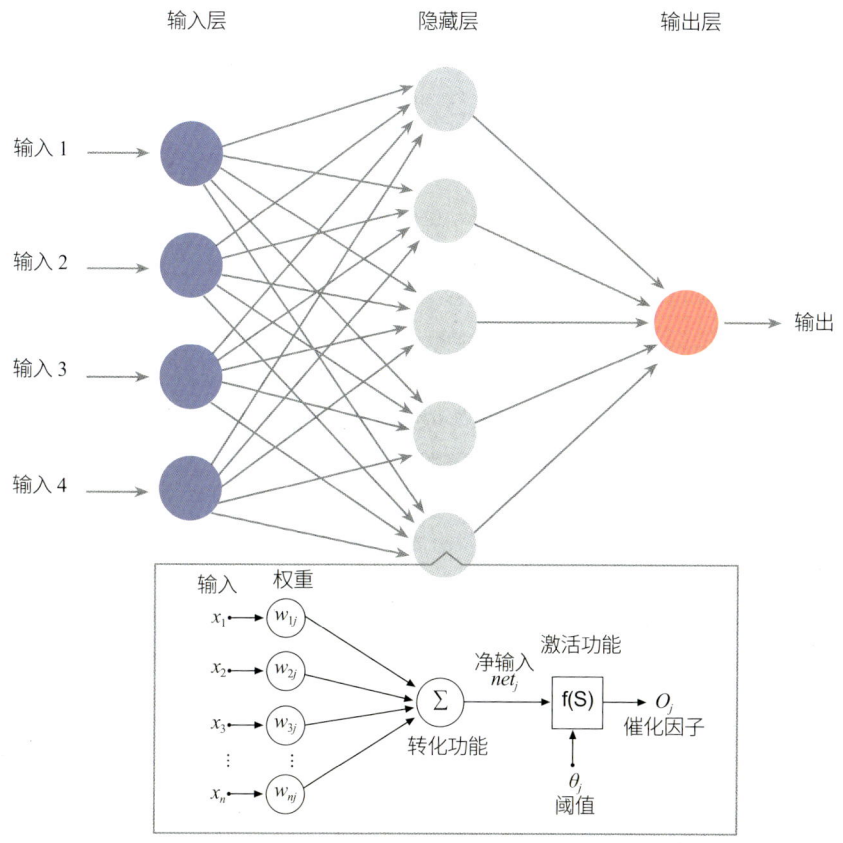

图 8-2 人工神经网络中的神经元

三、深度学习模型任务

深度学习方法可用于促进 CAD 系统中现有阶段的常见任务，如特征提取和分类，也可用于检测或分割任务，将其中感兴趣的区域分离以进行进一步分析。这些任务都将在以下部分中进行讨论。

（一）分割

首先是感兴趣区域分割或定位任务。感兴趣区域被分离或"裁剪"，提取整个图像或框架中的关键区域。通常，分割任务有 3 种不同的类型：目标检测、语义分割和实例分割。

在对象检测中，输出是一个矩形边界框，如图 8-3 所示，包含感兴趣的对象[具有左上角（x，y）坐标，以及宽度和高度]，以及模型所知对象的置信度度量（在训练时确定）。传统方法在滑动窗口上使用特征模块，如纹理[35]、梯度差异[36]或低维汇总[37]来分离感兴趣区。深度学习方法，如更快的基于区域的卷积神经网络（regional convolutional neural network，R-CNN）[38]、YOLO（You Only Look Once）[39]和 SSD（Single Shot Detection）[40]，它们使用区域候选网络或等效网络生成候选目标区域，并使用卷积神经网络（Convolutional Neural Network，CNN）对候选目标区域进行分类。这些方法最近在分离右心室心肌[41]、淋巴结转移瘤[42]甚至肺结节[43]方面取得了成功。

语义分割为图像中包含的每个像素提供了一个类别预测[44]，类似于图 8-3 所示的阴影区域，从而在识别图像的哪些部分比其他部分更重要方面提供了灵活性。从历史发展来看，医学技术人员最开始时采用手动执行语义分割，直到 21 世纪初，自动化技术才得以实现[45]。传统的语义分割方法包括使用基于图谱或模板的分割[46]和可变形模型[47]，它们已被用于海马[48]、前列腺[49]以及内侧颞叶[50]的定位。深度学习方法包括完全卷积网络[51]、UNET[52]、DeepLab[53]，以及基于混合条件随机场（Conditional Random Field，CNN-CRF）的方法[54]。尽管这些方法并非都应用于所有的 MRI 成像，但它们已普遍应用于分割脑损伤[55]、肝肿瘤[56]、脑肿瘤[57]，甚至某些脑区域的测量，如基底神经节和中脑[58]。

实例分割是最近发展起来的一个图像分割类别，旨在预测类标签和像素级实例模版用于定位对象或感兴趣区域的多个实例[59]。它不仅分离了属于特定类的像素，而且为区域的每个实例提供了唯一的标识符。目前多使用诸如 Mask R-CNN（R-CNN 的变异型）等方法以及 YOLACT 和 BlendMask 等方法来实现实例分割[60]。一旦进一步发展，这些方法在对多个感兴趣的目标和可移动的目标进行延时研究方面可能将会被证明是非常实用的。

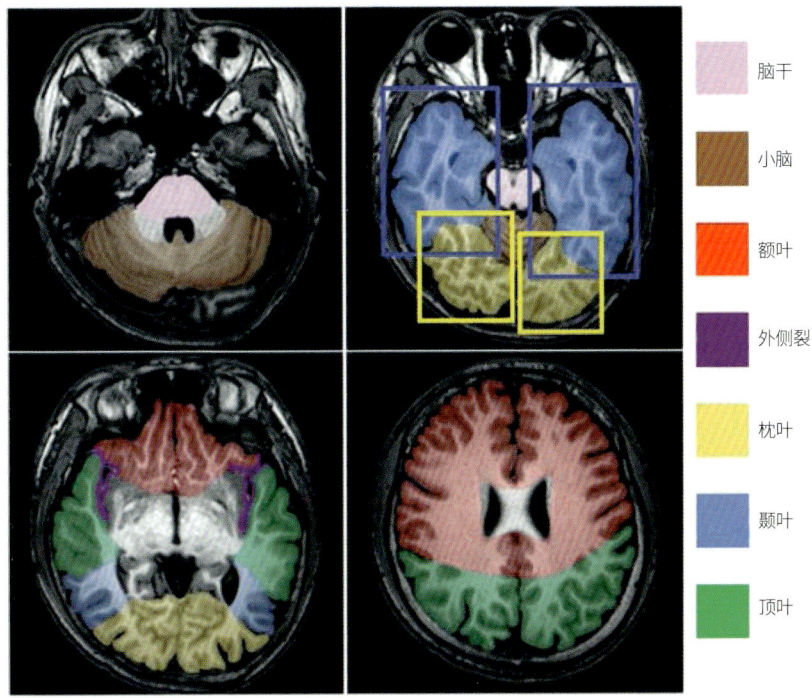

图 8-3 基于脑 MRI 的描绘大脑区域的技术示例

源自 Zhao, H., Wang, J., Lu, Z., Wu, Q., Lv, H.,Liu, H., Gong, X. (2015). Superficial siderosis of the central nervous systems induced by a single-episode of traumatic subarachnoid homerrhage: a study using mri-enhanced gradient eachi t2 star-weighted angoigraphy. PLoS One 10, e0116632

（二）特征提取

特征提取是一种无监督的降维方法，它提供了场景中关键细节的简洁表示，同时保留了使后续阶段更容易分类预测的属性。在进行分割时，纹理和梯度变异等传统方法已成功应用于特征提取，但它们也可用于导出对分类有用的特征[特别是 AD 的梯度变异直方图（Histogram of Gradients，HoG）[61]]。或者，如果输入维度或资源约束成为问题，则可以使用诸如 PCA 和线性判别分析等其他流行的降维方法来实现降维。导出一种较低维的表示，它使重建误差最小化，并且仍然保持其固有特性。

这些方法的例子包括自动编码器及其最近的更深层次的转化，如变分自动编码器和对抗自动编码器[62]。它们获得原始输入（编码部分）的压缩表示，并使用基于先验对每个后续输入进行下采样的隐藏层来检测重复结构[63]。或者，t 分布随机邻域嵌入（t-distributed Stochastic Neighbor Embedding，t-SNE）可以通过导出候选对概率分布来导出低维表示，该候选对概率分布被映射到最小化 Kullback-Leibler 散度的低维平面[64]。t-SNE 主要用于可视化高维数据，如 Gang 等[65]对肺癌胸部 X 射线分析所示。其将卷积自动编码器成功应用于研究大脑中与 AD 相关的部分[66]，并为 AD 的早期进展提供更好的预测[67]。

（三）分类

最后的任务涉及电脑辅助诊断阶段的最后一个阶段，即分类。通过已知样本和基本事实标签最小化在监督模型中发现的损失函数来形成决策边界。如"分类"部分所述，有许多常见的传统机器学习分类方法只需要少量的训练样本即可进行预测，如支持向量机、随机森林和逻辑回归。基于深度学习的方法也可以这样做，但需要更多的样本来训练有效的模型。常见的深度学习方法 CNN 使 AD 研究发生革命性变化[68]，该方法于 20 世纪 80 年代引入，计算成本高昂。可以通过使用图形处理单元（Graphical Processing Unit，GPU）来训练神经网络[69]，以及随后的 CNN[70]来降低这种成本带来了真正动力。如后文的"通用模型体系结构"部分所示，CNN 体系架构诸如 LeNet-5[71]最终进入了更多研究人员的研究范围，并见证了更多体系结构的兴起。其应用也扩展到手写数字之外，并已成为现代 AD 研究二进制和多类分类的基础。

四、通用模型体系结构

随着创新，深度神经网络从仅使用基本层发展，引入了新类型的层和新的架构，这同样带来了令人印象深刻的性能提高，以及深度学习方法在更新领域的进一步应用。以下各部分按时间顺序简要概述了每种通用模型体系结构。

（一）LeNet-5

在"分类"部分，LeNet-5 是首批为深度学习领域做出重大学术贡献的 CNN 架构。由 LeCun 等[71]于 1998 年提出，如图 8-4 所示，LeNet-5 使用了具有 7 层的 CNN，包括 3 个卷积层、2 个子采样层和 2 个完全连接层，以实现手写文档识别。卷积层使用滑动窗口在相应输入的部分上应用滤波器或内核来创建特征图，以不同的比例概述我们的简洁表示。子采样层通常用作传统阶段中的降维步骤。完全连接层将输入转换为与目标变量直接相关的适当维度（如是否患有 AD 或特定的进展阶段）。另一个相关的体系结构 AlexNet[72] 是通过使用线性整流函数（Rectified Linear Units，ReLU）作为激活函数和丢弃层而建立的。

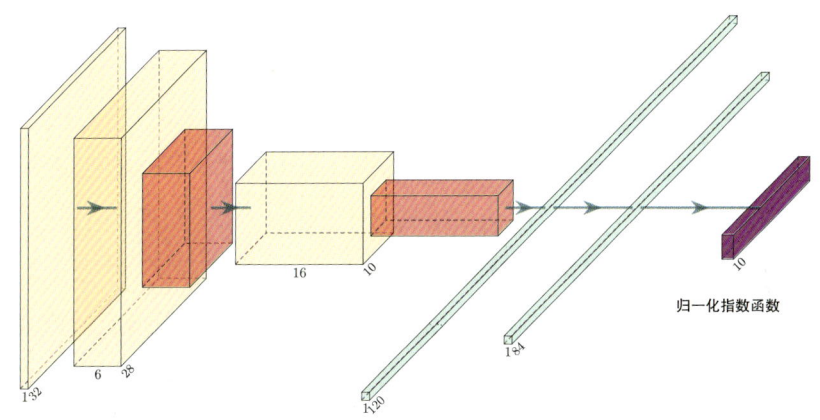

图 8-4 LeNet-5 架构使用 PlotNeuralNetv1 创建[73]
Harisiqbal88/plotneuralnet v1.0.0, https://doi.org/10.5281/zenodo.2526396

（二）UNET

UNET 是生物医学界非常流行的架构[52]。如"分割"部分所述，UNET 致力于解决感兴趣区域的分割，其中每个像素根据已知类别进行分类。如图 8-5 所示，被命名为 U 形。它从压缩或编码路径开始，使用卷积和 ReLU 图层块对输入进行缩减采样，然后是最大池化层。然后，扩展或解码路径使用具有递增参数的卷积和 ReLU 层块，以及将样本上采样到原始图像大小的转置卷积块来产生输出分割图。正如 Ronneberger 等[52] 在原始文章中提到的那样，UNET 也可以受益于数据增强方法，该方法通过以某种方式（旋转、重新缩放等）转换原始输入来添加额外的样本进行训练。

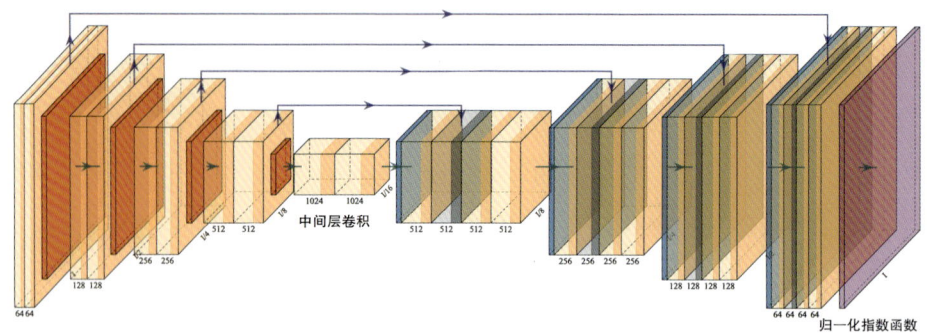

图 8-5　UNET 架构使用 PlotNeuralNetv1 创建 [73]
Harisiqbal88/plotneuralnet v1.0.0, https://doi.org/10.5281/zenodo.2526396

（三）视觉几何组

继 AlexNet 之后，研究人员意识到更深层的网络会产生更好的性能。Simonyan 和 Zisserman[74] 是视觉几何组（Visual Geometry Group，VGG）的成员，他们接受了这一见解，并于 2014 年创建了 VGG-16，深度大约是 AlexNet 的两倍。它包含堆叠的 13 个卷积层（具有较小的滤波器）和 3 个完全连接层，以获得更好的性能，但这是以额外的内存资源为代价的。VGG-16 之后是更深层次的变体 VGG-19，如图 8-6 所示，它也具有类似的效果。

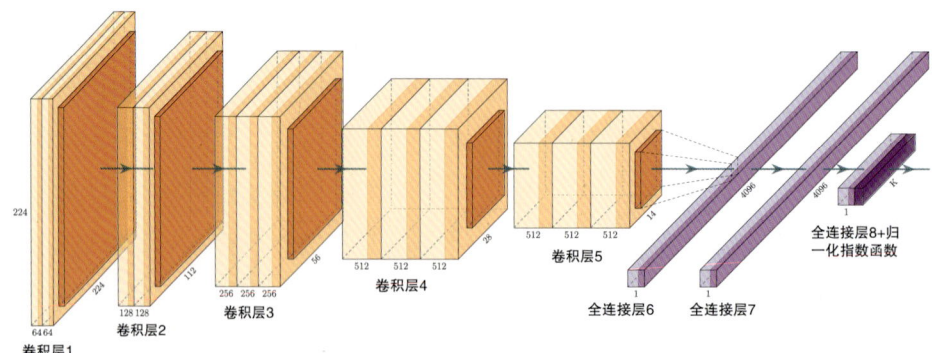

图 8-6　VGG-19 架构使用 PlotNeuralNetv1 创建 [73]
Harisiqbal88/plotneuralnet v1.0.0, https://doi.org/10.5281/zenodo.2526396

（四）ResNet

2015 年，微软研究院意识到，随着网络深度的增加，精确度会达到饱和点，并在一个点之后显著下降，也称为梯度消失问题。他们通过将跳跃连接或残差集成到更深的网络来解决这个问题（如图 8-6 所示），以及批量归一化，其中内部层被归一化并"重新集中"，这允许网络内更快的训练和有效的梯度流[75]。

（五）Inception-V4

VGG-16 和 VGG-19 所需的额外资源限制了其可扩展性。Szegedy 等[76]通过使用块或模块而不是堆叠卷积层来封装子网络解决了这一问题。通过堆叠包含具有不同滤波器的卷积层的块，然后进行级联和 1×1 卷积层用于降维，实现了与 VGG 相当的性能。然后使用改进的优化器、损失函数和对特定层的批量规范化，以及将 n 乘 n 卷积分解为 1 乘 n 和 n 乘 1 卷积[77]进一步扩展网络，随后区块之间的重组和一致性[76]产生了 Inception-V2、Inception-V3，最后是 Inception-V4，如图 8-6 所示。随后是变异体诸如 Xception[78]、ResNeXt-50[79]以及变体，如 DenseNet[80]，它们是目前最先进的架构体系。

第四节　使用深度学习的优势

多年来，CAD 系统中难以确定的行业级性能一直是人们的追求，许多人认为深度学习方法是实现这一追求的答案，这其中有很多原因。本节揭示了应该使用深度学习方法进行 AD-CAD 研究的主要原因。

一、端到端学习

这是第一个优点，也是最显著的益处之一，是不需要在流水线式的过程中进行特征工程。深度学习避免了手工制作特征的需要，反而是从原始数据本身自动发现适当的特征检测和分类所需的代表[81]。更少的制作时间意味着更少的开发时间和更少的成本消耗。

二、准确性提高

最有吸引力的优势是深度学习方法可以带来突出的结果。某些特定领域的传统方法已经达到了性能的上限，而基于深度学习的方法已被证明可以克服以往的局限[82]。性能的提高使深度学习成为一套流行的最新文献方法和现代CAD系统的组成部分。

三、迁移学习

迁移学习允许转移一个应用程序任务创建的预训练权重，并可在非必须具有相同的特征空间或分布的情况下，将其用作另一个任务的起点。迁移学习可以让你在有足够数据的数据库上进行训练，并将所获得的知识转移到新的网络中，从而在较小数据集上显著提高性能[83]。训练权重的导出也增加了先前训练模型的实用性，从而提高了模型的重复利用性，使部署更加高效。然而，正如Guo等[84]所指出的，这其中也存在一些隐忧。

四、稳健性

CAD系统中的数据丢失或对抗性攻击一直是一个长期存在的问题。Guo等[84]还表明，尽管深度学习方法对对抗性攻击也相当稳健，但其结果却因实施过程中使用的深度学习框架而异。研究人员最近发现，通过使用数据增强，深度学习对异常数据输入更具稳健性[85,86]，从而进一步验证了其在CAD系统中的应用。

五、可扩展性

最近对大数据应用的需求激增及其响应表明，深度学习方法的规模非常大，可以成功地在大量数据中发现复杂模式，以处理高维数据、语义索引和数据科学中的其他任务[87]。随着开始更好地了解深度学习方法的潜力，我们也将更好地挖掘深度学习和生物医学工程领域的额外优势。

第五节 使用深度学习的局限性

深度学习在 AD 中的应用存在一些局限性。首先，大多数深度学习模型通常需要大型数据集，这种情况经常不适用于 AD。另一个问题是数据丢失。在许多医学领域（如 AD），考虑到许多 AD 患者的身体虚弱和医疗状况，收集大量数据并不总是可行的。此外，大多数 AD 患者的年龄较大，有时很难从患者身上收集纵向数据，这对使用深度学习方法了解疾病的发展有所限制。

最后，与医学界相关的另一个问题是理解为什么深度学习方法会导致特定的预测。线性模型仍然具有的一个优势是，很容易解释为什么某些输入会转化为相应的预测。然而，对于更复杂的非线性模型（如基于深度学习的方法），情况却并非如此。尽管最近有关于实现模型解释的方法的工作进展，如敏感性分析、简单泰勒分解和分层相关性传播[88]，但基于深度学习的机器学习透明度仍然是一项艰巨的任务，也是一个新兴的探索领域。

第六节 结论

神经网络时代随着深度学习的兴起而重生。随着 GPU 驱动训练的兴起，模拟视觉皮质算法开始有所收获。CAD 系统中最先进的性能终于触手可及，工业商业系统的推出开始启动。与此同时，计算方面的成本似乎也不是基于深度学习方法的唯一限制。

尽管深度学习实现了最先进的性能、更强的稳健性、可扩展性、可重复性和部署潜力，但还是以 AD 和 CAD 系统的某些操作方面为代价的。深度学习方法的使用确实需要大的数据集才能获得足够的性能，较小的纵向研究是难以克服这些困难的，并且单纯为了医学理解而去解释模型也可能会很困难。尽管如此，这些限制也不应该影响 AD 相关的研究工作，反而需要更多的研究来解决我们提出的一些建议，以提供更多的价值，而不仅只是为临床医生和整个医学界提供一个答案。

参考文献

1. Dubois, B., Feldman, H. H., Jacova, C., DeKosky, S. T., Barberger-Gateau, P., Cummings, J., ... Jicha, G. (2007). Research criteria for the diagnosis of Alzheimer's disease: Revising the NINCDS-ADRDA criteria. The Lancet Neurology, 6, 734-746.

2. Arevalo-Rodriguez, I., Smailagic, N., Figuls, M. R. i, Ciapponi, A., Sanchez-Perez, E., Giannakou, A., ... Cullum, S. (2015). Mini-Mental State Examination (MMSE) for the detection of Alzheimer's disease and other dementias in people with mild cognitive impairment (MCI). Cochrane Database of Systematic Reviews, 2015(3), CD010783.

3. James, B. D., Power, M. C., Gianattasio, K. Z., Lamar, M., Oveisgharan, S., Shah, R. C., ... Bennett, D. A. (2020). Characterizing clinical misdiagnosis of dementia using medicare claims records linked to Rush Alzheimer's Disease Center (radc) cohort study data: Public health: Innovative methods in ADRD research. Alzheimer's & Dementia, 16, e044880.

4. WHO. (2019). Cause-specific mortality, 2000-2019. https://www.who.int/data/gho/data/themes/mortality-and-global-health-estimates/ghe-leading-causes-of-death [Online]. Accessed 15.05.21.

5. Xu, Y., Chen, K., Zhao, Q., Li, F., & Guo, Q. (2018). Short-term delayed recall of auditory verbal learning test provides equivalent value to long-term delayed recall in predicting MCI clinical outcomes: A longitudinal follow-up study. Applied Neuropsychology: Adult, 27(1), 73-81.

6. Ausó, E., Gómez-Vicente, V., & Esquiva, G. (2020). Biomarkers for Alzheimer's disease early diagnosis. Journal of Personalized Medicine, 10, 114.

7. Subasi, A. (2020). Use of artificial intelligence in Alzheimer's disease detection. In Artificial intelligence in precision health (pp. 257-278).

8. Wang, H., & Raj, B. (2017). On the origin of deep learning, arXiv:1702.07800.

9. Tanveer, M., Richhariya, B., Khan, R. U., Rashid, A. H., Khanna, P., Prasad, M., & Lin, C. T. (2020). Machine learning techniques for the diagnosis of Alzheimer's disease: A review. ACM Transactions on Multimedia Computing, Communications, and Applications, 16, 30:130:35. Available from https://doi.org/10.1145/3344998.

10. Pellegrini, E., Ballerini, L., Hernandez, Md. C. V., Chappell, F. M., González-Castro, V., Anblagan, D., ... Wardlaw, J. M. (2018). Machine learning of neuroimaging for assisted diagnosis of cognitive impairment and dementia. A systematic review, Alzheimer's & Dementia: Diagnosis, Assessment & Disease Monitoring, 10, 519-535. Available from https://doi.org/10.1016/j.dadm.2018.070.004.

11. Jo, T., Nho, K., & Saykin, A. J. (2019). Deep learning in Alzheimer's disease:

Diagnostic classification and prognostic prediction using neuroimaging data. Frontiers in Aging Neuroscience, 11, 220.

12. Ebrahimighahnavieh, M. A., Luo, S., & Chiong, R. (2020). Deep learning to detect Alzheimer's disease from neuroimaging: A systematic literature review. Computer Methods and Programs in Biomedicine, 187, 105242. Available from https://doi.org/10.1016/j.cmpb.2019.105242.

13. Shatte, A. B. R., Hutchinson, D. M., & Teague, S. J. (2019). Machine learning in mental health: A scoping review of methods and applications. Psychological Medicine 49, 1426-1448, publisher: Cambridge University Press. Available from https://doi.org/10.1017/S0033291719000151.

14. Miotto, R., Wang, F., Wang, S., Jiang, X., & Dudley, J. T. (2018). Deep learning for healthcare: Review, opportunities and challenges. Briefings in Bioinformatics, 19, 1236-1246, publisher: Oxford Academic. Available from https://doi.org/10.1093/bib/bbx044.

15. Bi, X., Li, S., Xiao, B., Li, Y., Wang, G., & Ma, X. (2020). Computer aided Alzheimer's disease diagnosis by an unsupervised deep learning technology. Neurocomputing, 392, 296-304. Available from https://doi.org/10.1016/j.neucom.2018.110.111.

16. Raghavendra, U., Acharya, U. R., & Adeli, H. (2019). Artificial intelligence techniques for automated diagnosis of neurological disorders. European Neurology, 82, 41-64, publisher: Karger Publishers PMID: 31743905. Available from https://doi.org/10.1159/000504292.

17. Karami, V., Nittari, G., & Amenta, F. (2019). Neuroimaging computer-aided diagnosis systems for Alzheimer's disease. International Journal of Imaging Systems and Technology, 29, 83-94. Available from https://doi.org/10.1002/ima.22300.

18. Hulbert, S., & Adeli, H. (2013). EEG/MEG-and imaging-based diagnosis of Alzheimer's disease. Reviews in the Neurosciences, 24, 563-576, De Gruyter section: Reviews in the Neurosciences. Available from https://doi.org/10.1515/revneuro-2013-0042.

19. Segovia, F., Bastin, C., Salmon, E., Górriz, J. M., Ramírez, J., & Phillips, C. (2014). Combining PET images and neuropsychological test data for automatic diagnosis of Alzheimer's disease. PLoS One, 9, e88687, publisher: Public Library of Science. Available from https://doi.org/10.1371/journal.pone.0088687.

20. Valenzuela, O., Jiang, X., Carrillo, A., & Rojas, I. (2018). Multi-objective genetic algorithms to find most relevant volumes of the brain related to Alzheimer's disease and mild cognitive impairment. International Journal of Neural Systems, 28, 1850022, publisher: World Scientific Publishing Co. Available from https://doi.org/10.1142/S0129065718500223.

21. Dessouky, M. M., Elrashidy, M. A., Taha, T. E., & Abdelkader, H. M. (2016). Computer-

aided diagnosis system for Alzheimer's disease using different discrete transform techniques. American Journal of Alzheimer's Disease & Other Dementiasr, 31, 282-293, SAGE Publications Inc. Available from https://doi.org/10.1177/1533317515603957.

22. Chaves, R., Ramírez, J., Górriz, J. M., López, M., Salas-Gonzalez, D., Álvarez, I., & Segovia, F. (2009). SVM-based computer-aided diagnosis of the Alzheimer's disease using t-test NMSE feature selection with feature correlation weighting. Neuroscience Letters, 461, 293-297. Available from https://doi.org/10.1016/j.neulet.2009.060.052.

23. Zhang, F., Tian, S., Chen, S., Ma, Y., Li, X., & Guo, X. (2019). Voxel-based morphometry: Improving the diagnosis of Alzheimer's disease based on an extreme learning machine method from the ADNI cohort. Neuroscience, 414, 273-279. Available from https://doi.org/10.1016/j.neuroscience.2019.050.014.

24. Khalid, S., Khalil, T., & Nasreen, S. (2014). A survey of feature selection and feature extraction techniques in machine learning. In Proceedings of the 2014 science and information conference (SAI), IEEE, London, UK (pp. 372-378). <https://ieeexplore.ieee.org/document/6918213> (Online; accessed 11.12.20).

25. Abdi, H., & Williams, L. J. (2010). Principal component analysis. WIREs Computational Statistics, 2, 433-459. Available from https://doi.org/10.1002/wics0.101.

26. Shaikh, T. A., & Ali, R. (2019). Automated atrophy assessment for Alzheimer's disease diagnosis from brain MRI images. Magnetic Resonance Imaging, 62, 167-173. Available from https://doi.org/10.1016/j.mri.2019.060.019.

27. Ruiz, E., Ramírez, J., Górriz, J. M., Casillas, J., & Initiative, tA. D. N. (2018). Alzheimer's disease computer-aided diagnosis: Histogram-based analysis of regional mri volumes for feature selection and classification. Journal of Alzheimer's Disease, 65, 819-842, publisher: IOS Press. Available from https://doi.org/10.3233/JAD-170514.

28. Podgorelec, V. (2012). Analyzing EEG signals with machine learning for diagnosing Alzheimer's disease. Elektronika ir Elektrotechnika, 18(8), 61-64. Available fromhttps://doi.org/10.5755/j01.eee.18.8.2627.

29. Shakarami, A., Tarrah, H., & Mahdavi-Hormat, A. (2020). A CAD system for diagnosing Alzheimer's disease using 2D slices and an improved AlexNet-SVM method. Optik, 212, 164-237. Available from https://doi.org/10.1016/j.ijleo.2020.164237.

30. Lahmiri, S., & Shmuel, A. (2019). Performance of machine learning methods applied to structural MRI and ADASs cognitive scores in diagnosing Alzheimer's disease. Biomedical Signal Processing and Control, 52, 414-419. Available from https://doi.org/10.1016/j.bspc.2018.080.009.

31. Ding, Y., Sohn, J. H., Kawczynski, M. G., Trivedi, H., Harnish, R., Jenkins, N. W., ... Franc, B. L. (2018). A deep learning model to predict a diagnosis of Alzheimer disease

by using 18F-FDG PET of the brain. Radiology, 290, 456-464, Radiological Society of North America. Available from https://doi.org/10.1148/radiol.2018180958.

32. Krupinski, E. A. (2020). Evaluating AI clinically it's not just ROC AUC! Radiology (p. 203782), Radiological Society of North America. Available from https://doi.org/10.1148/radiol.2020203782.

33. Frisoni, G. B., Bocchetta, M., Chételat, G., Rabinovici, G. D., De Leon, M. J., Kaye, J., ... Black, S. E. (2013). Imaging markers for Alzheimer disease: Which vs how. Neurology, 81, 487-500.

34. Russakovsky, O., Deng, J., Su, H., Krause, J., Satheesh, S., Ma, S., ... Bernstein, M. (2015). Imagenet large scale visual recognition challenge. International Journal of Computer Vision, 115, 211-252.

35. De Oliveira, M., Balthazar, M., D'abreu, A., Yasuda, C., Damasceno, B., Cendes, F., & Castellano, G. (2011). MR imaging texture analysis of the corpus callosum and thalamus in amnestic mild cognitive impairment and mild Alzheimer disease. American Journal of Neuroradiology, 32, 60-66.

36. Abbasi, S., & Tajeripour, F. (2017). Detection of brain tumor in 3D MRI images using local binary patterns and histogram orientation gradient. Neurocomputing, 219, 526-535.

37. Barra, V., & Boire, J.-Y. (2000). Tissue segmentation on MRimages of the brain by possibilistic clustering on a 3D wavelet representation. Journal of Magnetic Resonance Imaging: An Official Journal of the International Society for Magnetic Resonance in Medicine, 11, 267-278.

38. Ren, S., He, K., Girshick, R., & Sun, J. (2016). Faster R-CNN: Towards real-time object detection with region proposal networks. IEEE Transactions on Pattern Analysis and Machine Intelligence, 39, 1137-1149.

39. Redmon, J., Divvala, S., Girshick, R., & Farhadi, A. (2016). You only look once: Unified, real-time object detection. In Proceedings of the IEEE conference on computer vision and ppattern recognition (pp. 779-788).

40. Liu, W., Anguelov, D., Erhan, D., Szegedy, C., Reed, S., Fu, C.-Y., & Berg, A. C. (2016). SSD: Single shot multibox detector. In Proceedings of the European conference on computer vision, Springer (pp. 21-37).

41. Luo, G., An, R., Wang, K., Dong, S., & Zhang, H. (2016). A deep learning network for right ventricle segmentation in short-axis MRI. In Proceedings of the 2016 computing in cardiology conference (CinC), IEEE (pp. 485-488).

42. Lu, Y., Yu, Q., Gao, Y., Zhou, Y., Liu, G., Dong, Q., ... Zhang, Z. (2018). Identification of metastatic lymph nodes in MR imaging with faster region-based convolutional

neuralnetworks. Cancer Research, 78, 5135-5143.
43. George, J., Skaria, S., & Varun, V. (2018). Using YOLO based deep learning network for real time detection and localization of lung nodules from low dose CT scans. In Medical imaging 2018: computer-aided diagnosis, proceedings volume 10575, International Society for Optics and Photonics (p. 105751I).
44. Xie, C., Wang, J., Zhang, Z., Zhou Y., Xie, L., & Yuille, A. (2017). Adversarial examples for semantic segmentation and object detection. In Proceedings of the IEEE international conference on computer vision (pp. 1369-1378).
45. Dill, V., Franco, A. R., & Pinho, M. S. (2015). Automated methods for hippocampus segmentation: The evolution and a review of the state of the art. Neuroinformatics, 13, 133-150.
46. Cabezas, M., Oliver, A., Lladó, X., Freixenet, J., & Cuadra, M. B. (2011). A review of atlas-based segmentation for magnetic resonance brain images. Computer Methods and Programs in Biomedicine, 104, e158-e177.
47. Cootes, T. F., Edwards, G. J., & Taylor, C. J. (2001). Active appearance models. IEEE Transactions on Pattern Analysis and Machine Intelligence, 23, 681-685.
48. Crum, W. R., Scahill, R. I., & Fox, N. C. (2001). Automated hippocampal segmentation by regional fluid registration of serial MRI: Validation and application in Alzheimer's disease. NeuroImage, 13, 847-855.
49. Toth, R., & Madabhushi, A. (2012). Multifeature landmark-free active appearance models: Application to prostate MRI segmentation. IEEE Transactions on Medical Imaging, 31, 1638-1650.
50. Xie, L., Wisse, L. E., Pluta, J., de Flores, R., Piskin, V., Manjón, J. V., ... Wolk, D. A. (2019). Automated segmentation of medial temporal lobe subregions on in vivo T1-weighted MRI in early stages of Alzheimer's disease. Human Brain Mapping, 40, 3431-3451.
51. Long, J., Shelhamer, E., & Darrell, T. (2015). Fully convolutional networks for semantic segmentation. In Proceedings of the IEEE conference on computer vision and pattern recognition (pp. 3431-3440).
52. Ronneberger, O., Fischer, P., & Brox, T. (2015). U-net: Convolutional networks for biomedical image segmentation. In Proceedings of the international conference on medical image computing and computer-assisted intervention, Springer (pp. 234-241).
53. Chen, L.-C., Papandreou, G., Kokkinos, I., Murphy, K., & Yuille, A. L. (2017). Deeplab: Semantic image segmentation with deep convolutional nets, atrous convolution, and fully connected CRFs. IEEE Transactions on Pattern Analysis and Machine Intelligence, 40, 834-848.

54. Lin, G., Shen, C., Van Den Hengel, A., & Reid, I. (2016). Efficient piecewise training of deep structured models for semantic segmentation. In Proceedings of the IEEE conference on computer vision and pattern recognition (pp. 3194-3203).
55. Kamnitsas, K., Chen, L., Ledig, C., Rueckert, D., & Glocker, B. (2015). Multi-scale 3D convolutional neural networks for lesion segmentation in brain MRI. Ischemic Stroke Lesion Segmentation, 13, 46.
56. Christ, P. F., Ettlinger, F., Grün, F., Elshaera, M. E. A., Lipkova, J., Schlecht, S. ... Bilic, P. (2017). Automatic liver and tumor segmentation of CT and MRI volumes using cascaded fully convolutional neural networks, arXiv: 1702.05970.
57. Pereira, S., Alves, V., & Silva, C.A. (2018). Adaptive feature recombination and recalibration for semantic segmentation: Application to brain tumor segmentation in MRI. In Proceedings of international conference on medical image computing and computer-assisted intervention, Springer (pp. 706-714).
58. Milletari, F., Ahmadi, S.-A., Kroll, C., Plate, A., Rozanski, V., Maiostre, J., ... Bötzel, K. (2017). Hough-CNN: Deep learning for segmentation of deep brain regions in MRI and ultrasound. Computer Vision and Image Understanding, 164, 92-102.
59. Liu, S., Qi, L., Qin, H., Shi, J., & Jia, J. (2018). Path aggregation network for instance segmentation. In Proceedings of the IEEE conference on computer vision and pattern recognition (pp. 8759-8768).
60. Kim, M., Woo, S., Kim, D., & Kweon, I. S. (2021). The devil is in the boundary: Exploiting boundary representation for basis-based instance segmentation. In Proceedings of the IEEE/CVF winter conference on applications of computer vision (pp. 929-938).
61. Sarwinda, D., & Bustamam A. (2018) 3D-HoG features-based classification using MRI images to early diagnosis of Alzheimer's disease. In Proceedings of the 2018 IEEE/ACIS 17th international conference on computer and information science (ICIS), IEEE (pp. 457-462).
62. Wang, H.-P., Peng, W.-H., & Ko, W.-J. (2020). Learning priors for adversarial autoencoders. APSIPA Transactions on Signal and Information Processing, 9.
63. Wang, Y., Yao, H., & Zhao, S. (2016). Auto-encoder based dimensionality reduction. Neurocomputing, 184, 232-242.
64. Maaten, L. v d, & Hinton, G. (2008). Visualizing data using t-sne. Journal of Machine Learning Research, 9, 2579-2605.
65. Gang, P. Zhen, W., Zeng, W., Gordienko, Y., Kochura, Y., Alienin, O. ... Stirenko, S. (2018). Dimensionality reduction in deep learning for chest X-ray analysis of lung cancer. In Proceedings of the 2018 tenth international conference on advanced

computational intelligence (ICACI), IEEE (pp. 878-883).
66. Martinez-Murcia, F. J., Ortiz, A., Gorriz, J.-M., Ramirez, J., & Castillo-Barnes, D. (2019). Studying the manifold structure of Alzheimer's disease: A deep learning approach using convolutional autoencoders. IEEE Journal of Biomedical and Health Informatics, 24, 17-26.
67. Basu S., Wagstyl, K., Zandifar, A., Collins, L., Romero, A., & Precup, D. (2019). Early prediction of Alzheimer's disease progression using variational autoencoders. In Proceedings of the international conference on medical image computing and computer-assisted intervention, Springer (pp. 205-213).
68. LeCun, Y., Boser, B., Denker, J. S., Henderson, D., Howard, R. E., Hubbard, W., & Jackel, L. D. (1989). Backpropagation applied to handwritten zip code recognition. Neural Computation, 1, 541-551.
69. Oh, K.-S., & Jung, K. (2004). GPU implementation of neural networks. Pattern Recognition, 37, 1311-1314.
70. Chellapilla, K., Puri, S., & Simard, P. High performance convolutional neural networks for document processing (2006).
71. LeCun, Y., Bottou, L., Bengio, Y., & Haffner, P. (1998). Gradient-based learning applied to document recognition. Proceedings of the IEEE, 86, 2278-2324.
72. Krizhevsky, A., Sutskever, I., & Hinton, G. E. (2017). Imagenet classification with deep convolutional neural networks. Communications of the ACM, 60, 84-90.
73. Iqbal, H. (2018). Harisiqbal88/plotneuralnet v1.0.0. Available from https://doi.org/10.5281/zenodo.2526396.
74. Simonyan, K., & Zisserman, A. (2014). Very deep convolutional networks for largescale image recognition, arXiv:1409.1556.
75. He, K., Zhang, X., Ren, S., & Sun, J. (2016). Deep residual learning for image recognition. In Proceedings of the IEEE conference on computer vision and pattern recognition (pp. 770-778).
76. Szegedy, C., Ioffe, S., Vanhoucke, V., & Alemi, A. (2017). Inception-v4, inception-ResNet and the impact of residual connections on learning. In Proceedings of the AAAI conference on artificial intelligence, Vol. 31.
77. Szegedy, C., Vanhoucke, V., Ioffe, S., Shlens, J., & Wojna, Z. (2016). Rethinking the inception architecture for computer vision. In Proceedings of the IEEE conference on computer vision and pattern recognition (pp. 2818-2826).
78. Chollet, F. (2017). Xception: Deep learning with depthwise separable convolutions. In Proceedings of the IEEE conference on computer vision and pattern recognition (pp. 1251-1258).

79. Xie, S., Girshick, R., Dollár, P., Tu, Z., & He, K. (2017). Aggregated residual transformations for deep neural networks. In Proceedings of the IEEE conference on computer vision and pattern recognition (pp. 1492-1500).
80. Huang, G., Liu, Z., Van Der Maaten, L., & Weinberger, K. Q. (2017). Densely connected convolutional networks. In: Proceedings of the IEEE conference on computer vision and pattern recognition (pp. 4700-4708).
81. LeCun, Y., Bengio, Y., & Hinton, G. (2015). Deep learning. Nature, 521, 436-444.
82. Guo, Y., Liu, Y., Oerlemans, A., Lao, S., Wu, S., & Lew, M. S. (2016). Deep learning for visual understanding: A review. Neurocomputing, 187, 27-48.
83. Pan, S. J., & Yang, Q. (2009). A survey on transfer learning. IEEE Transactions on Knowledge and Data Engineering, 22, 1345-1359.
84. Guo, Q., Chen, S., Xie, X., Ma, L., Hu, Q., Liu, H. ... Li, X. (2019). An empirical study towards characterizing deep learning development and deployment across different frameworks and platforms. In Proceedings of the 2019 34th IEEE/ACM international conference on automated software engineering (ASE), IEEE (pp. 810-822).
85. Hendrycks, D., Mu, N., Cubuk, E. D., Zoph, B., Gilmer, J., & Lakshminarayanan, B. (2019). Augmix: A simple data processing method to improve robustness and uncertainty, arXiv:1912.02781.
86. Gao, X., Saha R. K., Prasad, M. R., & Roychoudhury, A. (2020). Fuzz testing based data augmentation to improve robustness of deep neural networks. In Proceedings of the 2020 IEEE/ACM 42nd international conference on software engineering (ICSE), IEEE (pp. 1147-1158).
87. Najafabadi, M. M., Villanustre, F., Khoshgoftaar, T. M., Seliya, N., Wald, R., & Muharemagic, E. (2015). Deep learning applications and challenges in big data analytics. Journal of Big Data, 2, 1-21.
88. Montavon, G., Samek, W., & Müller, K.-R. (2018). Methods for interpreting and understanding deep neural networks. Digital Signal Processing, 73, 1-15.

第三部分
痴呆的治疗

第九章 阿尔茨海默病伴抑郁的治疗

Ahmed A. Moustafa，Lily Bilson，Wafa Jaroudi 编
袁淑兰，赵江浩 译
肖卫民 校

第一节 引言

根据统计，每年用于治疗阿尔茨海默病（AD）患者的费用估计高达1720亿美元。找到能够减轻AD患者照顾负担的有效治疗手段，对于整个社会、患者自身及其家庭而言都极为重要。多项研究也表明，抑郁症可能是导致AD等多种神经系统疾病的危险因素[1-4]。

关于AD合并抑郁症的患病率，在多个研究中存在较大差异。Barca等[5]的报告称，在痴呆症患者中，抑郁的患病率可能高达86%。而在其他的研究中，AD患者中表现出抑郁症状的比例为17%~87%[6,7]。还有研究报告，AD中抑郁症的患病率估计在26%~50%[8,9]，其中最明显的抑郁表现是持续的情绪低落或正向情感缺失[9]。考虑到发病率高，为AD合并抑郁的患者提供合适的治疗显得至关重要，有助于减缓患者的记忆功能下降，这一点已由多项研究所证实。

第二节 治疗

本节探讨用于AD合并抑郁的多种现有治疗策略。已有多项研究采用不同的治疗方法来减轻痴呆患者的抑郁症状[10]，其中包括多种药物和非药物治疗方法[11]。本节主要探讨药物疗法和行为疗法对AD合并抑郁的治疗。

一、药物治疗

目前已有大量研究探讨了利用多种药物治疗痴呆合并抑郁的效果[12]，其中

主要包括抗抑郁药物、抗焦虑药物及抗胆碱药物。这些药物有的可以单独使用，有的则需要联合使用。例如，抗焦虑药和催眠药常常作为抗抑郁疗法的替代或补充[13]。也有研究显示，抗胆碱药能够缓解痴呆患者的抑郁症状[14,15]。

然而，对于抗抑郁药治疗痴呆相关抑郁的有效性仍存在争议，虽然许多研究强调其重要性，但仍缺乏确凿证据证明其综合疗效[16]。比如，选择性5-羟色胺再摄取抑制剂（Selective Serotonin Reuptake Inhibitor，SSRI）是经常被推荐的治疗方法，且多数患者能够很好地耐受，但是建议密切监测SSRI的疗效和可能产生的不良反应。有多项研究指出，包括舍曲林、氟西汀、西酞普兰、曲唑酮、莫氟西汀等在内的多种抗抑郁药物均能有效缓解痴呆相关的抑郁症状[17-22]，但也有一些研究给出了不同的结论[13]。早期研究发现，老年抑郁患者可以采用三环类抗抑郁药来缓解抑郁症状[23,24]。例如，Menon 等[20]推荐使用SSRI类抗抑郁药，因为抑郁与5-羟色胺系统的紊乱有关，他们认为这是最有效的。一项最近的研究比较了几种抗抑郁药和血管类药物在治疗痴呆患者抑郁症状方面的有效性，包括舍曲林、艾司西酞普兰和尼可地尔[25]。该研究发现，与其他药物相比，艾司西酞普兰在抗抑郁方面更有效。这与Gellis等[11]的报告相一致，后者发现西酞普兰和舍曲林可能比其他抗抑郁药更能有效治疗痴呆相关的抑郁症状。

与过去的研究不同，Evers等[13]发现，在所有被诊断为痴呆相关抑郁的患者中，有近42%的患者并未接受任何抗抑郁药物治疗。同时也有报告提到了老年抑郁症治疗中存在抗抑郁药物滥用和误用等情况[26]。2011年Nelson和Devanand[27]指出，抗抑郁药物对减轻痴呆患者的抑郁症状只有轻微的效果。一项荟萃分析发现，7项研究中只有2项报告证明抗抑郁药在治疗痴呆相关抑郁症方面比安慰剂更好[28]。还有人认为，抗抑郁药物通过改善海马功能来控制痴呆和记忆力下降[29]。

综上所述，治疗AD相关抑郁有多种药物治疗方法，包括SSRI以及抗焦虑药。然而，这些药物对AD患者抑郁症的疗效并不是决定性的。在接下来的内容中，我们将讨论现有的治疗AD抑郁症的行为疗法。

二、行为治疗

目前针对痴呆合并抑郁有多种行为疗法，包括体育锻炼、认知训练、回忆疗法及认知行为疗法（Cognitive Behavioral Therapy，CBT）等。

Williams 等针对 45 例居住在疗养院的中度至重度 AD 伴抑郁症状的患者进行了一项为期 16 周的综合锻炼研究[30,31]。参与研究的患者被分为 3 组：第一组接受综合锻炼；第二组仅进行步行训练；第三组则进行社会交谈训练。所有参与的患者均为在辅助下方可行走的患者，能够独立行走的患者被排除。为了评估患者的抑郁程度，研究使用了康奈尔痴呆抑郁量表（CSDD），将得分≥7 分的患者纳入研究。在评估中，"情绪"被定义为持续的情感状态，使用痴呆情绪评估量表和阿尔茨海默病情绪量表进行情绪评估。"情感"则被定义为情绪的外在表现，通过观察情感量表进行测量，这个量表之前已经在 AD 研究中使用过[32]。第一组的训练内容包括两个项目：首先进行 10 分钟的力量、平衡和灵活性训练，然后是步行训练，并逐周增加训练次数和步行时间；第二组的患者根据个人日常能力给予恒定的步行速度训练，逐周增加步行时间，最长达 30 分钟；第三组作为对照组，只进行相同时间的随意交谈。研究结果显示，3 组患者在治疗后的 CSDD 得分从基线的 12.4 分降至 9.77 分，其中有 35% 的患者在治疗后得分 < 7 分。在整个参与者样本中，从基线到研究结束，除了一项结果指标外，其余所有指标的评分均显著降低，对照组显然有一定的有益效果。针对在疗养院中患有重度 AD 合并抑郁症的患者，规范的运动锻炼计划已被证明具有明显的益处。这一结果与 Regan 等[33]2005 年的研究一致，后者在 2005 年研究发现，与不进行锻炼的人相比，参与体育活动的痴呆症患者往往报告的抑郁症状较少。由于锻炼对于长期患病的人来说难以实施，因此，应研究以椅子为基础的锻炼作为活动锻炼的替代方法的益处。

2017 年 Stewart 等[34]进行了一项非药物的心理社交团体干预研究，即探讨认知刺激疗法（Cognitive Stimulation Therapy，CST）在改善痴呆患者认知功能、生活质量和幸福感方面的疗效。该研究评估了 6 组共计 40 名参与者进行 CST 后对认知、生活质量及抑郁的影响。CST 的特点在于将回忆疗法、现实定向和验证疗法相结合，构建出一个系统化的心理社会项目。在该项目中，患者的意见被高度重视，并对其进行认知上的挑战。该疗法分为14个主题活动，每次约45分钟，每周2次，为期7周。这些认知任务主要涉及执行功能、多感官刺激和使用回忆来帮助定向。活动的内容丰富，包括体育游戏、声音感知、儿时回忆、食物体验、时事关注、面部和场景识别、词汇联想、创意活动、物品分类、方位感知、货币使用、数字和词汇游戏以及团队游戏。CST的核心原则涵盖了心理刺激、创新思考、敏感地应用定向技巧、适时使用回忆帮助定向、提供记忆触发点、确保会话之间的连续性和一致性、内隐学习、语言刺激、以人为本、尊重、参与、包容、提供选择、趣味性、最大化发挥潜能以及建立人际关系。为了评估疗效，研究者在干预前及干预后7周两个时间点对参与者进行了评估。参与者的年龄范围为50~94岁，平均年龄为78.8岁。通过观察和访谈的方式使用CSDD评估患者的抑郁状况，并记录与情绪有关的体征、行为和思维紊乱、生理症状及周期性功能变化。结果显示，干预前后的CSDD得分存在显著差异，参与者的抑郁状况得到缓解，认知状况得到改善，更加健谈，情绪更加愉快，并与其他参与者建立了深厚的友情。总的来说，CST被证实是一种有效的可缓解痴呆患者抑郁的方法。回忆疗法为痴呆患者提供了记忆辅助，如果能够成功回忆，那么记忆的增强很可能与抑郁症状的减轻有关。最近的一项研究也证实了这一预测[35]。然而，近期的一项综述对回忆疗法在AD中缓解抑郁症状的效果存在一些疑问。Woods等[36]对22项关于回忆疗法对痴呆影响的研究进行了回顾，报告了不一致的结果。

2000年，Marriott等[37]研究了家庭干预能否减轻痴呆照顾者的主观负担，以及是否对患者本身产生临床益处。该研究的主要结局是家庭干预能否减轻照顾者负担，次要结局是该干预能否对患者的认知和非认知症状产生影响，其中包括抑郁症状。研究采用随机对照试验将家庭干预与两个对照组进行比较，干预包括3个部分——照顾者教育、情绪管理及应对技能培训，每2周1次，共计14次。在其中2组（1个实验组和1个对照组）的参与者上进行了坎伯威家属访谈（Camberwell Family Interview，CFI），访谈采用半结构化方式进行并进行录音，以评估被访者的情感表达，过程通常需要大约 90 分钟。在治疗前、治疗后及治疗后 3 个月进行随访，对照顾者进行以下评估：一般健康问卷和贝克抑郁自评量表（BDL）。在相同的时间间隔内，对患者进行了以下评估：简易精神状态检查量表（MMSE）、康奈尔痴呆抑郁量表（CSDD）、MOUSEPAD（用于评估痴呆症中的多种精神症状和行为紊乱）以及临床痴呆评分（CDR）。结果证实了主要的假设，即干预组中的照顾者在治疗后及 3 个月随访时在压力和抑郁的测量上与 2 个对照组相比，均有显著的改善。研究发现，仅进行 CFI 的对照组没有效果，表明单次访谈不足以减轻照顾者的负担。对于次要假设有一定的支持，即家庭干预在治疗后对行为紊乱有显著效果，但随访时没有持续。2 种行为干预均显著减少了患者和照顾者的抑郁症状。这些结果具有重要的临床意义，这意味着帮助照顾者更好地应对自己的情绪状态、清晰地看待如何应对挑战性情境的干预在实践中是有益的。不仅是照顾者，更好地应对情境和提高情境掌控感带来的积极影响，对患者同样也有积极的作用。

尽管 CBT 通常被广泛应用于治疗严重抑郁症患者[38-41]，但在伴随抑郁的痴呆症患者中应用相对较少。Teri 等近期研究发现，CBT 有助于缓解痴呆患者的抑郁症状[42,43]。此外，还有一些更新的研究也支持这一观点。例如，Walker[44] 报告了 1 例个案研究，一位痴呆症患者通过 CBT 治疗，其中包括改变与痴呆和认知衰退相关的信念疗法，获得了显著的益处。Forstmeier 等[45] 最近指出，CBT 中的某些要素，如参与愉快的活动和进行生活回忆（即经历不同生活事件的不同阶段以增强记忆），能有效减轻痴呆患者的抑郁症状。还有一些关于使用 CBT 治疗痴呆患者照顾者抑郁症状的研究，但超出了本文的范围，有兴趣的读者可以参考 Hopkinson 等[46] 的相关文献。最新的研究还发现，与正念减压疗法相比，正念认知疗法更能有效缓解痴呆患者的抑郁症状[47]。

另一项研究采用了认知训练方法，旨在改善轻度认知障碍患者的认知功能退化和抑郁症状[48]。Sukontapol 等[48] 发现，与对照组相比，认知训练可以有效减轻抑郁症状。另外，Smith-Ray 等[49] 研究指出，经过 10 周的认知训练（每天使用 Posit Science Brain Health 问卷 2 小时），有痴呆症风险的老年人的抑郁症状显著减轻。若想了解关于认知训练对老年人及存在痴呆症风险者的影响的更多信息，可以参考 Naismith 和 Mowszowski[50] 的综述。至于如何通过认知训练来管理痴呆患者的抑郁症，Chan 等[51] 在 2020 年的综述中有详细说明。

有少数研究采用了 Lewinsohn 的"愉快事件训练法"，旨在帮助患者理解他们的行为与情感之间的关系，并协助他们减轻负面情绪。这种训练方法的优势在于，可以在家中或疗养院由护理人员进行训练。Teri 等[52] 在 2003 年的研究中发现，"愉快事件训练法"对于缓解痴呆患者的抑郁症状十分有效。但是，Lichtenberg 等[53] 在 2005 年的另一研究中指出，该方法未能显示出明显的积极疗效。

在治疗抑郁症状的方法中，除了常规手段，一些研究也对其他治疗方式进行了探索。例如，Onega 等[54] 在 2018 年的研究中指出，光照疗法对于减轻抑郁症状具有明显效果，特别是对于患有严重痴呆的患者。此外，关于宠物如何为年轻人和老年人带来抑郁症状的缓解，已有诸多研究为此提供了证据[55,56]。相应地，Baek 等[57] 在 2020 年的研究中同样确认，宠物辅助治疗对于痴呆患者的抑郁症状管理具有积极的效果。

有研究探索了行为治疗与药物治疗的联合方式对痴呆伴随抑郁症状的影响。Rodrigues 等[58] 在 2018 年的研究中专门探究了抗抑郁药物与社交参与联合作用对痴呆患者抑郁症状的影响。文中所指的社交参与度主要从两个方面来评估：一个是社交网络的规模，例如，患者拥有的朋友和家人数量以及与他们的互动频率；另一个是他们所感知的社交孤立程度，也就是孤独感。结果显示，正是社交参与度而非药物治疗起到了减轻抑郁症状的作用。另外，Giovagnoli 等[59] 在 2018 年的研究中发现，相较于单独使用美金刚，加入音乐疗法能更有效地缓解痴呆患者的抑郁症状。此外，根据 Lam 等[60] 在 2020 年进行了一项综述，他们在 82 项研究中得出音乐疗法对痴呆患者的抑郁和焦虑症状都有显著的治疗效果，这一发现也得到了 Moreno-Morales 等[61] 综述支持。Jung 等[62] 在 2020 年的研究中证实，一种结合了认知训练、艺术疗法和音乐疗法的综合行为治疗方案，对管理痴呆患者的抑郁症状具有明显效果。

总之，AD 患者中的抑郁症状有多种非药物治疗手段。其中包括运动疗法、认知行为疗法、基于家庭的干预等。虽然这些方法中的部分在缓解 AD 抑郁症状方面已被证明有效，但并非所有的方法都能达到预期效果。

第三节 结论

总之，通过现有的文献总结，对于痴呆合并抑郁的患者，行为疗法比药物治疗（如SSRI类药物）效果更佳。推荐的非药物干预措施包括减少与社会的隔离、正向主动行为激活（即与积极情绪相关的活动）、制定合理的锻炼计划以及增加愉快的体力活动等。同时也存在其他的治疗观点。例如，2014 年 Borisovskaya 等人研究了 AD 患者的认知、神经精神症状的治疗策略，其中包括躁动、精神异常、焦虑和抑郁等，建议治疗应从非药物干预开始，必要时再增加药物治疗[63]。

我们的研究还表明，行为异常和抑郁症状是可以相互影响的，因此改善行为障碍可以减少抑郁症状，反之亦然。比如，使用回忆疗法和 CBT 改善痴呆患者认知功能障碍往往也会减少抑郁症状发作。同样，通过缓解压力改善抑郁症状也可以延缓认知功能下降。未来的工作还应该关注到照顾者。例如，研究照顾者的情绪压力是如何影响痴呆患者的抑郁症状的[64,65]。

参考文献

1. Bennett, S., & Thomas, A. J. (2014). Depression and dementia: Cause, consequence or coincidence? Maturitas, 79(2), 184-190. Available from https://doi.org/10.1016/j.maturitas.2014.05.009.
2. Linnemann, C., & Lang, U. E. (2020). Pathways connecting late-life depression and dementia. Frontiers in Pharmacology, 11, 279. Available from https://doi.org/10.3389/fphar.2020.00279.
3. Modrego, P. J., & Ferrandez, J. (2004). Depression in patients with mild cognitive impairment increases the risk of developing dementia of Alzheimer type: A prospective cohort study. Archives of Neurology, 61(8), 1290-1293. Available from https://doi.org/10.1001/archneur.61.8.1290.

4. Steck, N., Cooper, C., & Orgeta, V. (2018). Investigation of possible risk factors for depression in Alzheimer's disease: A systematic review of the evidence. Journalof Affective Disorders, 236, 149-156. Available from https://doi.org/10.1016/j.jad.2018.04.034.
5. Barca, M. L., Selbaek, G., Laks, J., & Engedal, K. (2008). The pattern of depressive symptoms and factor analysis of the Cornell Scale among patients in Norwegian nursing homes. International Journal of Geriatric Psychiatry, 23(10), 1058-1065. Available from https://doi.org/10.1002/gps.2033.
6. Cummings, J. L., Miller, B., Hill, M. A., & Neshkes, R. (1987). Neuropsychiatric aspects of multi-infarct dementia and dementia of the Alzheimer type. Archives of Neurology, 44(4), 389-393.
7. Merriam, A. E., Aronson, M. K., Gaston, P., Wey, S. L., & Katz, I. (1988). Thepsychiatric symptoms of Alzheimer's disease. Journal of the American Geriatrics Society, 36(1), 7-12.
8. Starkstein, S. E., Chemerinski, E., Sabe, L., Kuzis, G., Petracca, G., Teson, A., & Leiguarda, R. (1997). Prospective longitudinal study of depression and anosognosia in Alzheimer's disease. British Journal of Psychiatry, 171, 47-52.
9. Teng, E., Ringman, J. M., Ross, L. K., Mulnard, R. A., Dick, M. B., Bartzokis, G., ... Alzheimer's Disease Research Centers of California-Depression in Alzheimer's Disease. (2008). Diagnosing depression in Alzheimer disease with the National Institute of Mental Health provisional criteria. American Journal of Geriatric Psychiatry, 16(6), 469-477. Available from https://doi.org/10.1097/JGP.0b013e318165dbae.
10. Orgeta, V., Qazi, A., Spector, A., & Orrell, M. (2015). Psychological treatments for depression and anxiety in dementia and mild cognitive impairment: Systematic review and meta-analysis. British Journal of Psychiatry, 207(4), 293-298. Available from https://doi.org/10.1192/bjp.bp.114.148130.
11. Gellis, Z. D., McClive-Reed, K. P., & Brown, E. (2009). Treatments for depression in older persons with dementia. Annals of Longterm Care, 17(2), 29-36.
12. Huang, Y. Y., Dou, K. X., Zhong, X. L., Shen, X. N., Chen, S. D., Li, H. Q., ... Yu, J. T. (2020). Pharmacological treatment of neuropsychiatric symptoms of dementia: A network meta-analysis protocol. Annals of Translational Medicine, 8(12), 746. Available from https://doi.org/10.21037/atm-20-611.
13. Evers, M. M., Samuels, S. C., Lantz, M., Khan, K., Brickman, A. M., & Marin, D. B. (2002). The prevalence, diagnosis and treatment of depression in dementia patients in chronic care facilities in the last six months of life. International Journal of Geriatric Psychiatry, 17(5), 464-472. Available from https://doi.org/10.1002/gps.634.

14. Birks, J. (2006). Cholinesterase inhibitors for Alzheimer's disease. Cochrane Database of Systemic Reviews (1), CD005593. Available from https://doi.org/10.1002/14651858.CD005593.
15. Mowla, A., Mosavinasab, M., Haghshenas, H., & Borhani Haghighi, A. (2007). Does serotonin augmentation have any effect on cognition and activities of daily living in Alzheimer's dementia? A double-blind, placebo-controlled clinical trial. Journal of Clinical Psychopharmacology, 27(5), 484-487. Available from https://doi.org/10.1097/jcp.0b013e31814b98c1.
16. Nagata, T., Shinagawa, S., Nakajima, S., Noda, Y., & Mimura, M. (2020). Pharmacological management of behavioral disturbances in patients with Alzheimer's disease. Expert Opinion on Pharmacotherapy, 21(9), 1093-1102. Available from https://doi.org/10.1080/14656566.2020.1745186.
17. Caballero, J., Hitchcock, M., Beversdorf, D., Scharre, D., & Nahata, M. (2006). Longterm effects of antidepressants on cognition in patients with Alzheimer's disease. Journal of Clinical Pharmacy and Therapeutics, 31(6), 593-598. Available from https://doi.org/10.1111/j.1365-2710.2006.00778.x.
18. Herrmann, N., & Lanctot, K. L. (2007). Pharmacologic management of neuropsychiatric symptoms of Alzheimer disease. The Canadian Journal of Psychiatry, 52(10), 630-646. Available from https://doi.org/10.1177/070674370705201004.
19. Lyketsos, C. G., DelCampo, L., Steinberg, M., Miles, Q., Steele, C. D., Munro, C., ... Rabins, P. V. (2003). Treating depression in Alzheimer disease: Efficacy and safety of sertraline therapy, and the benefits of depression reduction: The DIADS. Archives of General Psychiatry, 60(7), 737-746. Available from https://doi.org/10.1001/archpsyc.60.7.737.
20. Menon, A. S., Gruber-Baldini, A. L., Hebel, J. R., Kaup, B., Loreck, D., Itkin Zimmerman, S., ... Magaziner, J. (2001). Relationship between aggressive behaviors and depression among nursing home residents with dementia. International Journal of Geriatric Psychiatry, 16(2), 139-146.
21. Sink, K. M., Holden, K. F., & Yaffe, K. (2005). Pharmacological treatment of neuropsychiatric symptoms of dementia: A review of the evidence. The Journal of the American Medical Assocoiation, 293(5), 596-608. Available from https://doi.org/10.1001/jama.293.5.596.
22. Starkstein, S. E., & Mizrahi, R. (2006). Depression in Alzheimer's disease. Expert Review of Neurotherapeutics, 6(6), 887-895. Available from https://doi.org/10.1586/14737175.6.6.887.
23. Reifler, B. V., Teri, L., Raskind, M., Veith, R., Barnes, R., White, E., & McLean, P. (1989).

Double-blind trial of imipramine in Alzheimer's disease patients with and without depression. The Americal Journal of Psychiatry, 146(1), 45-49. Available from https://doi.org/10.1176/ajp.146.1.45.

24. Teri, L., Reifler, B. V., Veith, R. C., Barnes, R., White, E., McLean, P., & Raskind, M. (1991). Imipramine in the treatment of depressed Alzheimer's patients: impact on cognition. Journal of Gerontology, 46(6), P372-P377.

25. Takemoto, M., Ohta, Y., Hishikawa, N., Yamashita, T., Nomura, E., Tsunoda, K., ... Abe, K. (2020). The efficacy of sertraline, escitalopram, and nicergoline in the treatment of depression and apathy in Alzheimer's disease: The Okayama depression and apathy project (ODAP). Journal of Alzheimer's Disease, 76(2), 769-772. Available from https://doi.org/10.3233/JAD-200247.

26. Steffens, D. C., Skoog, I., Norton, M. C., Hart, A. D., Tschanz, J. T., Plassman, B. L., ... Breitner, J. C. (2000). Prevalence of depression and its treatment in an elderly population: The Cache County study. Archives of General Psychiatry, 57(6), 601-607.

27. Nelson, J. C., & Devanand, D. P. (2011). A systematic review and meta-analysis of placebo-controlled antidepressant studies in people with depression and dementia. Journal of the American Geriatrics Society, 59(4), 577-585. Available from https://doi.org/10.1111/j.1532-5415.2011.03355.x.

28. Lenze, E. J. (2011). Treating depression in older adults with dementia. Journal of the American Geriatrics Society, 59(4), 754-755. Available from https://doi.org/10.1111/j.1532-5415.2011.03357.x.

29. Dafsari, F. S., & Jessen, F. (2020). Depression-an underrecognized target for prevention of dementia in Alzheimer's disease. Translational Psychiatry, 10(1), 160. Available from https://doi.org/10.1038/s41398-020-0839-1.

30. Williams, C. L., & Tappen, R. M. (2007). Effect of exercise on mood in nursing home residents with Alzheimer's disease. American Journal of Alzheimer's Disease & Other Dementias, 22(5), 389-397. Available from https://doi.org/10.1177/1533317507305588.

31. Williams, C. L., & Tappen, R. M. (2008). Exercise training for depressed older adults with Alzheimer's disease. Aging and Mental Health, 12(1), 72-80. Available from https://doi.org/10.1080/13607860701529932.

32. Lawton, M. P., Van Haitsma, K., & Klapper, J. (1996). Observed affect in nursing home residents with Alzheimer's disease. The Journal of Gerontology B Series, Psychological Sciences and Social Sciences, 51(1), P3 P14. Available from https://doi.org/10.1093/geronb/51b.1.p3.

33. Regan, C., Katona, C., Walker, Z., & Livingston, G. (2005). Relationship of exercise and other risk factors to depression of Alzheimer's disease: The LASER-AD study.

International Journal of Geriatric Psychiatry, 20(3), 261-268. Available from https://doi.org/10.1002/gps.1278.

34. Stewart, D. B., Berg-Weger, M., Tebb, S., Sakamoto, M., Roselle, K., Downing, L., ... Hayden, D. (2017). Making a difference: A study of cognitive stimulation therapy for persons with dementia. Journal of Gerontological Social Work, 60(4), 300-312. Available from https://doi.org/10.1080/01634372.2017.1318196.

35. Moon, S., & Park, K. (2020). The effect of digital reminiscence therapy on people with dementia: A pilot randomized controlled trial. BMC Geriatrics, 20(1), 166. Available from https://doi.org/10.1186/s12877-020-01563-2.

36. Woods, B., O'Philbin, L., Farrell, E. M., Spector, A. E., & Orrell, M. (2018). Reminiscence therapy for dementia. Cochrane Database of Systemic Reviews (3), CD001120. Available from https://doi.org/10.1002/14651858.CD001120.pub3.

37. Marriott, A., Donaldson, C., Tarrier, N., & Burns, A. (2000). Effectiveness of cognitivebehavioural family intervention in reducing the burden of care in carers of patients with Alzheimer's disease. British Journal of Psychiatry, 176, 557-562.

38. Ahern, E., Kinsella, S., & Semkovska, M. (2018). Clinical efficacy and economic evaluation of online cognitive behavioral therapy for major depressive disorder: A systematic review and meta-analysis. Expert Review of Pharmacoeconomics & Outcomes Research, 18(1), 25-41. Available from https://doi.org/10.1080/14737167.2018.1407245.

39. Rubin-Falcone, H., Weber, J., Kishon, R., Ochsner, K., Delaparte, L., Dore, B., ... Miller, J. M. (2018). Longitudinal effects of cognitive behavioral therapy for depression on the neural correlates of emotion regulation. Psychiatry Research: Neuroimaging, 271, 82-90. Available from https://doi.org/10.1016/j.pscychresns.2017.11.002.

40. Vara, M. D., Herrero, R., Etchemendy, E., Espinoza, M., Banos, R. M., Garcia-Palacios, A., ... Botella, C. (2018). Efficacy and cost-effectiveness of a blended cognitive behavioral therapy for depression in Spanish primary health care: study protocol for a randomised non-inferiority trial. BMC Psychiatry, 18(1), 74. Available from https://doi.org/10.1186/s12888-018-1638-6.

41. Zhang, Z., Zhang, L., Zhang, G., Jin, J., & Zheng, Z. (2018). The effect of CBT and its modifications for relapse prevention in major depressive disorder: A systematic review and meta-analysis. BMC Psychiatry, 18(1), 50. Available from https://doi.org/10.1186/s12888-018-1610-5.

42. Teri, L., & Gallagher-Thompson, D. (1991). Cognitive-behavioral interventions for treatment of depression in Alzheimer's patients. Gerontologist, 31(3), 413-416.

43. Teri, L., Logsdon, R. G., Uomoto, J., & McCurry, S. M. (1997). Behavioral treatment of

depression in dementia patients: a controlled clinical trial. The Journal of Gerontology B Series, Psychological Sciences and Social Sciences, 52(4), P159-P166.
44. Walker, D. A. (2004). Cognitive behavioural therapy for depression in aperson with Alzheimer's disease. Behavioural and Cognitive Psychotherapy, 32, 495-500.
45. Forstmeier, S., Maercker, A., Savaskan, E., & Roth, T. (2015). Cognitive behavioural treatment for mild Alzheimer's patients and their caregivers (CBTAC): Study protocol for a randomized controlled trial. Trials, 16, 526. Available from https://doi.org/10.1186/s13063-015-1043-0.
46. Hopkinson, M. D., Reavell, J., Lane, D. A., & Mallikarjun, P. (2018). Cognitive behavioral therapy for depression, anxiety, and stress in caregivers of dementia patients: A systematic review and meta-analysis. Gerontologist, 59(4), e343-e362. Available from https://doi.org/10.1093/geront/gnx217.
47. Cheung, D. S. K., Kor, P. P. K., Jones, C., Davies, N., Moyle, W., Chien, W. T., ... Lai, C. (2020). The use of modified mindfulness-based stress reduction and mindfulness-based cognitive therapy programme for family caregivers of people living with dementia: A feasibility study. Asian Nursing Research (Korean Society of Nursing Science), 14(4)), 221-230. Available from https://doi.org/10.1016/j.anr.2020.08.009.
48. Sukontapol, C., Kemsen, S., Chansirikarn, S., Nakawiro, D., Kuha, O., & Taemeeyapradit, U. (2018). The effectiveness of a cognitive training program in people with mild cognitive impairment: A study in urban community. Asian Journal of Psychiatry, 35, 18-23. Available from https://doi.org/10.1016/j.ajp.2018.04.028.
49. Smith-Ray, R. L., Irmiter, C., & Boulter, K. (2016). Cognitive training among cognitively impaired older adults: A feasibility study assessing the potential improvement in balance. Frontiers in Public Health, 4, 219. Available from https://doi.org/10.3389/fpubh.2016.00219.
50. Naismith, S. L., & Mowszowski, L. (2016). Moving beyond mood: Is it time to recommend cognitive training for depression in older adults? In B. T. Baune, & P. J. Tully (Eds.), Cardiovascular diseases and depression (pp. 365-394). Cham: Springer.
51. Chan, J. Y. C., Chan, T. K., Kwok, T. C. Y., Wong, S. Y. S., Lee, A. T. C., & Tsoi, K. K. F. (2020). Cognitive training interventions and depression in mild cognitive impairment and dementia: A systematic review and meta-analysis of randomized controlled trials. Age Ageing, 49(5), 738-747. Available from https://doi.org/10.1093/ageing/afaa063.
52. Teri, L., Gibbons, L. E., McCurry, S. M., Logsdon, R. G., Buchner, D. M., Barlow, W. E., ... Larson, E. B. (2003). Exercise plus behavioral management in patients with Alzheimer disease: a randomized controlled trial. The Journal of the American Medical Assocoiation, 290(15), 2015-2022. Available from https://doi.org/10.1001/

jama.290.15.2015.

53. Lichtenberg, P. A., Kemp-Havican, J., Macneill, S. E., & Schafer Johnson, A. (2005). Pilot study of behavioral treatment in dementia care units. Gerontologist, 45(3), 406-410.

54. Onega, L. L., Pierce, T. W., & Epperly, L. (2018). Bright light therapy to treat depression in individuals with mild/moderate or severe dementia. Issues in Mental Health Nursing, 39(5), 1-4. Available from https://doi.org/10.1080/01612840.2018.1437648.

55. Ambrosi, C., Zaiontz, C., Peragine, G., Sarchi, S., & Bona, F. (2019). Randomized controlled study on the effectiveness of animal-assisted therapy on depression, anxiety, and illness perception in institutionalized elderly. Psychogeriatrics, 19(1), 55-64. Available from https://doi.org/10.1111/psyg.12367.

56. Mota Pereira, J., & Fonte, D. (2018). Pets enhance antidepressant pharmacotherapy effects in patients with treatment resistant major depressive disorder. Journal of Psychiatric Research, 104, 108-113. Available from https://doi.org/10.1016/j.jpsychires.2018.07.004.

57. Baek, S. M., Lee, Y., & Sohng, K. Y. (2020). The psychological and behavioural effects of an animal-assisted therapy programme in Korean older adults with dementia. Psychogeriatrics, 20(5), 645-653. Available from https://doi.org/10.1111/psyg.12554.

58. Rodrigues, J., Capuano, A. W., Barnes, L. L., Bennett, D. A., & Shah, R. C. (2018). Effect of antidepressant medication use and social engagement on the level of depressive symptoms in community-dwelling, older African Americans and Whites with dementia. Journal of Aging Health, 31(7), 1278-1296. Available from https://doi.org/10.1177/0898264318772983, 898264318772983.

59. Giovagnoli, A. R., Manfredi, V., Schifano, L., Paterlini, C., Parente, A., & Tagliavini, F. (2018). Combining drug and music therapy in patients with moderate Alzheimer's disease: A randomized study. Neurological Sciences, 39(6), 1021-1028. Available from https://doi.org/10.1007/s10072-018-3316-3.

60. Lam, H. L., Li, W. T. V., Laher, I., & Wong, R. Y. (2020). Effects of music therapy on patients with dementia A systematic review. Geriatrics (Basel), 5(4), 62. Available from https://doi.org/10.3390/geriatrics5040062.

61. Moreno-Morales, C., Calero, R., Moreno-Morales, P., & Pintado, C. (2020). Music therapy in the treatment of dementia: A systematic review and meta-analysis. Frontiers in Medicine (Lausanne), 7, 160. Available from https://doi.org/10.3389/fmed.2020.00160.

62. Jung, Y. H., Lee, S., Kim, W. J., Lee, J. H., Kim, M. J., & Han, H. J. (2020). Effect of integrated cognitive intervention therapy in patients with mild to moderate Alzheimer's disease. Dementia and Neurocognitive Disorders, 19(3), 86-95. Available from https://

doi.org/10.12779/dnd.2020.19.3.86.

63. Borisovskaya, A., Pascualy, M., & Borson, S. (2014). Cognitive and neuropsychiatric impairments in Alzheimer's disease: Current treatment strategies. Current Psychiatry Reports, 16(9), 470. Available from https://doi.org/10.1007/s11920-014-0470-z.

64. Kor, P. P. K., Liu, J. Y., & Chien, W. T. (2019). Effects on stress reduction of a modifiedmindfulness-based cognitive therapy for family caregivers of those with dementia: Study protocol for a randomized controlled trial. Trials, 20(1), 303. Available from https://doi.org/10.1186/s13063-019-3432-2.

65. Kor, P. P. K., Liu, J. Y. W., & Chien, W. T. (2020). Effects of a modified mindfulnessbased cognitive therapy for family caregivers of people with dementia: A randomized clinical trial. Gerontologist, gnaa125. Available from https://doi.org/10.1093/geront/gnaa125, September 4.

第十章　用于音乐干预治疗的负面情绪易感性痴呆量表的开发

Sandra Garrido，Wafa Jaroudi，Ahmed A. Moustafa　编
钟伙花，王　凤，倪卓新，詹云浩　译
陈仰昆　校

第一节　引言

根据统计，20%的阿尔茨海默病（AD）患者、30%的路易体痴呆（DLB）患者、33%的额颞叶痴呆（FTD）患者[1,2]以及63%的轻度认知障碍（MCI）患者都存在抑郁症状或已患有重度抑郁症（MDD）[3]。有大量证据表明，痴呆与抑郁之间不仅存在高度共病性，还存在双向关系。研究指出，晚年的抑郁症状可使患痴呆的风险增加3倍[4]。而患有MDD的MCI患者转变为AD的风险则增加了2倍[5]。抑郁的存在显著加速了痴呆患者的认知和功能衰退，同时也提高了他们进入养老机构的可能性[6]。

由于抑郁和痴呆常同时发生且关系密切，故有学者认为，反复的抑郁症状可能导致大脑变得更易于受到痴呆相关的退行性过程的影响[7]。某些研究甚至提出，若抑郁的患病率降低25%，全球可能减少约827 000例AD的发病[8]。抑郁症状严重影响了患者的生活质量，同时也给护理人员和医疗系统带来了巨大的压力[9,10]。激越也是痴呆患者的常见症状，具体表现包括重复动作、不安、游荡和攻击性等，其中高达80%的痴呆患者会表现出上述症状[11,12]。这些症状不仅会增加患者和护理者的压力，还会导致患者功能的进一步下降和生活质量的降低[13]。

痴呆患者常合并多种并发症，并且通常因身体其他健康问题而使用大量的药物，使得药物在治疗痴呆相关精神行为异常上受到质疑[14]。例如，常用的抗抑郁

药、抗焦虑药和抗精神病药与包括恶心和失眠在内的不良反应有关[15]。有证据表明，这些药物并不一定有效减轻症状，并可能与诸如精神错乱甚至导致死亡等严重不良临床事件有关[16,17]。因此，通常推荐首先使用非药物治疗手段来治疗痴呆患者的心理和行为症状[18]。然而，由于缺乏非药物治疗的标准化及循证指南，故药物治疗依然被广泛应用[19]。

研究表明，音乐疗法对痴呆症患者的生活质量和情绪有积极的影响。许多研究表明，积极形式的音乐治疗可以改善痴呆患者的抑郁、激越和认知功能[20,21]。例如，Raglio 等[22]在 2015 年的研究中明确指出，音乐疗法能够有效地缓解痴呆患者的激越症状。

音乐疗法对痴呆患者带来的益处显而易见，但由于音乐干预需要专业治疗师或音乐家在现场演奏，使得音乐疗法往往受到成本过高和实际操作难度大的限制而无法开展[23]。因此，虽然许多养老机构都试图实施某种形式的音乐项目，但他们通常无法频繁地使用专业音乐治疗师的方案[24,25]。因此，人们对在正式音乐治疗场所之外使用预录音乐用于治疗目的的兴趣日益浓厚。这种方案不仅相对易于获取，而且成本效益显著。无论是在住宅还是家庭护理环境中，大多数人都能随时享受到预录音乐的益处。越来越多的研究显示，与那些个人没有特别喜好甚至可能不喜欢的音乐相比，自选音乐和与个人经历紧密相关的音乐更能有效地调节情绪[23]。因此，人们的兴趣已开始转向在养老背景下使用"个性化播放列表"——即根据个体的音乐品味创建的预录音乐播放列表。

然而，研究表明，为痴呆症患者等易感人群播放音乐比仅选择个人"最喜欢的音乐"需要更多的关注。例如，一些研究报告显示，虽然大多数参与者受益于使用基于喜欢的个性化播放列表，但需明确并非普遍都能取得良好治疗效果。一些参与者的反应是中性的，甚至有些会出现情绪的恶化[26,27]。研究表明，音乐的特征（如节奏和调式）和个体因素（如近期或终身抑郁史以及痴呆症的严重程度）都会影响个性化播放列表的情绪治疗效果[24,25,28]。之前的其他研究表明，健康的参与者听音乐时，内向人格因素可能预示不良治疗效果[29]。如前所述，文献还表明，在某些情况下，音乐干预可能会增加痴呆症患者的焦虑，并且可能触发患者对音乐的强烈记忆和压抑情绪[30,31]。

这些发现证明了评估音乐干预潜在人群的适用性的重要性，以及音乐干预应该根据个体情况特别谨慎实施。这在不涉及训练有素的音乐治疗师的音乐节目的情况下尤其重要。例如，护理人员或志愿者可能希望为痴呆症患者使用音乐节目。虽然音乐治疗的负面反应并非经常出现，有时甚至会有良好的治疗效果，但对有抑郁史的人来说音乐干预治疗可能是有害的[32]。音乐治疗师接受过训练，可以应对与音乐有关的不良反应，如过度刺激、情绪泛滥或引发痛苦记忆[31]，而未经训练的护理人员可能不太能够处理这些负面反应。因此，在对痴呆症患者实施音乐干预治疗之前，有必要确定高危人群，以确保建立适当的监测和支持系统。

截至到目前，还没有工具可以帮助老年护理机构的护理人员或音乐治疗师识别可能需要特别照顾的人群。虽然前面讨论的因素可以帮助识别高风险的参与者，但使用之前建立的量表来评估音乐节目的潜在参与者的这些因素会给护理人员带来相当大的负担。目前的研究旨在通过开发和评估一种筛选工具来解决这一问题，该筛选工具主要用于识别可能容易受到音乐干预而出现不良反应的人群。

第二节　方法

一、条目研发

基于文献和已有量表构建负面情绪易感性痴呆量表（Vulnerability to Negative Affect in Dementia Scale，VNADS）的首个量表条目池，此量表旨在反映先前被发现与音乐负面反应相关的因素。因此，作为量表研发的第一步，我们抽取既往量表的条目形成了一个量表条目池。抽取条目的量表包括广泛焦虑性量表、患者健康问卷、反刍、反思性问卷，以及专门为 VNADS 开发的 2 个条目[33-35]。在消除了不同量表中概念上重复的条目后，使用了先前开发的量表中载荷最重的条目。最终的量表包含 24 个条目，评分范围从 1（非常不同意）到 5（非常同意）。

二、条目预测试

第 1 版 VNADS 首先在 384 名认知健康参与者中进行了预测试,用以验证 24 条目量表的结构及有效性。样本从普通人群中挑选,而非用于预测试的痴呆患者。这样做的原因是在对痴呆患者进行正式测试之前,通过大样本对量表的总体结构进行验证。受试者年龄在 18 岁及以上,通过在各种网站、博客、讨论页面和社交媒体平台上的推广参与线上调查。其他用于验证的量表包括 Leiden 抑郁敏感性指数量表[36]、老年焦虑量表(Geriatric Anxiety Inventory,CAI)[37]、21 项抑郁焦虑压力量表(DASS-21)[38]以及 Kessler 10 量表(K10)[39]。进行相关分析以检验与先前量表的关系,并进行主成分分析和可靠性分析。

三、痴呆症患者测试替代版 VNADS

基于预测试结果形成改良版的 VNADS,并形成由家庭成员或照顾者完成的替代版 VNADS。替代版 VNADS 特意调整了措辞,使其更好地反映观察者对痴呆患者过去或现在的行为及情感状态的观察。改良版的 VNADS 是一个包含音乐聆听及会话模拟的在线调查,对 48 名(男性 18 名,女性 30 名)60 岁及以上(平均年龄为 64.9 岁,标准差为 2.7)的痴呆症患者及其照顾者共同进行了测试。这些参与者是通过在相关网站、社交媒体页面上的广告,以及向澳大利亚新南威尔士州的痴呆患者团体发送的邮件列表中招募来的。这些参与者中 48.1% 诊断为 AD,13.5% 诊断为非特异性痴呆,7.7% 诊断为血管性痴呆(VaD),3.8% 诊断为 FTD,3.8% 诊断为 MCI,23.1% 诊断为其他类型痴呆。认知障碍分级采用痴呆严重程度评定量表(Dementia Severity Rating Scale,DSRS)[40]进行评估。在完成 DSRS 和 VNADS(替代版)后,调查者指导参与者从 5 首歌曲的列表中选择 3 首歌曲。这些歌曲来自可能符合参与者年龄段品味的多种风格,包括古典、乡村、民谣、流行和爵士乐。所选歌曲的目的是引起听众的悲伤,其调式多为小调,节奏相对缓慢,都是西方传统音乐中典型的悲伤音乐。在线调查需要先回答一个问题,以确认他们能够听这首歌。参与者(或其照顾者)得到以下指令:"听这首歌你感觉怎么样(或者痴呆症患者代表他们回答这个问题)?移动滑块以显示音乐的效果。"随后，参与者在滑块上对音乐的效果进行评分，滑块可以从消极"1"移动到积极"5"，中间部分为中性。同时还对音乐的熟悉程度进行了评分，因为熟悉程度也可在音乐效果上发挥作用[41]。为了抵消音乐熟悉程度的消极影响，参与者可以在调查结束前从更快乐的歌曲列表中选择一首歌曲，并对他们的反应进行类似的评分。最后，再次进行因素分析，以探索量表的结构以及其在识别可能对音乐产生负面情感反应的个体中的应用价值。

第三节　结果

一、版本 1 的预测试

采用 Kaiser 归一化法对 VNADS 条目进行主成分分析，其中 4 个成分的特征值 > 1。然而屏幕图显示的模型主要由 1 个主要成分和 3 个次要成分构成，最后一个成分不易解释，因其组成项目与第一个成分的组成项目有强烈的相关性。在最终模型中保留了 3 个成分，累计解释了 56.6% 的方差。综合考虑后，最终的量表包含三个成分，分别为：①抑郁；②多虑；③情绪。信度分析结果显示，量表整体的 Cronbach's α 系数为 0.93，删除第 22 项后，该系数略微提高至 0.94。因此，从量表中移除第 22 项。

根据作者的建议，计算了经修订后的 VNADS 的其余 23 项以及其他量表的总分。通过 Pearson 相关系数分析，发现 VNADS 与 LIEDS（$r=69$, $P < 0.001$）、DASS 压力子量表（$r=69$, $P < 0.001$）、DASS 焦虑子量表（$r=62$, $P < 0.001$）、DASS 抑郁子量表（$r=71$, $P < 0.001$）、K10（$r=78$, $P < 0.001$）以及 GAI（$r=74$, $P < 0.001$）呈显著的正相关。这意味着 VNADS 与这些可能预测音乐节目产生负面反应的量表具有很强的相关性。

二、VNADS 试验（指标）

使用的是未加权最小二乘法配合方差最大旋转法固定提取 3 个因子，对 VNADS（指标）23 个项目进行了验证性因素分析。其中删除通用性值低于 5

和交叉承载系数差异小于 2 的项目，留下 10 个子项目（表 10-1）。再次进行因子分析，结果确定了 3 个因子被标记为：①抑郁；②多虑；③情绪。这 3 个因子解释了数据中 69.66% 的方差。这 10 个项目的信度分析显示 Cronbach's α 为 89。

表 10-1　修订后的 VNADS（指标）项目的内容

项目序数		抑郁	多虑	情绪
1	最近 2 周，他/她感到沮丧、悲观或者绝望	0.745	—	0.499
2	在他/她的一生中，经常感到不快乐、沮丧或绝望	0.838	—	—
3	在过去的 2 周里，他/她觉得自己很失败，或者让别人失望	0.764	—	—
4	在他/她的一生中，经常感到自己不好，就像是一个失败者或让别人失望	0.802	—	—
5	在过去 2 周，他/她一直无法停止担忧	—	—	0.577
6	在他/她的脑海中经常回想自身在过去某些场景下是如何表现的	—	0.853	—
7	他/她经常重新审视过去所做的事情	—	0.785	—
8	他/她经常反思生活中那些不应该再关心的片段	—	0.895	—
9	他/她发现很难不去想以前生活中事件的创伤记忆	—	0.678	—
10	他/她经常流泪，或者感觉比以前更想哭	—	—	0.689

根据这 10 个项目的得分，将参与者分为"无风险到低风险"和"中风险到高风险"组。由于得分 3 表示选择"中立"，因此如果参与者得分为 33 分或以下，说明他们同意的项目不超过 1 个，则将参与者归类为"无风险至低风险"；如果参与者得分为 34 或以上，代表他们同意 2 个或更多的项目，则将它们归类为"中风险至高风险"。然后进行 Mann-Whitney 检验，以对哀伤音乐的反应作为因变量，VNADS 风险组作为自变量。结果表明，与"中风险至高风险"组（$n=10$，

中位数 =2）相比，"无风险至低风险"组（n=31，中位数 =4）对音乐的情绪反应评分更高，能够对音乐产生更明显的情绪反应，结果具有显著的统计学意义（U=94，z=–1.98，P=0.044）。同时以对快乐音乐的反应作为因变量进行类似的分析，发现组间无统计学差异。这些结果表明，VNADS（指标）的 10 项版本对于鉴定那些听悲伤音乐时可能产生负面情感反应的痴呆症患者是有效的。

第四节　讨论

本章报告的两项研究旨在开发并初步测试一个简短的问卷，以识别可能对音乐产生负面情感反应的痴呆症患者。第一项研究针对认知健康的参与者，采用了一个 24 项的问卷。结果显示问卷具有很高的内部一致性，并与其他经验证的、涉及相似领域的长问卷具有中到强的相关性。在第二项研究中，利用 VNADS 的简化版（10 项）成功识别了可能对音乐产生负面反应的个体。此版本中的项目主要涉及 3 个关联维度：①抑郁；②多虑；③情绪。

这些结果与之前的研究一致，无论是对痴呆患者还是年轻的成年人[24-26]，均发现患有抑郁或多虑的人在听悲伤音乐时更容易产生负面情感[32,42,43]。尽管 VNADS 的长版本考察了对音乐的强烈情感反应，但这些项目的因子负荷相对较弱。这表明与其说对音乐的强烈情感反应更能预测对音乐的不良反应，不如说总体心理健康和多虑这种终生思维模式更为关键。多虑往往与抑郁相伴，表现为对负面情境的过度思考[35,44]。多虑过度或抑郁的人对负面刺激更为敏感，对负面情感恢复也更为困难[45,46]。因此，这类人群在听悲伤音乐时更容易产生负面反应[47]。相对而言，对音乐的强烈情感反应可能与心理"净化"机制有关，虽然开始可能是负面的，但最终却带来了积极的心理效益[48]。这意味着，即使对音乐有强烈的情感反应，也并不代表音乐对个体不利[49]。事实上，即便是容易对"悲伤"音乐产生负面反应的个体，他们仍可从音乐中受益。但为了更好地选择和使用音乐，识别这些个体是关键，这样才能更有针对性地管理任何可能出现的负面反应。

本文报道的研究并未在受控条件下执行，因此具有一定局限性。特别是第二项研究，它采取模拟实验方法并基于一个规模较小的样本。鉴于其并非在实验室设置中进行，可能会有研究者难以控制的外部变量对结果造成了影响。未来研究应当在面对面的环境中对该量表进行测试，采用多种测量方式深入评估音乐听觉的效果，并扩大涉及痴呆症患者及其护理者的样本规模。

此次研究中所采用的实验模式并不支持完全个性化的音乐听觉。虽然音乐选择考虑到了个人的音乐类别偏好，但先前的研究[50]已指出，与个人相关的音乐更易引起正面反应。此外，本研究在代理测量方面也有所不足。已有研究[51]显示自我报告与代理测量之间常出现偏差。在痴呆症患者中寻找测量心理结构的标准方法始终是这类研究的挑战。未来，可以考虑将轻至中度受损患者的 VNADS 自报告与代理版本进行对比，或加入行为测量来做对照。

尽管存在上述局限，但 VNADS 仍是一款宝贵的工具，它能帮助识别那些在参与音乐或其他艺术项目时可能需要额外关注或支持的个体。VNADS 的精简版只有 10 个项目，不会引起受访者的问卷疲劳，因此为护理人员或研究者在未来研究提供了一个实用的评估工具。

基　　金：本研究由 NHMRC-ACR 痴呆研究发展奖学金资助给第一作者。

利益冲突：作者声明本章的出版不存在利益冲突。

致　　谢：无。

参考文献

1. Whitfield, D. R., Vallortigara, J., Alghamdi, A., Hortobagyi, T., Ballard, C., Thomas, A. J., ... Francis, P. T. (2015). Depression and synaptic zinc regulatino in Alzheimer disease, dementia with Lewy bodies, and Parkinson disease dementia. The American Journal of Geriatric Psychiatry, 23(2), 141-148.
2. Chakrabarty, T., Sepehry, A. A., Jacova, C., & Hsiung, G.-Y. R. (2015). The prevalence of depressive symptoms in frontotemporal dementia: A meta-analysis. Dementia and

Geratric Cognitive Disorders, 39, 257-271.
3. Panza, F., Frisardi, V., Capurso, C., D'Introno, A., Colacicco, A., Imbimbo, B., ... Solfrizzi, V. (2010). Late-life depression, mild cognitive impairment, and dementia: Possible continuum? American Journal of Geriatric Psychiatry, 18, 98-116.
4. Brommelhoff, J., Gatz, M., Johansson, B., McArdle, J., Fratiglioni, L., & Pedersen, N. (2009). Depression as a risk factor or prodromal feature for dementia? Findings in a population-based sample of Swedish twins. Psychology and Aging, 24, 373-384.
5. Ownby, R., Crocco, E., Acevedo, A., John, V., & Loewensteing, D. (2006). Depression and risk for Alzheimer disease: Systematic review, meta-analysis, and metaregression analysis. Archives of General Psychiatry, 63, 530-538.
6. Potter, G., & Steffens, D. (2007). Contribution of depression to cognitive impairment and dementia in older adults. The Neurologist, 13, 105-117.
7. Aznar, S., & Knudsen, G. M. (2011). Depression and Alzheimer's disease: Is stress the initiating factor in a common neuropathological cascade? Journal of Alzheimer's Disease, 23, 177-193.
8. Bames, D. E., & Yaffe, K. (2011). The projected effect of risk factor reduction on Alzheimer's disease prevalence. Lancet Neurology, 10, 819-828.
9. Banerjee, S., Samsi, K., Petrie, C. D., Alvir, J., Treglia, M., Schwam, E. M., & del Valle, M. (2009). What do we know about quality of life in dementia? A review of the emerging evidence on the predictive and explanatory value of disease specific measures of health related quality of life in people with dementia. International Journal of Geriatric Psychiatry, 24(1), 15-24.
10. Curran, E. M., & Loi, S. (2012). Depression and dementia. Medical Journal of Australia, 1 (Suppl 4), 40-44.
11. Cerejeira, J., Lagarto, L., & Mukaetova-Ladinska, E. B. (2012). Behavioral and psychological symptoms of dementia. Frontiers in Neurology, 3(73). Available from https://doi.org/10.3389/fneur.2012.00073.
12. Sourial, R., McCusker, J., Cole, M., & Abrahamowicz, M. (2001). Agitation in demented patients in an acute care hospital: Prevalence, disruptiveness and staff burden. International Psychogeriatrics, 13, 183-197. Available from https://doi.org/10.1017/S1041610201007578.
13. Kales, H. C., Gitlin, L. N., & Lyketsos, C. G. (2014). Management of neuropsychiatric symptoms of dementia is clinical settings: Recommendations from a multidisciplinary panel. Journal of American Geriatric Society, 62, 762-769.
14. Gottfries, C.-G. (2001). Late life depression. European Archives of Psychiatry and Clinical Neuroscience, 251(Suppl. 2), 57-61.

15. Caltagirone, C., Bianchetti, A., Di Luca, M., Mecocci, P., Padovani, A., Pirfo, E., ... Musicco, M. (2005). Guidelines for the treatment of Alzheimer's disease from the Italian Association of Psychogeriatrics. Drugs & Aging, 22(Suppl. 1), 1-26.
16. Farina, N., Morrell, L., & Banerjee, S. (2017). What is the therapeutic value of antidepressants in dementia? A narrative review. International Journal of Geriatric Psychiatry, 32(1), 32-49.
17. Sacchetti, E., Turrina, C., & Valsecchi, P. (2010). Cerebrovascular accidents in elderly people treated with antipsychotic drugs. Drug Safety, 33, 273-288.
18. Arzemia, M., Elseviers, M., Petrovic, M., Van Bortel, L., & Stichele, R. V. (2011). Geriatric drug utilisation of psychotropics in Belgian nursing homes. Human Psychopharmacology, 26, 12-20. Available from https://doi.org/10.1002/hup.1160.
19. Hansen, R. A., Gartlehner, G., Lohr, K. N., & Kaufer, D. I. (2007). Functional outcomes of drug treatment in Alzheimer's disease. Drugs & Aging, 24, 155-167. Available from https://doi.org/10.2165/00002512-200724020-00007.
20. O'Connor, D. W., Ames, D., Gardner, B., & King, M. (2009). Psychosocial treatments of behavior symptoms in dementia: A systematic review of reports meeting quality standards. International Psychogeriatrics, 21(2), 225-240.
21. Van der Steen, J. T., Smaling, H. J. A., van der Wouden, J. C., Bruinsma, M. S., Scholten, R. J. P. M., & Vink, A. C. (2018). Music-based therapeutic interventions for people with dementia. Cochrane Database of Systematic Reviews (7), CD00347. Available from https://doi.org/10.1002/14651858.CD003477.pub4.
22. Raglio, A., Bellandi, D., Baiardi, P., Gianotti, M., Ubezio, M. C., Zanacchi, E., ... Stramba-Badiale, M. (2015). Effect of active music therapy and individualized listening to music on dementia: A multicenter randomized controlled trial. Journal of theAmerican Geriatrics Society, 63(8), 1534-1539. Available from https://doi.org/10.1111/jgs.13558.
23. Nair, B. R., Browne, W., Marley, J., & Heim, C. (2013). Music and dementia. Degenerative Neurological and Neuromuscular Disease, 3, 47-51.
24. Garrido, S., Dunne, L., Perz, J., Chang, E., & Stevens, C. (2018a). The use of music in aged care facilities: A mixed methods study. Journal of Health Psychology, 15, 765-776.
25. Garrido, S., Stevens, C., Chang, E., Dunne, L., & Perz, J. (2018b). Music and dementia: Individual differences in response to personalized playlists. Journal of Alzheimer's Disease, 64(3), 933-941. Available from https://doi.org/10.3233/JAD-180084.
26. Martin, P. K., Schroeder, R. W., Smith, J. M., & Jones, B. (2016). The Roth project Music and memory: Surveying the observed benefit of personalized music in individuals with diagnosed or suspected dementia. Alzheimer's & Dementia, 12(7 Suppl.), P988. Available from https://doi.org/10.1016/j.jalz.2016.06.2028.

27. Ziv, N., Granot, A., Hai, S., Dassa, A., & Haimov, I. (2007). The effect of background stimulative music on behaviour in Alzheimer's patients. Journal of Music Therapy, 44(4), 329-343.
28. Garrido, S., Stevens, C., Chang, E., Dunne, L., & Perz, J. (2019). Music and dementia: Musical features and affective responses to personalized playlists. American Journal of Alzhiemers and Other Dementias, 34(4), 247-253. Available from https://doi.org/10.1177/1533317518808011.
29. Garrido, S., Bangert, D., & Schubert, E. (2016). Musical prescriptions for mood improvements: A mixed methods study. The Arts in Psychotherapy, 51, 46-53.
30. Garland, K., Beer, E., Eppingstall, B., & O'Connor, D. W. (2007). A comparison of two treatments of agitated behaviour in nursing home redidents with dementia: Simulated family presence and preferred music. American Journal of Geriatric Psychiatry, 15(6),514-521.
31. Moore, K. S. (2014). Five problems music can create. Retrieved from https://www.psychology-today.com/us/blog/your-musical-self/201408/5-problems-music-can-create; Accessed 28.11.19.
32. Garrido, S., & Schubert, E. (2015). Music and people with tendencies to depression. Music Perception, 32(4), 313-321. Available from https://doi.org/10.1525/MP.2015.32.4.313.
33. Kroenke, K., Lowe, B., Spitzer, R. L., & Williams, J. B. (2006). A brief measure for assessing generalized anxiety disorder: The GAD-7. Archives of Internal Medicine, 166(10), 1092-1097.
34. Spitzer, R. L., Kroenke, K., & Williams, J. B. (1999). Patient health questionnaire study group. Validity and utility of a self-report version of PRIME-MD: The PHQ primary care study. JAMA: The Journal of the American Medical Association, 282, 1737-1744.
35. Trapnell, P. D., & Campbell, J. D. (1999). Private self-consciousness and the five-factor model of personality: Distinguishing rumination from reflection. Journal of Personality and Social Psychology, 76(2), 284-304.
36. Van der Does, A. J. W., & Williams, J. W. G. (2003). Leiden Index of Depressive Sensitivity -Revised (LEIDS-R). Leiden University. Retrieved from https://www.dousa.nl/publications_depression.htm#LEIDS.
37. Pachana, N., Byrne, G., Siddle, H., Koloski, N., Harley, E., & Arnold, E. (2007). Development and validation of the geriatric anxiety inventory. International Psychogeriatrics, 19, 103-114.
38. Lovibond, S. H., & Lovibond, P. F. (1995). The structure of negative emotional states: Comparison of the Depression Anxiety Stress Scales (DASS) with the beck depression

and anxiety inventories. Behaviour Research and Therapy, 33(3), 335-343. Available from https://doi.org/10.1016/0005-7967(94)00075-U.

39. Kessler, R. C., Barker, P. R., Colpe, L. J., Epstein, J. F., Gfroerer, J. C., Hiripi, E., ... Zaslavsky, A. M. (2003). Screening for serious mental illness in the general population. Archives of General Psychiatry, 60(2), 184-189.

40. Clark, C. M., & Ewbank, D. C. (1996). Performance of the dementia severity rating scale: A caregiver questionnaire for rating severity in Alzheimer disease. Alzheimer Disease and Associated Disorders, 10(1), 31-39.

41. Sung, H. C., Chang, A. M., & Lee, W. L. (2010). A preferred music listening intervention to reduce anxiety in older adults with dementia in nursing homes. Journal of Clinical Nursing, 19(78), 1056-1064. Available from https://doi.org/10.1111/j.1365-2702.2009.03016.x.

42. Chen, L., Zhou, S., & Bryant, J. (2007). Temporal changes in mood repair through music consumption: Effects of mood, mood salience, and individual differences. Media Psychology, 9, 695-713.

43. Wilhelm, K., Gilllis, I., Schubert, E., & Whittle, E. L. (2013). On a blue note: Depressed people's reasons for listening to music. Music and Medicine, 5(2), 76-83.

44. Nolen-Hoeksema, S., & Morrow, J. (1993). Effects of rumination and distraction on naturally occurring depressed mood. Cognition & Emotion, 7(6), 561-570.

45. Gotlib, I. H., Krasnoperova, E., Neubauer Yue, D., & Joormann, J. (2004). Attentional biases for negative interpersonal stimuli in clinical depression. Journal of Abnormal Psychology, 113(1), 127-135.

46. Platt, B., Murphy, S. E., & Lau, J. Y. F. (2015). The association between negative attentional biases and symptoms of depression in a community sample of adolescents. PeerJ, 3, e1372.

47. Foland-Ross, L. C., Hamilton, J. P., Joormann, J., Berman, M. G., Jonides, J., & Gotlib, I. H. (2013). The neural basis of difficulties disengaging from negative irrelevant material in major depression. Psychological Science, 24(3), 334-344.

48. Garrido, S., & Schubert, E. (2013). Adaptive and maladaptive attraction to negative emotion in music. Musicae Scientiae, 17(2), 145-164. Available from https://doi.org/10.1177/1029864913478305.

49. Zhan, J., Tang, F., Mei, H., Jin, F., Jing, X., Chang, L., & Jing, L. (2017). Regulating rumination by anger: Evidence for the mutual promotion and counteraction (MPMC) theory of emotionality. Frontiers in Psychology, 8, 1871. Available from https://doi.org/10.3389/fpsyg.2017.01871.

50. Gerdner, L. A. (2012). Individualized music for dementia: Evolution and application of

evidence-based protocol. World Journal of Psychiatry, 2(2), 26-32.
51. Howland, M., Allan, K. C., & Sajatovic, M. (2017). Patient-rated versus proxy-rated cognitive and functional measures in older adults. Patient Related Outcome Measures, 8, 33-42. Available from https://doi.org/10.2147/PROM.S126919.

第十一章 运用音乐改善痴呆人群的精神健康

Ahmed A. Moustafa, Eid Abo Hamza, Wafa Jaroudi, Sandra Garrido 编
李爱萍,袁一棉 译
刘勇林 校

第一节 引言

音乐治疗是一种基于循证方法,相较于以倾听音乐提高生活质量[1],更倾向于参与音乐,如唱歌[2,3]、演奏乐器[2-4]以及歌曲创作[5]。音乐治疗的实施需要一位经过培训和注册的音乐治疗师,他能使用既定的疗法为痴呆患者定制"音乐治疗"计划。音乐疗法不仅可以通过唱歌等活动提高患者的身体和语言机能[6],也使他们与具有个人意义的歌曲联系起来从而改善患者之间的人际交往[7]。此外,音乐疗法通过缓解抑郁[2,8]和激越[1]症状,已被用于提高痴呆个体的心理健康。因此,音乐治疗也能改善痴呆个体的认知功能和记忆力下降[8]。

除了音乐治疗,音乐还能在正式治疗场合之外有效地适用于改善痴呆症患者的精神健康。研究表明,即使没有受过培训的音乐治疗师在场参与,基于循证依据的音乐聆听项目也可以减少患者的激越[9,10]和焦虑。音乐干预也可以提高痴呆患者的沟通能力,增加其参与度和警觉性,使其与护理人员的联系更加紧密[11]。本章将进一步探讨音乐疗法和非治疗师主导的音乐干预手段,以及它们如何改善一些痴呆患者的心理和认知健康。

第二节 音乐疗法

痴呆患者的抑郁、焦虑和激越等心理学症状的管理是复杂的。多种并发症的存在意味着药物治疗并不总是理想的[12]。故而,来自世界各地的多个决策机

构建议将非药物治疗作为管理痴呆症状的一线方法[13,14]。因此，音乐疗法已成为管理痴呆患者心理学症状（如抑郁、焦虑和激越）的一种普遍通用的替代治疗方法。下文将分别讨论音乐疗法对焦虑和激越以及心境和抑郁的影响。

一、焦虑和激越

音乐疗法能够获益的最强有力的证据之一是，其能减少痴呆患者激越症状。例如，Raglio 等[15]评估了音乐疗法对伴有 6 个月以上行为障碍的重度痴呆患者的有效性。共 60 名试验者被分为对照组和实验组。实验组患者接受为期 1 个多月的 3 轮（每 12 次音乐治疗为 1 轮）音乐治疗，方法是让患者参与即兴音乐创作。在整个研究过程中对受试者采用以下方法进行评估：简易精神状态检查量表（MMSE）、日常生活能力 Barthel 指数和神经精神问卷调查。音乐治疗是非语言的，主要通过声音、乐曲和即兴创作作用于受试者的行为，以及通过演奏乐器表达情感。Ragli 等[15]发现，音乐治疗计划有助于改善和管理痴呆患者的行为学和心理学症状，尤其是激越[15]。这些研究发现，仅仅在实施音乐治疗 1 个月后，患者的行为障碍症状就有所改善，提示音乐治疗在痴呆患者中的有效性。

同样地，Ridder 等[16]探讨了音乐疗法是否可以减轻中重度痴呆患者的激越型的行为学和心理学症状。他们也对音乐疗法是否能够提高生活质量以及影响抗精神病药物的使用感兴趣。该研究的音乐治疗项目以个人为中心，这意味着他们对不同的个体采取不同的方法，通过唱歌、演奏乐器、跳舞或其他活动，如交谈和散步等多种形式进行即兴创作。该研究样本量为 42 名试验者，其中音乐治疗组 21 例，对照组或标准护理组 21 例。经过 6 周的音乐治疗后，与对照组或标准护理组患者相比，音乐治疗组患者的激越程度下降。对于抗精神病药物的使用情况，音乐治疗组患者的药物使用没有任何显著改变，而未接受音乐治疗患者使用的抗精神病药物有所增加[16]。这些发现进一步证实音乐疗法可以减少激越，并提高患者的生活质量和心理健康。

Sung 等[17]研究证明，小组音乐治疗同样有效，他们评估了小组音乐干预如何影响痴呆患者的焦虑和激越程度。该研究由两个实验小组构成，包括受试组的27名参与者，对照组的28名参与者。Sung等[17]的音乐干预治疗让受试组作为一个小组演奏打击乐器，如手鼓和手铃，每周两次，每次30分钟，持续6周，治疗中使用受试者熟知的音乐和歌曲，并考虑了其音乐偏好。相较于对照组，受试组在参加音乐表演后的焦虑感显著降低。同时，受试组的激越症状有所减轻，但与对照组相比，这种改善并不显著。不过，Sung等[17]认为，这种情况可能与患者没有表现出激越行为有关，后者可能限制了参与者激越症状的显著改善或减少[17]，就像焦虑症状那样。另外，对照组参与者的焦虑和激越情绪也有所减轻[17]。Sung等[17]认为，这一研究发现与受试组中的个体有关，随着时间的推移，这些受试个体的情绪和心境有所改善，从而影响了居住在同一家养老机构的对照组个体。他们提出，移情在改善痴呆患者的情绪方面发挥着作用，也就是说，情绪改善的受试者将他们的积极情绪投射到环境中的其他人身上，从而改善其他人的情绪。

其他研究更详细地分析了音乐影响痴呆患者的机制。例如，McDermott等[18]采用访谈方式来探讨痴呆患者对音乐的感知，以及他们的家人、护理人员和音乐治疗师等其他人，如何感知音乐治疗的效果。研究结果表明，音乐疗法可以让痴呆患者映射和联结周围的世界及他们过往的经历，是改善行为障碍（如激越）和燃起对生活的信心的一种方式。痴呆患者的照顾人员指出，音乐疗法对痴呆患者具有放松情绪的作用，并改善他们的居住环境。音乐的选择与患者的性格、生活经历、文化认同和生活年代有关，使他们能够与治疗期间倾听的音乐建立联结[18]。这些发现表明，音乐干预通过允许个体进行沟通交流、表达感受、减少激越，并与自己和身份重新联结，从而产生心理社会效应。

二、心境和抑郁

几项研究探讨了音乐疗法对同时伴有抑郁症状的痴呆患者的影响。例如，Ashida[19]调查了作为一种回忆形式的音乐疗法对20例痴呆患者抑郁症状的影响。与Bevins等[20]以及Ridder等[16]其他研究者的试验类似，该音乐疗法让参与者演奏乐器，如鼓、吉他，或让参与者根据自己临场的即时想法，或看着窗外，或对着天气即兴歌唱。研究发现，音乐治疗可以减少抑郁情绪，提高沟通技巧。此外，音乐治疗减少了社交退缩，帮助试验者更多地参与社交活动，这表明他们的情绪得到了改善[19]。

另一项研究也评估了音乐疗法对减轻抑郁的影响。Chu 等[8]研究了各种音乐治疗手段对减轻痴呆患者抑郁的有效性，包括选择歌曲、聆听音乐和演奏乐器等。在为期 6 周的音乐治疗中，心理学家密切监测试验者的自杀意念以及抑郁症状的变化。还有研究对唾液样本进行了分析，以检测皮质醇水平，它既表明应激水平升高，也可能提示抑郁症状的发展[21,22]。对试验者的认知水平也定期应用 MMSE 进行测评。该研究报道经过音乐治疗后，抑郁症状减轻，认知能力改善，尤其是轻度和中度痴呆患者。然而，分析并未发现皮质醇水平有任何提高[8]。因此，强有力的证据表明，音乐疗法可以减轻痴呆患者的抑郁症状，改善认知能力。研究发现，音乐涉及节奏和歌词，其可以刺激认知功能，如短期记忆、注意力、计算和语言能力[8]。音乐疗法会刺激语言程序，而语言程序通常会受到抑郁症状的影响[23]。然而，音乐疗法对重症痴呆患者效果欠佳[24,25]。这可能是因为重症痴呆与更广泛的脑损伤和一些认知问题有关。广泛的疾病表现限制了音乐刺激认知功能（如记忆）的能力或潜力，这些功能在痴呆晚期会下降。

还有一些研究探讨了音乐疗法对心境的影响。Bevins 等[20]评估了音乐治疗对既有痴呆又有智力残疾(如 Down/唐氏综合征)患者的有效性。受试者接受 3 项评估，而后参与 18 次音乐疗法干预。音乐干预课程主要包括受试者通过音乐分享感受、演奏乐器、表演式的音乐交流。受试者和照顾者都参加了半结构化访谈。该研究称，通过小组音乐治疗发现，参与音乐课程的受试者既愉悦又兴奋。另有报道称，归因于音乐治疗课程，大多数受试者的沟通能力和心境也有所改善[20]。

第三节 非治疗师主导的音乐干预

除了音乐疗法，非音乐治疗师主导的音乐干预也可以对痴呆患者的心理健康产生积极影响。这些干预措施包括在老年护理机构使用背景音乐，以及在护理院使用经标准化的个性化播放曲目和现场音乐活动。

一、幸福感、焦虑、心境

几项研究调查了音乐干预对痴呆患者精神健康的影响。例如，Van der Vleuten 等[26]探讨了现场音乐表演对痴呆患者的幸福感和生活质量的影响。在样本量为 54 名轻度和重度痴呆患者的试验中，大多数参与者都享受现场音乐表演，并感受到观赏表演对他们幸福感的积极作用。研究结果表明，现场音乐表演可能对轻度痴呆患者产生的积极影响更持久，而对重度痴呆症患者来说，可能只是一种即时的快乐或愉悦。这一发现与其他研究一致表明，音乐疗法提升幸福感的有效性与痴呆患者的病程阶段及症状严重程度相关[24,25]。

由于有证据表明音乐偏好会影响对幸福感的体验和效果[18]，Sung 等[27]探讨了聆听偏好音乐如何影响痴呆患者的焦虑。他们将 29 人分配到试验组，将 23 人分配到对照组，来比较两组聆听偏好音乐的情况。两组参与者都接受了标准的护理，如参加社交活动和身体锻炼，但试验组额外参加了每周 2 次、为期 6 周的音乐聆听课程。用音乐偏好量表测评参与者的音乐偏好，使用痴呆症焦虑评分量表测评参与者的焦虑症状和体征。与 McDermott 等[18]研究一致，Sung 等[27]发现，聆听偏好音乐可以显著减少参与者的焦虑。Sung 等[27]认为，偏好音乐在减轻焦虑症状方面的有效性与受试者个体对音乐的熟悉程度相关。例如，音乐所强加的记忆和环境氛围，这些都会激发痴呆患者的积极情绪。研究结果强调，对痴呆患者实施音乐干预之前考虑个人音乐偏好很重要。

二、音乐干预的负面影响与正面影响

虽然主流观点倾向于将音乐视为痴呆患者的"万金油"，但研究表明，音乐干预可能对痴呆患者产生或积极或消极的影响。例如，Ziv 等[28]探讨了背景音乐对阿尔茨海默病（AD）患者积极行为和消极行为的影响。在这项研究中，28 例患有中度 AD 的受试者聆听了他们熟悉的愉悦欢快的音乐。研究人员观察受试者的行为，并将其分为积极、消极或中性。积极行为表现为健谈、大笑、微笑、安抚他人和歌唱。消极行为包括激越表现、攻击、抱怨、行为重复、哭泣和打扰他人。中性行为包括睡眠和凝望天空。音乐课程每周1次，为期3周。研究结果表明，当受试者聆听音乐时，其积极行为增加，消极行为减少。有9名受试者，无论他们是否聆听背景音乐，消极行为均中止。然而，在28名受试者中，也有9名受试者对背景音乐没有反应，2名受试者在聆听背景音乐时出现负面行为[28]。

同样地，在一项循证支持的程序化的个体化播放曲目的音乐干预研究中，Garrido 等[11]发现大多数参与聆听的患者其积极行为增加。但有报道称，有4种不同类型的受试者在11种聆听状态下出现心境恶化。根据既往精神状况识别那些可能容易受到负面影响的痴呆患者，为需要额外照顾的他们选择音乐，并监测他们聆听的反应，这些是该研究强调的重点[8,11]。

尽管可能存在潜在的负面影响，但研究表明，养老院并未认识到谨慎的必要性，也并不完全具备有效实施音乐干预所需的技能。为了调查音乐干预在老年护理机构中的实施情况[24,25]，对多个疗养院的工作人员进行了在线问卷调查和访谈。结果表明，大多数老年护理机构将不符合循证标准的音乐干预纳入他们的环境设置。音乐干预项目很少有专业的音乐治疗师参与，尽管对音乐干预的看法主要是正面积极的，但是也有一些个体表现出了负面反应[24,25]。当音乐过于响亮或重复时，或音乐引发令人痛苦的记忆时，负面消极反应可能会出现[24,25]。可用资源、员工的参与程度和专业知识的局限性被认为是有效执行音乐干预措施的重大障碍。事实上，员工的知识可能会对音乐干预措施的有效性产生相当大的影响。Sung 等[29]探讨了214名护士对痴呆症患者接受音乐治疗的态度和期望。问卷调查的结果显示，护士们对在疗养院中使用音乐和音乐疗法治疗痴呆症患者持积极态度。正如 Garrido 等[24,25]研究中所发现的，护理人员在使用或实施音乐干预方面没有接受过太多的培训和教育[29]。作者建议，这应该是老年护理机构护理人员培训的一部分。

第四节 音乐疗法和干预措施作用机制的理论

尽管已经有一些理论，但音乐疗法和其他音乐干预措施的确切作用机制并不完全清楚。一些人认为，社会过程是痴呆症患者音乐治疗和音乐干预有效性的潜在因素之一。与音乐疗法一样，研究已经确定了社会过程如何影响非治疗师主导的干预的反应。Sherratt 等[30]探讨了与预先录制的音乐相比，作为现场音乐组成部分的社交互动如何影响参与者的行为。研究人员记录并观察了参与者在四种条件下的行为指标：没有音乐、商业录制的磁带音乐、音乐家演唱的磁带音乐和同一音乐家演唱的现场表演。四种条件下的歌曲选择都是一样的。结果显示，参与者对现场音乐条件的参与度最高。这表明，在音乐体验中融入社交互动可以增强痴呆症患者的幸福感。此外，音乐作为音乐治疗的重要组成部分，它可以调节唤醒水平，增加环境中其他人的参与度[7]。除了与音乐相关的社交过程，人们还认为音乐疗法和音乐干预也会影响边缘系统[31]，而边缘系统在恐惧和压力等情绪中起着关键作用[32-34]。正如之前的一些研究所[31]报告的那样，通过调动边缘系统，音乐疗法可能减轻压力和焦虑。还有理论认为，音乐可以调节唤醒水平，进而会影响认知功能[35]。

第五节 结论和未来的研究

本章回顾的研究表明，音乐疗法和非治疗师主导的音乐干预措施在帮助缓解痴呆症患者的激越、焦虑和抑郁等心理症状方面具有巨大潜力。本综述强调使用与痴呆症患者个人相关的音乐的重要性，同时应注意治疗相关负面反应的潜在可能性。专业音乐治疗师接受过个性化音乐治疗和管理负面反应的培训。然而，在正式音乐治疗环境之外进行音乐干预时，护理人员需要接受进一步的培训，以便最有效地实施音乐治疗。幸运的是，目前有可供在老年护理机构中指导开展音乐干预的循证指南[36,37]。研究表明，遵循这些方案的结果比采用更特殊的方法的结果更为正面[1]。然而，在老年护理机构实施音乐干预仍然存在持续的挑战，因护理人员通常负担过重，几乎没有时间进行额外的培训或在护理环境中实施新的项目。此外，在老年护理机构中，往往存在一种情感或心理需求次于生理需求的文化认同。因此，政府政策和市场力量都在推动"全人"和"以人为本"的痴呆症护理方法[38]。因为音乐反映了我们作为个体的身份，可以使痴呆症患者重新建立自我意识，所以音乐干预在这些护理模式中起着重要作用[39]。未来的研究需要考虑音乐和音乐疗法如何进一步融入痴呆症患者的护理实践中。

参考文献

1. Garrido, S., Dunne, L., Chang, E., Perz, J., Stevens, C., & Haertsch, M. (2017). The use of music playlists for people with dementia: A critical synthesis. Journal of Alzheimer's Disease, 60, 1129-1142.

2. Lam, H. L., Li, W. T. V., Laher, I., & Wong, R. Y. (2020). Effects of music therapy on patients with dementia A systematic review. Geriatrics (Basel), 5(4), 62. Available from https://doi.org/10.3390/geriatrics5040062.

3. Perez-Eizaguirre, M., & Vergara-Moragues, E. (2020). Music therapy interventions in palliative care: A systematic review. Journal of Palliative Care. available from https://doi.org/10.1177/0825859720957803.

4. Leggieri, M., Thaut, M. H., Fornazzari, L., Schweizer, T. A., Barfett, J., Munoz, D. G., & Fischer, C. E. (2019). Music intervention approaches for Alzheimer's disease: A review of the literature. Frontiers in Neuroscience, 13, 132. Available from https://doi.org/10.3389/fnins.2019.00132.

5. Clark, I. N., Stretton-Smith, P. A., Baker, F. A., Lee, Y. C., & Tamplin, J. (2020). It's feasible to write a song": A feasibility study examining group therapeutic songwriting for people living with dementia and their family caregivers. Frontiers in Psychology, 11, 1951. Available from https://doi.org/10.3389/fpsyg.2020.01951.

6. Davidson, J., & Garrido, S. (2015). Singing and psychological needs. In G. Welsh, D. Howard, & J. Nix (Eds.), The Oxford handbook of singing. Oxford: Oxford University Press.

7. Ridder, H. M. O. (2011). How can singing in music therapy influence social engagement for people with dementia? Insights from the polyvagal theory. In F. Baker, & S. Uhlig (Eds.), Voicework in music therapy: Research and practice (pp. 130-146). London:

Jessica Kingsley Publishers.
8. Chu, H., Yang, C. Y., Lin, Y., Ou, K. L., Lee, T. Y., O'Brien, A. P., & Chou, K. R. (2014). The impact of group music therapy on depression and cognition in elderly persons with dementia: A randomized controlled study. Biological Research for Nursing, 16(2), 209-217. Available from https://doi.org/10.1177/1099800413485410.
9. Park, H., & Specht, J. (2009). Effect of individualized music on agitation in individuals with dementia who live at home. Journal of Gerontological Nursing, 35, 47-55.
10. Park, H. (2010). Effect of music on pain for home-dwelling persons with dementia. Pain Management Nursing, 11, 141-147.
11. Garrido, S., Dunne, L., Stevens, C., & Chang, E. (2020). Music playlists for people with dementia: Trialing a guide for caregivers. Journal of Alzheimer's Disease, 77(1), 219-226.
12. Sacchetti, E., Turrina, C., & Valsecchi, P. (2010). Cerebrovascular accidents in elderly people treated with antipsychotic drugs. Drug Safety, 33, 273-288.
13. Caltagirone, C., Bianchetti, A., Di Luca, M., Mecocci, P., Padovani, A., Pirfo, E., & Italian Association of Psychogeriatrics. (2005). Guidelines for the treatment of Alzheimer's disease from the Italian Association of Psychogeriatrics. Drugs & Aging, 22(Suppl. 1), 1-26.
14. Ouslander, J., Bartesl, S., & Beck, C. (2003). Consensus statement on improving the quality of mental health care in US nursing homes: Management of depression and behavioral symptoms associated with dementia. Journal of the American Geriatric Society, 51, 1287-1298.
15. Raglio, A., Bellelli, G., Traficante, D., Gianotti, M., Ubezio, M. C., Gentile, S., & Trabucchi, M. (2010). Efficacy of music therapy treatment based on cycles of sessions: A randomised controlled trial. Aging and Mental Health, 14(8), 900-904. Available from https://doi.org/10.1080/13607861003713158.
16. Ridder, H. M. O., Stige, B., Qvale, L. G., & Gold, C. (2013). Individual music therapy for agitation in dementia: An exploratory randomized controlled trial. Aging & Mental Health, 17(6), 667-678. Available from https://doi.org/10.1080/13607863.2013.790926.
17. Sung, H. C., Lee, W. L., Li, T. L., & Watson, R. (2012). A group music intervention using percussion instruments with familiar music to reduce anxiety and agitation of institutionalized older adults with dementia. International Journal of Geriatric Psychiatry, 27(6), 621-627. Available from https://doi.org/10.1002/gps.2761support/caregiving/stages-behaviors/depression.
18. McDermott, O., Orrell, M., & Ridder, H. M. (2014). The importance of music for people with dementia: The perspectives of people with dementia, family carers, staff and music

therapists. Aging & Mental Health, 18(6), 706-716. Available from https://doi.org/10.1080/13607863.2013.875124.

19. Ashida, S. (2000). The effect of reminiscence music therapy sessions on changes in depressive symptoms in elderly persons with dementia. Journal of Music Therapy, 37(3), 170-182. Available from https://doi.org/10.1093/jmt/37.3.170.

20. Bevins, S., Dawes, S., Kenshole, A., & Gaussen, K. (2015). Staff views of a music therapy group for people with intellectual disabilities and dementia: A pilot study. Advances in Mental Health and Intellectual Disabilities, 9(1), 40-48. Available from https://doi.org/10.1108/AMHID-04-2014-0005.

21. Pulopulos, M. M., Baeken, C., & De Raedt, R. (2020). Cortisol response to stress: The role of expectancy and anticipatory stress regulation. Hormones and Behavior, 117, 104587. Available from https://doi.org/10.1016/j.yhbeh.2019.104587.

22. Pulopulos, M. M., Hidalgo, V., Puig-Perez, S., Montoliu, T., & Salvador, A. (2020). Relationship between cortisol changes during the night and subjective and objective sleep quality in healthy older people. International Journal of Environmental Research and Public Health, 17(4), 1264. Available from https://doi.org/10.3390/ijerph17041264.

23. Potkins, D., Myint, P., Bannister, C., Tadros, G., Chithramohan, R., Swann, A., & Margallo-Lana, M. (2003). Language impairment in dementia: Impact on symptoms and care needs in residential homes. International Journal of Geriatric Psychiatry, 18(11), 1002-1006. Available from https://doi.org/10.1002/gps.1002.

24. Garrido, S., Dunne, L., Perz, J., Chang, E., & Stevens, C. J. (2018). The use of music in aged care facilities: A mixed-methods study. Journal of Health Psychology, 25(10-11), 1425-1438. Available from https://doi.org/10.1177/1359105318758861.

25. Garrido, S., Stevens, C., Chang, E., Dunne, L., & Perz, J. (2018). Music and dementia: Individual differences in response to personalized playlists. Journal of Alzheimer's Disease, 64(3), 933-941. Available from https://doi.org/10.3233/JAD-180084.

26. van der Vleuten, M., Visser, A., & Meeuwesen, L. (2012). The contribution of intimate live music performances to the quality of life for persons with dementia. Patient Education and Counseling, 89(3), 484-488. Available from https://doi.org/10.1016/j.pec.2012.05.012.

27. Sung, H. C., Chang, A. M., & Lee, W. L. (2010). A preferred music listening intervention to reduce anxiety in older adults with dementia in nursing homes. Journal of Clinical Nursing, 19(7-8), 10561064. Available from https://doi.org/10.1111/j.1365-2702.2009.03016.x.

28. Ziv, N., Granot, A., Hai, S., Dassa, A., & Haimov, I. (2007). The effect of background stimulative music on behavior in Alzheimer's patients. Journal of Music Therapy, 44(4),

329-343. Available from https://doi.org/10.1093/jmt/44.4.329.
29. Sung, H. C., Lee, W. L., Chang, S. M., & Smith, G. D. (2011). Exploring nursing staff's attitudes and use of music for older people with dementia in long-term care facilities. Journal of Clinical Nursing, 20(1112), 1776-1783. Available from https://doi.org/10.1111/j.1365-2702.2010.03633.x.
30. Sherratt, K., Thornton, A., & Hatton, C. (2004). Emotional and behavioural responses to music in people with dementia: An observational study. Aging & Mental Health, 8(3), 233-241. Available from https://doi.org/10.1080/13607860410001669769.
31. Moore, K. S. (2013). A systematic review on the neural effects of music on emotion regulation: Implications for music therapy practice. Journal of Music Therapy, 50(3), 198-242.
32. Rajmohan, V., & Mohandas, E. (2007). The limbic system. Indian Journal of Psychiatry, 49(2), 132-139. Available from https://doi.org/10.4103/0019-5545.33264.
33. Rolls, E. T. (2015). Limbic systems for emotion and for memory, but no single limbic system. Cortex; A Journal Devoted to the Study of the Nervous System and Behavior, 62, 119-157. Available from https://doi.org/10.1016/j.cortex.2013.12.005.
34. Rolls, E. T. (2019). The cingulate cortex and limbic systems for action, emotion, and memory. Handbook of Clinical Neurology, 166, 23-37. Available from https://doi.org/10.1016/B978-0-444-64196-0.00002-9.
35. Schafer, T., Sedlmeier, P., Stadtler, C., & Huron, D. (2013). The psychological functions of music listening. Frontiers in Psychology, 4, 511. Available from https://doi.org/10.3389/fpsyg.2013.00511.
36. Clements-Cortes, A., Pearson, C., & Chang, K. (2015). Creating effective music listening opportunities. Toronto: Baycrest. Retrieved from www.baycrest.org/care/culture-arts-innovation/therapeutic-arts/music-therapy/creating-effective-music-listeningopportunities.
37. Garrido, S., Dunne, L., Stevens, C., Chang, E., & Perz, J. (2019). Music playlists for people with dementia: A guide for carers, health workers and family. Retrieved from https://musicfordementia.github.io/.
38. Manthorpe, J., & Samsi, K. (2016). Person-centered dementia care: Current perspectives. Clinical Interventions in Aging, 11, 1733-1740. Available from https://doi.org/10.2147/CIA.S104618.
39. Evans, S. C., Garabedian, C., & Bray, J. (2017). 'Now he sings'. The My Musical Memories Reminscence Programme: Personalised interaction reminiscence sessions for people living with dementia. Dementia (Basel, Switzerland), 18(3), 1181-1198.

第十二章 多奈哌齐治疗阿尔茨海默病的疗效

Samuel L. Warren，Ahmed A. Moustafa 编
姚敏怡，丘东海 译
肖卫民 校

第一节 引言

阿尔茨海默病（AD）是一种神经退行性疾病，它存在多种病理改变，如淀粉样蛋白斑块沉积、认知功能障碍、神经纤维缠结和继发性炎症[1]。在 AD 中，这些异常的神经系统症状非常严重，并逐渐恶化到死亡。因此，迫切需要能够治疗 AD 进展性症状的干预措施。用于治疗 AD 症状的最常见的药物是胆碱酯酶抑制剂[2]。乙酰胆碱在 AD 进展期间常被耗尽，而胆碱酯酶抑制剂通过调节神经递质乙酰胆碱发挥作用。胆碱酯酶抑制剂被认为可以通过维持胆碱能功能进而防止和减缓 AD 的一些症状。因此，文献提示，使用胆碱酯酶抑制剂可以治疗 AD 的一些进展性症状（如认知功能下降）[3,4]。

多奈哌齐、利凡斯的明和加兰他敏是治疗 AD 最常见的胆碱酯酶抑制剂[5]。尽管以上胆碱酯酶抑制剂都有各自不同的治疗效果，但是这些药物都主要用于治疗 AD 的神经心理症状（如记忆和注意力）。一些研究表明，胆碱酯酶抑制剂可以改善 AD 患者的认知和日常功能[6,7]。例如，多奈哌齐、加兰他敏和利凡斯的明都被发现能改善 AD 患者的记忆功能[8]。也有证据表明，胆碱酯酶抑制剂可以影响 AD 的神经退行性症状。例如，一些研究表明，胆碱酯酶抑制剂可以帮助维持 AD 患者海马的结构和功能[9]。然而，这一有关神经退行性变的研究存在高度争议。由此可见，关于胆碱酯酶抑制剂的具体作用和疗效还存在一些争议。

虽然胆碱酯酶抑制剂有一定的益处，但这些药物的有效性取决于个体因素，

如年龄、疾病阶段（早期与晚期）和药物剂量。胆碱酯酶抑制剂的效果可能会因为不良事件而减弱，这可能会使一些人拒绝治疗。例如，部分患者在服用胆碱酯酶抑制剂时会出现恶心、呕吐和腹泻等不良反应[10]。因此，关于胆碱酯酶抑制剂的有效性和安全性存在争议。对于如何最好地使用胆碱酯酶抑制剂治疗AD也存在争议。本章将讨论使用多奈哌齐治疗AD的有效性和安全性，具体包含以下内容：①多奈哌齐的治疗效果；②多奈哌齐的不良反应；③多奈哌齐未来的研究方向；④多奈哌齐联合治疗 [多奈哌齐联合美金刚或认知刺激疗法（CST）]。旨在了解多奈哌齐对 AD 的影响以及未来研究的重点领域。

值得注意的是，本章专门讨论多奈哌齐而非其他胆碱酯酶抑制剂。对多奈哌齐特别关注，主要基于以下原因：①它是最流行的胆碱酯酶抑制剂；②它是已被批准可以用于治疗所有阶段 AD 的唯一药物；③与其他胆碱酯酶抑制剂（如利凡斯的明和加兰他敏）相比，它具有额外的益处[11,12]。这些益处包括改善神经心理效应、剂量和给药效应（例如，与利凡斯的明不同，其口服形式每天只需摄入 1 次），以及其有争议的成本效益[13,14]。

第二节　多奈哌齐在阿尔茨海默病中的作用

一、多奈哌齐对 AD 神经心理症状的影响

在 AD 研究中，胆碱酯酶抑制剂的开发和使用主要基于胆碱能假说。胆碱能假说最初认为是神经递质乙酰胆碱的缺失和功能障碍导致 AD 患者的认知功能下降[15]。然而，目前的理论认为，胆碱能下降是 AD 患者认知功能下降的危险因素或促成过程[16]。大脑胆碱能系统在处理注意力、神经可塑性和复杂的认知过程（如记忆）方面起着重要的作用[17]。因此，AD 的高阶症状和涉及胆碱能系统的任务之间存在明确的联系。例如，前脑基底部的神经退行性变与 AD 患者的胆碱性神经元和记忆功能的丢失有关[18,19]。在健康老年人中，胆碱能神经元通常会缓慢退化[20]；然而，当代的胆碱能假说表明，在 AD 患者中，老年斑和神经纤维缠结会显著增加胆碱能下降[16]。因此，当代的理论（如淀粉样蛋

白级联假说）认为，胆碱能下降是 AD 的症状（而非曾经认为的病因）[21]。尽管如此，迄今为止，胆碱酯酶抑制剂仍是唯一能有效治疗和延缓 AD 症状的药物（美金刚除外）。

在文献中，多奈哌齐能治疗 AD 的神经心理学症状已被广泛认同[8,22]。例如，由 Chang 等[23] 进行的研究发现，多奈哌齐对认知和功能衰退的症状有积极影响。通过对比多奈哌齐治疗组和对照组的简易精神状态检查量表（MMSE）、认知能力筛查工具以及临床痴呆评定量表评分（CDR）可以发现这些结果。Chan 等[23] 也发现，MMSE 和 CDR 评分与参与者退出治疗存在关联。患者的 MMSE 每增加 1 分，退出治疗的机会将减少 6%；与此同时，CDR 评分每增加 1 分，退出治疗的机会增加 10.5%。相应地，Chang 等[23] 提示早期进行多奈哌齐治疗可减缓 AD 患者认知和功能衰退的初始症状，且可能对于治疗退出具有保护性作用。

同时也观察到多奈哌齐剂量（从 5 mg 到 10 mg 或 23 mg）可进一步改善 AD 患者的神经心理症状。例如，Farlow 等[24] 的研究比较了多奈哌齐剂量 10 mg 和 23 mg 治疗 AD 的安全性和有效性。不同剂量的比较用于了解多奈哌齐更高剂量是否比标准剂量 10 mg 更能改善 AD 的症状。约 1451 名参与者被招募后分成两组，分别是 23 mg 实验组（$n=972$）和 10 mg 标准剂量组（$n=479$），并采用 SIB-认知量测、MMSE、日常生活能力（ADL）以及临床医生印象变化量表评分记录认知和心理测量。Farlow 等[24] 发现，23 mg 多奈哌齐组的认知评分较 10 mg 多奈哌齐组更好（SIB-认知测量）。他们也认为更高的多奈哌齐剂量对晚期 AD 患者更有效。因此，Farlow 等[24] 认为多奈哌齐可以治疗 AD 的认知症状，同时增加剂量（23 mg）可进一步改善这些症状。相应地，在更广泛的文献中观察到在 5 mg 和 10 mg 多奈哌齐之间存在相似的剂量效应[25,26]。

然而，一些研究发现多奈哌齐并不影响认知和功能。例如，Andersen 等[27] 研究多奈哌齐对 AD 神经心理症状的影响，得到结果为阴性。尤其是 Andersen 等[27] 发现，多奈哌齐治疗组或安慰剂组的认知评分无显著差异。然而，值得注意的是，参与者经历了显著的不良反应，包括厌食症和导致参与者退出的胃肠道问题（药物组发生率为 25%）。Andersen 等[27] 的研究发现，潜在的认知功能改善可能被多奈哌齐的不良反应所掩盖。在更广泛的文献中，有证据表明，虽然多奈哌齐可以改善认知和功能能力，但治疗的成功取决于多奈哌齐的剂量、个体的生理和 AD 的分期。因此，一些多奈哌齐研究结果为阴性，如 Andersen 等[27]，可能是因为多奈哌齐的不良反应大于研究人群中药物所带来的益处。

二、多奈哌齐的不良反应

显然，多奈哌齐可治疗 AD 的一些神经心理学症状。然而，药物剂量、疗效与多奈哌齐不良反应之间存在相关性，致使治疗能力受到限制。之前的多数研究（如果不是全部的话）报告了多奈哌齐的积极作用，也报道了许多不良反应效应。因此，重要的是要弄清楚治疗获益是否超过多奈哌齐的不良反应。此外，了解药物剂量的变化和环境因素如何影响治疗结果也很重要。

由多奈哌齐的不良反应导致参与者不适或退出很常见。比如，Griffith 等[28]研究中，有 64 名参与者经历了 151 次多奈哌齐引起的不良事件，如腹泻、高血压、尿路感染、头痛、头晕、厌食和恶心等，16 名参与者或将他们的多奈哌齐剂量从 10 mg 减少到 5 mg，或完全退出研究。在一篇关于这个话题的综述中，Adlimoghaddam 等[29]发现，多奈哌齐治疗组受试者的认知和功能得到改善，同时多奈哌齐治疗导致参与者的退出率也增加（特别是在较高药物剂量时）。因此，一些参与者可能由于多奈哌齐的不良反应而无法继续得到治疗。

尽管多奈哌齐的不良反应在研究中频繁出现，但仅出现在少数研究对象中，这一点很重要。而且，研究表明多奈哌齐的不良反应并不经常掩盖其治疗效果[30]。例如，Jia 等[31]的研究分析了多奈哌齐治疗轻度至中度 AD 患者的安全性。该研究[31]是一项关于服用 10 mg 多奈哌齐发生不良事件的深入双盲研究。大约 241 名受试者服用多奈哌齐 5 mg/d，持续 4 周；随后服用 10 mg/d，共 20 周。通过 MMSE、ADL 量表、APOE4 基因和心电图来评估参与者对多奈哌齐的反应。Jia 等[31]发现，最初的 241 名参与者中有 93 名报告了不良事件；然而，这些不良事件都没有导致住院或严重反应。研究还发现，服用 10 mg 多奈哌齐（与 5 mg 相比）的受试者 MMSE 较好。此外，我们观察到携带 *APOE4* 基因或合并心血管疾病的参与者发生不良事件的可能性增加。因此，Jia 等[31]得出结论是，10 mg 剂量的多奈哌齐是安全的，个体因素（例如，心血管健康及是否携带 *APOE4* 基因）影响不良事件的程度大于剂量效应。

因此，目前的证据表明，多奈哌齐的治疗效果较药物的不良反应更为突出。然而，尽管 10 mg 和 23 mg 多奈哌齐的剂量能减少 AD 患者认知和功能衰退的症状，但其疗效取决于对药物的信任和个体反应性。即使 AD 的某些症状得到改善，但因为药物的不良反应仍有可能减少多奈哌齐的继续治疗。因此，研究人员和临床医生在用多奈哌齐治疗 AD 时应慎之又慎。文献表明，多奈哌齐剂量从 5 mg 逐渐转变为 10 mg 时，研究对象的治疗反应最好。尽管如此，从文献中可以清楚地看到，10 mg 或 23 mg 剂量对个体并非总是适宜的，并可能导致退出治疗或生活质量（QOL）降低[32]。因此，研究者必须观察个体对多奈哌齐的反应并据此调整治疗方案。5 mg 剂量为多奈哌齐的推荐剂量，因其比高剂量（10 mg 或 23 mg 剂量）安全得多，并且仍能显著改善 AD 患者的认知、日常功能和 QOL。

三、多奈哌齐在 AD 中的潜在作用

如前所述，胆碱酯酶抑制剂研究主要集中在治疗 AD 的神经心理学症状上。然而，一些初步研究也表明多奈哌齐可以治疗 AD 的其他症状。例如，研究表明，多奈哌齐可用于治疗 AD 的一些神经退行性、代谢性和神经精神症状[33-35]。然而，这些症状的治疗仍然存在很大争议。本章将探讨多奈哌齐治疗 AD 的一些潜在作用，旨在突出多奈哌齐研究的新领域并激发进一步的研究。

胆碱能假说认为，胆碱能系统的功能与 AD 的神经退行性机制密切相关。因此，一些研究表明，多奈哌齐能延缓 AD 患者的神经退行性变[9,34]。例如，Ishiwata 等[36]的研究发现，多奈哌齐治疗可影响 AD 患者的神经退行性变症状。具体来说，Ishiwata 等[36]评估了 265 名参与者（80 名对照组和 185 名可能的 AD 参与者）的海马萎缩情况。该研究使用磁共振成像（MRI）和广泛的认知功能来检测海马萎缩和神经心理评分。通过收集的数据，Ishiwat 等[36]认为，多奈哌齐可以影响

AD 患者认知与海马萎缩存在相关性。而且，他们发现，多奈哌齐治疗组比对照组减缓了海马萎缩。因此，有证据表明多奈哌齐能减缓 AD 患者的神经退行性变；然而，有些研究报道了相反的证据[37]。因此，多奈哌齐与神经退行性变的关系需要进一步的研究。

AD 的神经退行性变症状也与 AD 的代谢异常密切相关。一些初步研究表明，多奈哌齐可能对 AD 患者的脑代谢有治疗作用。例如，Moon 等[35]研究了多奈哌齐治疗对 AD 患者海马萎缩和代谢下降症状的影响。大约 21 名参与者使用磁共振光谱和基于体素的形态学技术进行研究。受试者还接受了韩国 MMSE、AD 评估量表——认知、CDR 和老年抑郁量表的心理测试。关于神经退行性变，Moon 等[35]发现多奈哌齐治疗可增加认知能力和海马体积。相反，未接受多奈哌齐治疗的受试者认知评分更差，海马萎缩更严重。这些结果与之前 Ishiwata 等[36]的结果相似。Moon 等[35]也发现多奈哌齐治疗对代谢异常有保护作用。他们发现多奈哌齐治疗导致了 N-乙酰天冬氨酸/肌酸比值的增加以及肌醇/肌酸和胆碱/肌酸比值的降低。这些代谢比值很重要，因为它们表明多奈哌齐可对抗 AD 患者的淀粉样/tau 病（与 N-乙酰天冬氨酸有关）、神经退行性变和胆碱能下降（胆碱/肌酸比值）的症状。因此，Moon 等[35]认为，多奈哌齐可用于治疗 AD 患者的神经退行性变和代谢异常。

最后，一些初步研究表明多奈哌齐可改善 AD 的一些神经精神症状（如抑郁、冷漠、焦虑）。例如，Cummings 等[33]回顾了多奈哌齐治疗神经精神症状的疗效，他们发现多奈哌齐可改善 AD 的一些神经精神症状，如妄想、焦虑、激越和易怒。这些结果是由多奈哌齐组和对照组的神经精神量表（NPI）评分的差异决定的。同时研究者发现多奈哌齐能持续在晚期 AD 患者和临床患者中改善神经精神症状。因此，Cummings 等[33]表明，多奈哌齐可改善 AD 的神经精神症状，甚至可能是目前治疗痴呆的神经精神药物的安全替代药物。然而，Cummings 等[33]确实注意到多奈哌齐在作为 AD 神经精神症状的独立治疗前，需要进行大量的研究。此外，其他一些研究发现多奈哌齐并不影响 AD 的神经精神症状[12,14]。因此，多奈哌齐对 AD 神经精神症状的治疗作用还需要进一步研究。

总之，多奈哌齐可以治疗 AD 的神经变性、代谢和神经精神症状；然而，还需要进一步的研究和重复验证。多奈哌齐还有其他一些潜在作用在本章未讨论，需要进一步研究。例如，关于多奈哌齐和 AD 生物标志物（如 β 淀粉样蛋白）之间的关系的研究较少，需要进一步研究[7,38]。未来的研究应着眼于研究这些主题，以了解多奈哌齐治疗这些症状的有效性、疗效和安全性。

第三节　多奈哌齐的联合治疗

虽然多奈哌齐可以改善 AD 的某些症状，但胆碱能抑制剂并不是一种可以解决所有问题的治疗手段。因此，为了更好地治疗 AD，研究人员经常寻找其他干预手段来弥补多奈哌齐的不足。其中两种最常见的治疗方法为多奈哌齐联用 CST 和美金刚。本节探讨了这两种联合治疗的疗效和安全性，并将其与单独使用多奈哌齐的治疗效果进行比较。

一、认知刺激疗法联合多奈哌齐治疗

CST 是一种寻求维持和提高 AD 患者社会、认知和功能技能的心理干预[39]。接受 CST 干预的患者通常会在小组研讨会中完成指定任务和活动。这些小组任务被认为有益于提高和保持 AD 患者的社会和心理技能。例如，一些研究表明 CST 可以显著改善 AD 患者的社交技能、日常功能和生活质量[40]。英国国家健康与护理规范研究所建议治疗痴呆时使用 CST[41]。

CST 通常与多奈哌齐联合治疗，这两种干预措施均可以改善认知和日常生活功能。此外，CST 也被认为可以提高 AD 患者的生活质量。有证据表明，多奈哌齐和 CST 联合治疗 AD 的效果比它们单独使用时更好[42]。例如，Matsuda[43]的一项研究比较了单独使用多奈哌齐与多奈哌齐联合 CST 治疗的有效性，两组受试者均接受 5 mg 剂量的多奈哌齐，联合治疗组进行认知、会话、记忆和社交任务训练。Matsuda[43]发现，单独使用多奈哌齐的患者出现认知功能下降，而联合治疗组没有。由此可见，尽管多奈哌齐单独治疗确实减缓了 AD 中的认知下降，

但联合治疗更有效。

在另一项研究中,Chapman 等[44]也发现 CST 和多奈哌齐联合治疗比单独使用多奈哌齐更有效。Chapman 等[44]发现,联合治疗改善了患者的认知、日常功能、情绪(如减少了易怒)、QOL 和语言交流。这些测量是使用 MMSE、NPI、QOL 和其他量表进行定量评估。Chapman 等[44]认为,CST 可以作为多奈哌齐治疗的补充,从而减缓 AD 进展并改善情绪。但 Chapman 等[44]推测,之所以情绪会出现改善,是因为接受 CST 的个体在持续地从事能够防止衰退的心理任务。同时,他们也注意到两种治疗的效果具有滞后性,需要一段时间才能显现(大约 8 个月)。

总的来说,多奈哌齐和 CST 联合治疗 AD 比单独使用胆碱酯酶抑制剂的效果更好。然而,CST 的效果和改善程度仍存在一定的争议。需要进一步的研究来了解详细的相互作用。例如,多奈哌齐剂量对联合用药的影响(如 5 mg、10 mg、23 mg)。探究对比不同混合干预的组合将会对治疗 AD 很有帮助(例如,联合多奈哌齐、CST、美金刚的治疗)。然而有证据表明,CST 是 AD 的一种有效的治疗方法,尤其是在与多奈哌齐联合使用时。

二、多奈哌齐和美金刚的联合治疗

在 AD 的治疗中,胆碱酯酶抑制剂和美金刚联合使用的方案是比较常见的。美金刚是一种 N-甲基-D-天冬氨酸受体拮抗剂,通过调节神经递质谷氨酸来发挥作用[45]。谷氨酸调节很重要,因为在 AD 中该种神经递质浓度增加,可导致显著的神经元损伤。既往文献显示,美金刚和多奈哌齐联合是治疗 AD 最常见的搭配方式[3]。这种联合治疗方案在临床上也得到了广泛的应用[11]。本节将讨论多奈哌齐联合美金刚的药物治疗的效果。

有证据表明,美金刚和多奈哌齐的联合治疗优于单独的药物治疗(例如,单独使用多奈哌齐)。例如,Cao 等[46]的研究比较了多奈哌齐单独给药和与美金刚联合给药的治疗效果。该研究特别关注于调查 AD 和慢性阻塞性肺疾病的每种治疗方法的有效性和安全性。其使用了大约 310 例来自中国河北医科大学的患者的数据，这些患者接受了 10 mg 多奈哌齐的基线治疗。研究人员通过多种评估工具，如 MMSE、痴呆 QOL 评分、布里斯托日常生活活动量表、NPI 和一般健康问卷，记录了患者的认知和心理状况。研究结果显示，与单独使用多奈哌齐相比，多奈哌齐和美金刚联合治疗的效果更好，并且两组间在观察不良反应时没有显著差异。

Chen 等[47]对关于多奈哌齐和美金刚联合治疗的研究进行了一项荟萃分析，尝试从相关文献中探讨联合治疗研究的结论和评估质量。从 Cochrane、PsycINFO、PubMed、Ovid Medline 和 Embase 数据库的文献中检索出 11 篇文章，对患者的认知、心理（如精神错乱、情绪）、行为、整体功能和不良事件进行分析。Chen 等[47]发现，多奈哌齐联合美金刚治疗比单独给药更有效。同样地，Cao 等[46]发现美金刚和多奈哌齐联合治疗改善了 AD 患者的认知、行为、心理和生活技能。这些作用在疾病的后期阶段也持续存在，而单一的胆碱酯酶抑制剂治疗往往会导致认知功能的恶化。Chen 等[47]还发现，与多奈哌齐单药治疗相比，联合治疗不会增加不良事件的风险。

有证据表明，多奈哌齐和美金刚的联合治疗对改善阿尔茨海默病的神经心理症状效果更佳，且安全性与单独使用多奈哌齐相当。因此，研究者和临床医生在允许的情况下应考虑使用多奈哌齐和美金刚的联合治疗。但是，值得注意的是，由胆碱酯酶抑制剂引起的所有并发症（不良反应）在联合治疗期间仍会发生。研究人员和临床医生应该对接受联合药物治疗的个体进行观察，并对治疗进行相应地调整。

第四节 结论

本章评估了多奈哌齐在 AD 治疗中的应用。由于多奈哌齐作为胆碱酯酶抑制剂的历史性和普遍性，我们特别评估了多奈哌齐。在本章中，我们探讨了关于多奈哌齐在合理使用下，其剂量和不良反应的影响。同时对联合治疗和未来研究的方向进行了讨论。我们发现多奈哌齐对 AD 的认知和功能症状有轻度到中度的改善，这一结论得到了大量文献支持且无任何争议。然而，对于多奈哌齐在 AD 中的辅助作用，如神经退行性、代谢性和神经精神方面的治疗，确实存在很多争议。

在本章中，我们观察到多奈哌齐对 AD 的认知、功能、神经退行性（脑萎缩和体积）、神经精神和代谢症状发挥着正向作用。

然而，多奈哌齐、脑萎缩和 AD 神经精神症状之间的关系尚处于初步研究阶段，需要进一步的研究（由于研究结果相互矛盾）。我们还一致发现，多奈哌齐治疗的神经心理益处随着多奈哌齐剂量的增加而增加（从 5 mg 到 10 mg 或 23 mg）。但随着剂量的增加，其腹泻、恶心等不良事件的发生及严重程度也增加。为了减少多奈哌齐的不良反应，大多数研究将个体的服用剂量从低剂量逐渐过渡到中等剂量（例如，从 5 mg 滴定到 10 mg）或使用联合疗法（例如，多奈哌齐联合美金刚或 CST）以补充多奈哌齐的不足。因此，当调节剂量和使用滴定或联合治疗策略时，多奈哌齐的不良反应似乎不超过药物带来的益处。尽管如此，由于多奈哌齐与患者的生活质量相关，因此仍需要进一步改进其不良反应[32]。

多奈哌齐研究的最大问题之一是其对死亡率的影响。许多研究，尤其是涉及高剂量多奈哌齐的研究，有少量到中等数量的个体由于无法承受药物的不良反应而退出研究，剩余的仅是对药物反应良好的参与者，这会影响参与者的死亡率。因此，对多奈哌齐的准确表述和客观理解可能会受到参与者死亡率的干扰。未来的研究应该确定那些最容易受到多奈哌齐不良反应影响的患者，并寻求方法减少这些危险因素。研究人员也应该探索减少多奈哌齐治疗期间不良事件的方法。参与者死亡率的发生与多奈哌齐研究中个体因素的潜在问题密切相关。参与者的个人特质和环境变量会影响其对药物的反应和接受度。已经有一些研究表明，遗传优势和人口统计学特征对多奈哌齐的接受度具有重要影响。但这些研究都是新近的且缺乏深入探讨。因此，研究人员在进行多奈哌齐研究时应尝试探讨这些因素。同样重要的是，当参与者死亡发生时，研究人员需密切关注和披露真实的统计方法，以提高透明度。

总之，本章探讨了多奈哌齐在治疗 AD 中的疗效。我们发现了多奈哌齐能显著改善认知能力下降的因素，同时也有证据表明多奈哌齐能影响 AD 的其他因素（如神经退行性变）。本章旨在总结目前的文献，并指导和阐述未来的研究，以便能够更好地治疗和理解 AD。

反过来，我们认为多个领域需要广泛的研究和重复验证。第一，未来的研究应该探索联合治疗与高剂量多奈哌齐治疗相比的疗效。第二，未来的研究应探究如何控制和减少多奈哌齐的不良反应，尤其是涉及到服用高剂量多奈哌齐的人群。我们不应该阻止研究人员去探究高剂量多奈哌齐的使用，但是必须对高剂量多奈哌齐所带来递增的不良反应进行弥补。第三，未来的研究应寻求进一步探索个体变量对多奈哌齐治疗质量和接受度的影响。也就是说，研究人员应该探索基因、年龄和非痴呆疾病如糖尿病对多奈哌齐治疗质量和接受度的影响。我们强调的这些变量对治疗成功至关重要，但至今相关研究仍然缺乏。最后，应该探究如何在多奈哌齐治疗期间改善 AD 患者的生活质量。我们认为 AD 患者应该尽可能得到最好的治疗和生活质量。因此，所有这些研究领域都与本章的目标相一致，即改善 AD 患者的生活并提高多奈哌齐的疗效。

参考文献

1. Alzheimer's Association. (2018). 2018 Alzheimer's disease facts and figures. Alzheimer's & Dementia, 14(3), 367-429.
2. Singh, R., & Sadiq, N. M. (2020). Cholinesterase inhibitors. StatPearls Publishing. Available from http://www.ncbi.nlm.nih.gov/books/NBK544336/.
3. Zemek, F., Drtinova, L., Nepovimova, E., Sepsova, V., Korabecny, J., Klimes, J., & Kuca, K. (2014). Outcomes of Alzheimer's disease therapy with acetylcholinesterase inhibitors and memantine. Expert Opinion on Drug Safety, 13(6), 759-774. Available from https://doi.org/10.1517/14740338.2014.914168.
4. Zhang, X., Yu, R., Wang, H., & Zheng, R. (2020). Effects of rivastigmine hydrogen tartrate and donepezil hydrochloride on the cognitive function and mental behavior of patients with Alzheimer's disease. Experimental and Therapeutic Medicine, 20(2), 1789-1795. Available from https://doi.org/10.3892/etm.2020.8872.

5. Sharma, K. (2019). Cholinesterase inhibitors as Alzheimer's therapeutics (Review). Molecular Medicine Reports, 20(2), 1479-1487. Available from https://doi.org/10.3892/mmr.2019.10374.

6. Espiritu, A. I., & Cenina, A. R. F. (2020). The effectiveness and tolerability of the high dose donepezil at 23 mg tablet per day for Alzheimer's disease: A meta-analysis of randomized controlled trials. Acta Medica Philippina, 54(3), Article 3. Retrieved from. Available from https://actamedicaphilippina.upm.edu.ph/index.php/acta/article/view/1669.

7. Ma, Y., Ji, J., Li, G., Yang, S., & Pan, S. (2018). Effects of donepezil on cognitive functions and the expression level of β-amyloid in peripheral blood of patients with Alzheimer's disease. Experimental and Therapeutic Medicine, 15(2), 1875-1878.

8. Haake, A., Nguyen, K., Friedman, L., Chakkamparambil, B., & Grossberg, G. T. (2020). An update on the utility and safety of cholinesterase inhibitors for the treatment of Alzheimer's disease. Expert Opinion on Drug Safety, 19(2), 147-157. Available from https://doi.org/10.1080/14740338.2020.1721456.

9. Moss, D. E. (2020). Improving anti-neurodegenerative benefits of acetylcholinesterase inhibitors in Alzheimer's disease: Are irreversible inhibitors the future? International Journal of Molecular Sciences, 21(10), 3438. Available from https://doi.org/10.3390/ijms21103438.

10. Doody, R. S., Geldmacher, D. S., Farlow, M. R., Sun, Y., Moline, M., & Mackell, J. (2012). Efficacy and safety of donepezil 23 mg versus donepezil 10 mg for moderatetosevere Alzheimer's disease: A subgroup analysis in patients already taking or not taking concomitant memantine. Dementia and Geriatric Cognitive Disorders, 33(2 3), 164-173. Available from https://doi.org/10.1159/000338236.

11. Alzheimer's Association. (2020). Medications for memory. Alzheimer's Disease & Dementia. Retrieved from. Available from https://alz.org/alzheimers-dementia/treatments/medications-for-memory.

12. Kobayashi, H., Ohnishi, T., Nakagawa, R., & Yoshizawa, K. (2016). The comparative efficacy and safety of cholinesterase inhibitors in patients with mild-to-moderate Alzheimer's disease: A Bayesian network meta-analysis. International Journal of Geriatric Psychiatry, 31(8), 892-904. Available from https://doi.org/10.1002/gps.4405.

13. Benjamin, B., & Burns, A. (2007). Donepezil for Alzheimer's disease. Expert Review of Neurotherapeutics, 14737175.7.10.1243 7(10), 1243-1249. Available from https://doi.org/10.1586/.

14. Blanco-Silvente, L., Castells, X., Saez, M., Barceló, M. A., Garre-Olmo, J., VilaltaFranch, J., & Capellà, D. (2017). Discontinuation, efficacy, and safety of

cholinesterase inhibitors for Alzheimer's disease: A meta-analysis and meta-regression of 43 randomized clinical trials enrolling 16 106 patients. The International Journal of Neuropsychopharmacology, 20(7), 519-528. Available from https://doi.org/10.1093/ijnp/pyx012.

15. Bartus, R. T., Dean, R. L., Beer, B., & Lippa, A. S. (1982). The cholinergic hypothesis of geriatric memory dysfunction. Science (New York, N.Y.), 217(4558), 408-414. Available from https://doi.org/10.1126/science.7046051.

16. Craig, L. A., Hong, N. S., & McDonald, R. J. (2011). Revisiting the cholinergic hypothesis in the development of Alzheimer's disease. Neuroscience & Biobehavioral Reviews, 35(6), 1397-1409. Available from https://doi.org/10.1016/j.neubiorev.2011.03.001.

17. Teipel, S. J., Grinberg, L. T., Hampel, H., & Heinsen, H. (2009). Cholinergic system imaging in the healthy aging process and Alzheimer disease. In L. R. Squire (Ed.), Encyclopedia of neuroscience (pp. 857-868). London: Academic Press. Available from https://doi.org/10.1016/B978-008045046-9.02041-6.

18. Ferreira-Vieira, T. H., Guimaraes, I. M., Silva, F. R., & Ribeiro, F. M. (2016). Alzheimer's disease: Targeting the cholinergic system. Current Neuropharmacology, 14(1), 101-115. Available from https://doi.org/10.2174/1570159X13666150716165726.

19. Francis, P. T., Palmer, A. M., Snape, M., & Wilcock, G. K. (1999). The cholinergic hypothesis of Alzheimer's disease: A review of progress. Journal of Neurology, Neurosurgery & Psychiatry, 66(2), 137-147. Available from https://doi.org/10.1136/jnnp.66.2.137.

20. Davidson, P. S. R., & Winocur, G. (2010). Aging and cognition. In G. F. Koob, M. L. Moal, & R. F. Thompson (Eds.), Encyclopedia of behavioral neuroscience (pp. 20-26). London: Academic Press. Available from https://doi.org/10.1016/B978-0-08-045396-5.00031-2.

21. Armstrong, R. A. (2013). What causes Alzheimer's disease? Folia Neuropathologica, 51(3), 169-188. Available from https://doi.org/10.5114/fn.2013.37702.

22. Cacabelos, R. (2007). Donepezil in Alzheimer's disease: From conventional trials to pharmacogenetics. Neuropsychiatric Disease and Treatment, 3(3), 303-333.

23. Chang, Y.-P., Yang, C.-H., Chou, M.-C., Chen, C.-H., & Yang, Y.-H. (2015). Clinical compliance of donepezil in treating Alzheimer's disease in Taiwan. American Journal of Alzheimer's Disease & Other Dementias, 30(4), 346-351. Available from https://doi.org/10.1177/1533317514556875.

24. Farlow, M. R., Salloway, S., Tariot, P. N., Yardley, J., Moline, M. L., Wang, Q., ... Satlin, A. (2010). Effectiveness and tolerability of high-dose (23 mg/d) versus standard-dose (10

mg/d) donepezil in moderate to severe Alzheimer's disease: A 24-week, randomized, double-blind study. Clinical Therapeutics, 32(7), 1234-1251. Available from https://doi.org/10.1016/j.clinthera.2010.06.019.

25. Birks, J., & Harvey, R. J. (2006). Donepezil for dementia due to Alzheimer's disease. The Cochrane Database of Systematic Reviews (1), CD001190. Available from https://doi.org/10.1002/14651858.CD001190.pub2.

26. Yatabe, Y., Hashimoto, M., Kaneda, K., Honda, K., Ogawa, Y., Yuuki, S., & Ikeda, M. (2013). Efficacy of increasing donepezil in mild to moderate Alzheimer's disease patients who show a diminished response to 5 mg donepezil: A preliminary study. Psychogeriatrics: The Official Journal of the Japanese Psychogeriatric Society, 13(2), 88-93. Available from https://doi.org/10.1111/psyg.12004.

27. Andersen, F., Viitanen, M., Halvorsen, D. S., Straume, B., Wilsgaard, T., & Engstad, T. A. (2012). The effect of stimulation therapy and donepezil on cognitive function in Alzheimer's disease. A community based RCT with a two-by-two factorial design. BMC Neurology, 12, 59. Available from https://doi.org/10.1186/1471-2377-12-59.

28. Griffith, P., Lichtenberg, P., Goldman, R., & Payne-Parrish, J. (2006). Safety and efficacy of donepezil in African Americans with mild-to-moderate Alzheimer's disease. Journal of the National Medical Association, 98(10), 1590-1597.

29. Adlimoghaddam, A., Neuendorff, M., Roy, B., & Albensi, B. C. (2018). A review of clinical treatment considerations of donepezil in severe Alzheimer's disease. CNS Neuroscience & Therapeutics, 24(10), 876-888. Available from https://doi.org/10.1111/cns.13035.

30. Jackson, S., Ham, R. J., & Wilkinson, D. (2004). The safety and tolerability of donepezil in patients with Alzheimer's disease. British Journal of Clinical Pharmacology, 58(Suppl. 1), 1-8. Available from https://doi.org/10.1111/j.1365-2125.2004.01848.x.

31. Jia, J., Wei, C., Jia, L., Tang, Y., Liang, J., Zhou, A., ... Doody, R. S. (2017). Efficacy and safety of donepezil in Chinese patients with severe Alzheimer's disease: A randomized controlled trial. Journal of Alzheimer's Disease, 56(4), 1495-1504. Available from https://doi.org/10.3233/JAD-161117.

32. Rogers, S. L., Farlow, M. R., Doody, R. S., Mohs, R., & Friedhoff, L. T. (1998). A 24-week, double-blind, placebo-controlled trial of donepezil in patients with Alzheimer's disease. Donepezil Study Group. Neurology, 50(1), 136-145. Available from https://doi.org/10.1212/wnl.50.1.136.

33. Cummings, J., Lai, T. -J., Hemrungrojn, S., Mohandas, E., Kim, S. Y., Nair, G., & Dash, A. (2016). Role of donepezil in the management of neuropsychiatric symptoms in Alzheimer's disease and dementia with Lewy bodies. CNS Neuroscience &

Therapeutics, 22(3), 159-166. Available from https://doi.org/10.1111/cns.12484.

34. Dubois, B., Chupin, M., Hampel, H., Lista, S., Cavedo, E., Croisile, B., ... Dormont, D. (2015). Donepezil decreases annual rate of hippocampal atrophy in suspected prodromal Alzheimer's disease. Alzheimer's & Dementia, 11(9), 1041-1049. Available from https://doi.org/10.1016/j.jalz.2014.10.003.

35. Moon, C.-M., Kim, B.-C., & Jeong, G.-W. (2016). Effects of donepezil on brain morphometric and metabolic changes in patients with Alzheimer's disease: A DARTELbased VBM and 1H-MRS. Magnetic Resonance Imaging, 34(7), 1008-1016. Available from https://doi.org/10.1016/j.mri.2016.04.025.

36. Ishiwata, A., Mizumura, S., Mishina, M., Yamazaki, M., & Katayama, Y. (2014). The potentially protective effect of donepezil in Alzheimer's disease. Dementia and Geriatric Cognitive Disorders, 38(3 4), 170-177. Available from https://doi.org/10.1159/000358510.

37. Wang, L., Harms, M. P., Staggs, J. M., Xiong, C., Morris, J. C., Csernansky, J. G., & Galvin, J. E. (2010). Donepezil treatment and changes in hippocampal structure in very mild Alzheimer's disease. Archives of Neurology, 67(1), 99-106. Available from https://doi.org/10.1001/archneurol.2009.292.

38. Lu, J., Wan, L., Zhong, Y., Yu, Q., Han, Y., Chen, P., ... Guo, C. (2015). Stereoselective metabolism of donepezil and steady-state plasma concentrations of S-donepezil based on CYP2D6 polymorphisms in the therapeutic responses of Han Chinese patients with Alzheimer's disease. Journal of Pharmacological Sciences, 129(3), 188-195. Available from https://doi.org/10.1016/j.jphs.2015.10.010.

39. Kim, K., Han, J. W., So, Y., Seo, J., Kim, Y. J., Park, J. H., ... Kim, K. W. (2017). Cognitive stimulation as a therapeutic modality for dementia: A meta-analysisPsychiatry Investigation, 14(5), 626-639. Available from https://doi.org/10.4306/ pi.2017.14.5.626.

40. Cammisuli, D. M., Danti, S., Bosinelli, F., & Cipriani, G. (2016). Non-pharmacological interventions for people with Alzheimer's Disease: A critical review of the scientific literature from the last ten years. European Geriatric Medicine, 7(1), 57-64. Available from https://doi.org/10.1016/j.eurger.2016.01.002.

41. Pink, J., O'Brien, J., Robinson, L., & Longson, D. (2018). Dementia: Assessment, management and support: Summary of updated NICE guidance. BMJ (Clinical Research Edition), 361, k2438. Available from https://doi.org/10.1136/bmj.k2438.

42. Chen, J., Duan, Y., Li, H., Lu, L., Liu, J., & Tang, C. (2019). Different durations of cognitive stimulation therapy for Alzheimer's disease: A systematic review and metaanalysis. Clinical Interventions in Aging, 14, 1243-1254. Available from https://doi.org/ 10.2147/CIA.S210062.

43. Matsuda, O. (2007). Cognitive stimulation therapy for Alzheimer's disease: The effect of cognitive stimulation therapy on the progression of mild Alzheimer's disease in patients treated with donepezil. International Psychogeriatrics, 19(2), 241-252.
44. Chapman, S. B., Weiner, M. F., Rackley, A., Hynan, L. S., & Zientz, J. (2004). Effects of cognitive-communication stimulation for Alzheimer's disease patients treated with donepezil. Journal of Speech, Language, and Hearing Research, 47(5), 1149-1163.
45. Kishi, T., Matsunaga, S., Oya, K., Nomura, I., Ikuta, T., & Iwata, N. (2017). Memantine for Alzheimer's disease: An updated systematic review and meta-analysis. Journal of Alzheimer's Disease, 60(2), 401-425. Available from https://doi.org/10.3233/JAD-170424.
46. Cao, Y., Qian, L., Yu, W., Li, T., Mao, S., & Han, G. (2020). Donepezil plus memantine versus donepezil alone for treatment of concomitant Alzheimer's disease and chronic obstructive pulmonary disease: A retrospective observational study. Journal of International Medical Research, 48(2). Available from https://doi.org/10.1177/0300060520902895.
47. Chen, R., Chan, P.-T., Chu, H., Lin, Y.-C., Chang, P.-C., Chen, C.-Y., & Chou, K.-R. (2017). Treatment effects between monotherapy of donepezil versus combination with memantine for Alzheimer disease: A meta-analysis. PLoS One, 12(8), e0183586. Available from https://doi.org/10.1371/journal.pone.0183586.